Cardiac Electrophysiology and Catheter Ablation of Different Arrhythmias

Cardiac Electrophysiology and Catheter Ablation of Different Arrhythmias

Guest Editors

Hussam Ali
Antonio Frontera

MDPI

Basel • Beijing • Wuhan • Barcelona • Belgrade • Novi Sad • Cluj • Manchester

Guest Editors
Hussam Ali
Arrhythmia and EP Research Center
IRCCS MultiMedica
Milan
Italy

Antonio Frontera
Cardiac Arrhythmia Department
Great Metropolitan Hospital Niguarda
Milan
Italy

Editorial Office
MDPI AG
Grosspeteranlage 5
4052 Basel, Switzerland

This is a reprint of the Special Issue, published open access by the journal *Journal of Clinical Medicine* (ISSN 2077-0383), freely accessible at: https://www.mdpi.com/journal/jcm/special_issues/6KW8698261.

For citation purposes, cite each article independently as indicated on the article page online and as indicated below:

Lastname, A.A.; Lastname, B.B. Article Title. *Journal Name* **Year**, *Volume Number*, Page Range.

ISBN 978-3-7258-6382-2 (Hbk)
ISBN 978-3-7258-6383-9 (PDF)
https://doi.org/10.3390/books978-3-7258-6383-9

Contents

Journal of
Clinical Medicine

MDPI

Editorial

Closing Editorial for the Special Issue: Cardiac Electrophysiology and Catheter Ablation of Different Arrhythmias

Hussam Ali [1,*] and Antonio Frontera [2]

1 Arrhythmia & Electrophysiology Centre, IRCCS MultiMedica, Sesto San Giovanni, 20099 Milan, Italy
2 Cardiac Arrhythmia Department, Great Metropolitan Hospital Niguarda, 20162 Milan, Italy
* Correspondence: hussamali.ep@gmail.com

Cardiac electrophysiology and catheter ablation for diverse arrhythmic substrates continue to evolve rapidly, leveraging new techniques and energy sources. While significant advances in catheter ablation have enhanced safety and efficacy, many challenging arrhythmias and conditions still require further study and research in order to optimize patient outcomes.

As Guest Editors of the Special Issue "Cardiac Electrophysiology and Catheter Ablation of Different Arrhythmias", we focused on the management, diagnosis, intracardiac mapping, and ablation of cardiac arrhythmias. This Editorial highlights key findings from this Special Issue and outlines future research directions.

Although the implantable cardioverter–defibrillator (ICD) is an established strategy for preventing sudden cardiac death (SCD) in heart failure (HF) patients, it can lead to significant complications, comorbidity, and reduced quality of life [1]. In this light, research on the optimization of HF medical treatment, with the aim of improving hemodynamics and cardiac remodeling and reducing the burden of ventricular arrhythmias, is critical. In their comprehensive and highly relevant review, Zaher et al. summarize the literature data concerning the antiarrhythmic effects of optimized medical therapy and their impact on SCD prevention in HF patients with reduced ejection fraction [2]. The authors confirm that there is robust evidence that a protective role is played by beta-blockers, mineralocorticoid receptor antagonists, and Angiotensin receptor–Neprilysin inhibitors and show promising data regarding the use of Na-glucose cotransporter 2 inhibitors. Notably, while current guidelines for ICD implantation rely heavily on remote trials, future research must evaluate how contemporary medical therapies influence SCD risk. This may refine ICD indications for primary prevention in HF patients [3].

Similarly to HF patients, individuals with hypertrophic cardiomyopathy (HCM) are also at an increased risk of SCD, but there are fewer evidence-based data for risk stratification and low agreement between the available guidelines for primary prevention [4]. In their comprehensive review on the topic, Sclafani et al. analyzed the complex mechanisms and substrates of SCD in HCM patients. Unlike traditional reviews, the authors propose a dynamic, physiology-driven framework for SCD risk prediction that incorporates cellular, structural, and electrophysiological substrates [5]. Cellular abnormalities, such as ionic dysfunction, may occur early in the disease, preceding overt structural abnormalities, which might explain poor outcomes in some HCM patients who received an "apparently" favorable prognosis based on current criteria. Conversely, while myocardial scarring is a recognized risk factor, its architecture/myocardial disarray and associated functional substrates are complex and remain challenging to assess. The authors emphasize that future advancements in genetic, molecular, and cardiac imaging diagnostic tools may provide a more individualized substrate-driven assessment of SCD risk and ICD indications in HCM patients and may guide specific non-invasive treatments.

Ventricular arrhythmias are a major cause of SCD, particularly in the context of underlying electrical or structural heart disease. While catheter ablation is often considered a curative therapy for idiopathic ventricular tachycardia, its role is usually adjunctive to ICD therapy in the presence of structural heart disease [6]. In this Special Issue, Schlatzer et al. present their "real-world" experience regarding catheter ablation of ventricular arrhythmias in 120 patients at a Swiss tertiary care center [7]. Their data confirm high acute success rates (>90%) for catheter ablation (CA) for both premature ventricular beats and ventricular tachycardias. On the other hand, related complications (<10%) were mainly observed in patients with structural heart disease. In this light, the preventive role of CA in patients with structural heart disease and its potential substitution for ICD therapy require further assessment in large randomized clinical trials.

Another patient cohort with an increased SCD risk comprises those with ventricular pre-excitation (Wolff–Parkinson–White, WPW), mainly due to the rapid conduction over their accessory pathway during atrial arrhythmias. Though CA has been proven to be a safe and curative therapy in most WPW patients, its timing and related complications should be carefully assessed in children [8]. In this regard, Sanzo et al. present important findings from their retrospective study including 153 pediatric WPW patients [9]. At a long-term follow-up of about 5 years, the spontaneous loss of pre-excitation was observed in 28% of patients. Interestingly, left-truncated Kaplan–Meier analysis estimated that pre-excitation would persist only in about one half and one third of patients at the age of 1 and 16 years, respectively. Predictors of the spontaneous resolution of pre-excitation included an intermittent WPW pattern and the absence of symptoms. Notably, no malignant arrhythmic events were reported in the study cohort. Accordingly, these findings support a more conservative approach in children with WPW since spontaneous pre-excitation loss occurs frequently in the early years, obivating the need for invasive treatments.

Atrial fibrillation (AF) is the most common sustained arrhythmia, with a substantial impact on morbidity, mortality, stroke risk, quality of life, and health system capacity. Despite impressive advancements in CA as a promising therapy, numerous challenges are still present, with suboptimal ablation outcomes observed in many AF patients [10].

While an in-depth and comprehensive understanding of AF mechanisms, particularly persistent forms, is still lacking, most of the current research and trials are orientated towards ablation "burning" rather than mapping "understanding". In their review paper, Ye et al. navigate the fascinating field of AF mapping using high-density epicardial mapping [11]. The authors highlighted the importance of accurate unipolar atriogram analysis, mapping during both sinus rhythm and AF, and the role of Bachmann's bundle and endo-epi asynchrony in AF maintenance. Though epicardial mapping and signal fingerprinting may be limited to cardiac surgery and research studies, combining them with rapidly evolving artificial intelligence may improve our understanding of AF mechanisms and substrates, offering novel ablation targets for a tailored approach [12]. We congratulate the authors' group, guided by Prof. De Groot, on their continuous research focusing on signal analysis and decoding AF mechanisms.

An additional innovative AF mapping technology is electrocardiographic flow (ECF) mapping, which allows a temporospatial display of complex atrial propagation patterns during AF, helping to localize active drivers or "hot spots" [13]. In their analysis of two previous studies, Nilsson et al. show the utility of this approach in phenotyping the AF substrate and predicting recurrences over a 12-month follow-up after AF ablation. Patients with untreated non-pulmonary vein sources, identified through ECF, had higher rates of AF recurrence [14]. Future research is needed to assess the utility and feasibility of

ECF mapping in daily practice, particularly in guiding individualized ablation in persistent AF substrates.

Atypical (non-cavotricuspid isthmus-dependent) atrial flutters may present a proarrhythmic effect from previous AF ablation. Although less complex than AF substrates, atypical flutters can be challenging and often require advanced skills and high-density mapping [15]. In a retrospective study including 19 patients, Johner et al. elegantly displayed the electrophysiological features and substrates of 25 atypical atrial flutters using a 3D mapping system (Rhythmia) [16]. More than 50% of circuits were dual-loop re-entry circuits, mostly involving a perimitral loop with a second roof-dependent loop. Interestingly, dual-loop circuits showed wider isthmuses and faster conduction velocities. Ablation at the common isthmus of a dual-loop re-entry more frequently terminated the arrhythmia than targeting uncommon isthmuses, which often led to a change in tachycardia rate or activation sequence. This timely article highlights the importance of high-density mapping combined with conventional pacing maneuvers as multisite atrial entrainment in accurately delineating the entire tachycardia circuit and identifying the optimal ablation target.

Due to the progressive nature of AF (i.e., AF begets AF), the timing of CA could play a critical role. In their retrospective study, Farghaly et al. assessed the impact of CA timing in 130 AF patients undergoing RF pulmonary vein isolation, with a 16-month median follow-up [17]. The early-ablation group (within one year of AF diagnosis) had higher rates of freedom from atrial arrhythmia recurrence (84.4% vs. 60.8% in the late-ablation group, $p = 0.039$). Moreover, early ablation was associated with lower rates of cardiovascular hospitalizations (18% vs. 42%, $p = 0.023$) and AF progression (0.0% vs. 11.3%). According to multivariate analysis, late ablation and AF recurrence during the blanking period were independent predictors of recurrences. These findings were confirmed in a recent meta-analysis including more than 40.000 AF patients over 2 years of follow-up [18]. Early ablation was associated with lower recurrence rates in both paroxysmal and persistent AF, particularly in younger patients (<55 years) [18].

One of the challenging aspects of CA in AF is the creation of transmural durable lesions, with the aim of permanently isolating the pulmonary veins without compromising procedure safety. Over the last several years, advancements in CA technologies and energies, 3D mapping systems, and operator experience have contributed toward addressing this challenge [19]. Interestingly, Sprenger et al. used a complex machine learning model to predict ablation or lesion size indexes for local-impedance drop-guided ablation, showing significant differences in application duration through the different metrics used [20]. Although this study was retrospective and requires affirmation through future studies, it highlighted the promising utility of machine-learning in predicting ablation lesion quality using multi-parametric data.

Pulsed-field ablation (PFA) is an emerging ablation technology that has rapidly attracted attention in clinical practice due to its remarkable efficacy and safety profile. Beyond its fast and efficient workflow during AF ablation, the key advantage of PFA lies in its cardiac selectivity, which helps to minimize collateral damage and enhance procedural safety [21]. In this Special Issue, Mahrous et al. assessed left atrial function following PFA of AF in a limited number of patients over a six-month follow-up [22]. Their findings demonstrated improved echocardiographic parameters of left atrial function after ablation, indicating favorable atrial remodeling. Notably, these preliminary data have been corroborated in patients with persistent AF undergoing more extensive PFA beyond pulmonary vein isolation (such as posterior wall isolation) without any negative impact on left atrial compliance and function [23].

In summary, this Special Issue discusses several pressing topics in the rapidly evolving field of cardiac electrophysiology and catheter ablation, including ventricular arrhythmias, sudden cardiac death, and atrial fibrillation. We extend our sincere thanks to all the authors, reviewers, and *Journal of Clinical Medicine* staff for their valuable contributions and support in bringing this Special Issue to fruition.

Funding: This research received no external funding.

Conflicts of Interest: The authors declare no conflicts of interest.

References

1. Ezzat, V.A.; Lee, V.; Ahsan, S.; Chow, A.W.; Segal, O.; Rowland, E.; Lowe, M.D.; Lambiase, P.D. A systematic review of ICD complications in randomised controlled trials versus registries: Is our 'real-world' data an underestimation? *Open Heart* **2015**, *2*, e000198. [CrossRef] [PubMed] [PubMed Central]
2. Zaher, W.; Della Rocca, D.G.; Pannone, L.; Boveda, S.; de Asmundis, C.; Chierchia, G.B.; Sorgente, A. Anti-Arrhythmic Effects of Heart Failure Guideline-Directed Medical Therapy and Their Role in the Prevention of Sudden Cardiac Death: From Beta-Blockers to Sodium-Glucose Cotransporter 2 Inhibitors and Beyond. *J. Clin. Med.* **2024**, *13*, 1316. [CrossRef] [PubMed] [PubMed Central]
3. Goldenberg, I.; Ezekowitz, J.; Albert, C.; Alexis, J.D.; Anderson, L.; Behr, E.R.; Daubert, J.; Di Palo, K.E.; Ellenbogen, K.A.; Dzikowicz, D.J.; et al. Reassessing the need for primary prevention implantable cardioverter-defibrillators in contemporary patients with heart failure. *Heart Rhythm* **2025**, *22*, 1040–1051. [CrossRef] [PubMed]
4. Scolari, F.L.; Garbin, H.I.; de Carvalho, G.D.; Rodrigues, F.T.; de Menezes, R.A.; Correia, E.B.; Bittencourt, M.I. Low agreement among guidelines for primary prevention implantable cardioverter-defibrillator recommendations in hypertrophic cardiomyopathy. *Am. J. Cardiol.* **2025**, *236*, 86–91. [CrossRef] [PubMed]
5. Sclafani, M.; Falasconi, G.; Tini, G.; Musumeci, B.; Penela, D.; Saglietto, A.; Arcari, L.; Bucciarelli-Ducci, C.; Barbato, E.; Berruezo, A.; et al. Substrates of Sudden Cardiac Death in Hypertrophic Cardiomyopathy. *J. Clin. Med.* **2025**, *14*, 1331. [CrossRef] [PubMed] [PubMed Central]
6. Cronin, E.M.; Bogun, F.M.; Maury, P.; Peichl, P.; Chen, M.; Namboodiri, N.; Aguinaga, L.; Leite, L.R.; Al-Khatib, S.M.; Anter, E.; et al. 2019 HRS/EHRA/APHRS/LAHRS expert consensus statement on catheter ablation of ventricular arrhythmias: Executive summary. *Europace* **2020**, *22*, 450–495. [CrossRef] [PubMed]
7. Schlatzer, C.; Berg, J.; Duru, F.; Brunckhorst, C.; Saguner, A.M.; Haegeli, L.M. Real World Data from Catheter Ablation of Ventricular Tachycardias and Premature Ventricular Complexes in a Tertiary Care Center. *J. Clin. Med.* **2024**, *13*, 2310. [CrossRef] [PubMed] [PubMed Central]
8. Brugada, J.; Katritsis, D.G.; Arbelo, E.; Arribas, F.; Bax, J.J.; Blomström-Lundqvist, C.; Calkins, H.; Corrado, D.; Deftereos, S.G.; Diller, G.P.; et al. 2019 ESC Guidelines for the management of patients with supraventricular tachycardia. The Task Force for the management of patients with supraventricular tachycardia of the European Society of Cardiology (ESC). *Eur. Heart J.* **2020**, *41*, 655–720. [CrossRef] [PubMed]
9. Sanzo, A.; Seganti, A.; Demarchi, A.; Fino, R.S.; Raso, I.; Codazzi, A.C.; Petracci, B.; Bongiorno, A.; Rordorf, R.; Mannarino, S. Spontaneous Resolution of Ventricular Pre-Excitation During Childhood: A Retrospective Study. *J. Clin. Med.* **2025**, *14*, 2367. [CrossRef] [PubMed]
10. Cappato, R.; Levy, S.; Providencia, R.; Ali, H.; Ardashev, A.; Barra, S.; Creta, A.; Farkowski, M.; Heeger, C.H.; Kanagaratnam, P.; et al. Internal reviewers. Concise Guidelines of the European Cardiac Arrhythmias Society (ECAS) on "Catheter Ablation of Atrial Fibrillation". *J. Cardiovasc. Electrophysiol.* **2025**, *36*, 1076–1099. [CrossRef] [PubMed] [PubMed Central]
11. Ye, Z.; Jia, Y.; van Schie, M.S.; Knops, P.; Yildirim, V.; Taverne, Y.J.H.J.; de Groot, N.M.S. High-Density and Resolution Epicardial Mapping of the Atria: Translational Research with Clinical Impact. *J. Clin. Med.* **2024**, *13*, 6386. [CrossRef] [PubMed] [PubMed Central]
12. Seitz, J.; Mohr Durdez, T.; Lotteau, S.; Bars, C.; Pisapia, A.; Gitenay, E.; Monteau, J.; Reist, M.; Serdi, M.; Dayot, A.; et al. Artificial intelligence-adjudicated spatiotemporal dispersion: A patient-unique fingerprint of persistent atrial fibrillation. *Heart Rhythm* **2024**, *21*, 540–552. [CrossRef] [PubMed]
13. Haines, D.E.; Kong, M.H.; Ruppersberg, P.; Haeusser, P.; Avitall, B.; Szili-Torok, T.; Verma, A. Electrographic flow mapping for atrial fibrillation: Theoretical basis and preliminary observations. *J. Interv. Card. Electrophysiol.* **2023**, *66*, 1015–1028. [CrossRef] [PubMed] [PubMed Central]
14. Nilsson, K.R.; Anerao, A.; Kong, M.H.; Derejko, P.; Szili-Török, T.; Goyal, S.; Turagam, M.; Verma, A.; Castellano, S. Electrographic Flow Mapping Provides Prognosis for AF Ablation Outcomes Across Two Independent Prospective Patient Cohorts. *J. Clin. Med.* **2025**, *14*, 693. [CrossRef] [PubMed] [PubMed Central]

15. Ko Ko, N.L.; Sriramoju, A.; Khetarpal, B.K.; Srivathsan, K. Atypical atrial flutter: Review of mechanisms, advances in mapping and ablation outcomes. *Curr. Opin. Cardiol.* **2022**, *37*, 36–45. [CrossRef] [PubMed]
16. Johner, N.; Namdar, M.; Shah, D.C. Anatomical and Electrophysiological Characteristics of Dual-Loop Re-Entry in Atypical Atrial Flutter: Implications for Mapping and Catheter Ablation. *J. Clin. Med.* **2024**, *13*, 2847. [CrossRef] [PubMed] [PubMed Central]
17. Farghaly, A.A.A.; Ali, H.; Lupo, P.; Foresti, S.; De Ambroggi, G.; Atta, S.; Abdel-Galeel, A.; Tohamy, A.; Cappato, R. Early versus Late Radiofrequency Catheter Ablation in Atrial Fibrillation: Timing Matters. *J. Clin. Med.* **2024**, *13*, 4643. [CrossRef] [PubMed] [PubMed Central]
18. Karakasis, P.; Tzeis, S.; Pamporis, K.; Schuermans, A.; Theofilis, P.; Milaras, N.; Tsiachris, D.; Efremidis, M.; Antoniadis, A.P.; Fragakis, N. Impact of catheter ablation timing according to duration of atrial fibrillation history on arrhythmia recurrences and clinical outcomes: A meta-analysis. *Europace* **2025**, *27*, euaf110. [CrossRef] [PubMed]
19. Morales, G.; Hunter, T.D.; Rajendra, A.; Boo, L.M.; Osorio, J. Real-world trends in atrial fibrillation ablation indicate increasing durability of pulmonary vein isolation at repeat ablation. *Pacing Clin. Electrophysiol.* **2023**, *46*, 535–542. [CrossRef] [PubMed]
20. Sprenger, L.; Moser, F.; Maslova, V.; Zaman, A.; Nonnenmacher, M.; Willert, S.; Frank, D.; Lian, E. Prediction of Ablation Index and Lesion Size Index for Local Impedance Drop-Guided Ablation. *Ournal Clin. Med.* **2025**, *14*, 832. [CrossRef] [PubMed] [PubMed Central]
21. Tabaja, C.; Younis, A.; Hussein, A.A.; Taigen, T.L.; Nakagawa, H.; Saliba, W.I.; Sroubek, J.; Santangeli, P.; Wazni, O.M. Catheter-Based Electroporation: A novel technique for catheter ablation of cardiac arrhythmias. *JACC Clin. Electrophysiol.* **2023**, *9*, 2008–2023. [CrossRef] [PubMed]
22. Mahrous, N.; Blaschke, F.; Schöppenthau, D.; Hindricks, G.; Boldt, L.H.; Parwani, A.S. LA PULSE: Evaluating Left Atrial Function Pre- and Post-Atrial Fibrillation Ablation Using PULSEd Field Ablation. *J. Clin. Med.* **2024**, *14*, 68. [CrossRef] [PubMed] [PubMed Central]
23. Zaher, W.; Marcon, L.; Della Rocca, D.G.; Thayse, K.; Tran-Ngoc, E.; Ebinger, K.R.; Vetta, G.; Pannone, L.; Boveda, S.; de Asmundis, C.; et al. Pulsed-field ablation beyond pulmonary vein for persistent atrial fibrillation: Efficacy and impact on left atrial function. *J. Interv. Card. Electrophysiol.* **2025**. ahead of print. [CrossRef] [PubMed]

Journal of
Clinical Medicine

MDPI

Review

Anti-Arrhythmic Effects of Heart Failure Guideline-Directed Medical Therapy and Their Role in the Prevention of Sudden Cardiac Death: From Beta-Blockers to Sodium-Glucose Cotransporter 2 Inhibitors and Beyond

Wael Zaher [1], Domenico Giovanni Della Rocca [2], Luigi Pannone [2], Serge Boveda [3], Carlo de Asmundis [2], Gian-Battista Chierchia [2] and Antonio Sorgente [1,2,*]

1 Department of Cardiology, Centre Hospitalier EpiCURA, Route de Mons 63, 7301 Hornu, Belgium; wael.zaher@ulb.be

2 Heart Rhythm Management Centre, Postgraduate Program in Cardiac Electrophysiology and Pacing, Universitair Ziekenhuis Brussel-Vrije Universiteit Brussel, European Reference Networks Guard-Heart, Laarbeeklan 101, Jette, 1090 Brussels, Belgium; domenicodellarocca@hotmail.it (D.G.D.R.); lui.pannone@gmail.com (L.P.); carlodeasmundis@me.com (C.d.A.); jeanbaptiste.chierchia@uzbrussel.be (G.-B.C.)

3 Heart Rhythm Management Department, Clinique Pasteur, 31076 Toulouse, France; sboveda@clinique-pasteur.com

* Correspondence: sorgente.antonio@gmail.com

Abstract: Sudden cardiac death (SCD) accounts for a substantial proportion of mortality in heart failure with reduced ejection fraction (HFrEF), frequently triggered by ventricular arrhythmias (VA). This review aims to analyze the pathophysiological mechanisms underlying VA and SCD in HFrEF and evaluate the effectiveness of guideline-directed medical therapy (GDMT) in reducing SCD. Beta-blockers, angiotensin receptor–neprilysin inhibitors, and mineralocorticoid receptor antagonists have shown significant efficacy in reducing SCD risk. While angiotensin-converting enzyme inhibitors and angiotensin receptor blockers exert beneficial impacts on the renin-angiotensin-aldosterone system, their direct role in SCD prevention remains less clear. Emerging treatments like sodium-glucose cotransporter 2 inhibitors show promise but necessitate further research for conclusive evidence. The favorable outcomes of those molecules on VA are notably attributable to sympathetic nervous system modulation, structural remodeling attenuation, and ion channel stabilization. A multidimensional pharmacological approach targeting those pathophysiological mechanisms offers a complete and synergy approach to reducing SCD risk, thereby highlighting the importance of optimizing GDMT for HFrEF. The current landscape of HFrEF pharmacotherapy is evolving, with ongoing research needed to clarify the full extent of the anti-arrhythmic benefits offered by both existing and new treatments.

Keywords: heart failure with reduced ejection fraction; sudden cardiac death; ventricular arrhythmias; guideline-directed medical therapy; pharmacological management

1. Introduction

Heart failure (HF), and, more specifically, heart failure with reduced ejection fraction (HFrEF), stands as a public health challenge characterized by substantial morbidity and mortality, notably attributed to sudden cardiac death (SCD). The incidence of SCD in the HF population is fivefold greater than in the general population, accounting for 40–50% of all deaths, which is a considerable proportion of potentially preventable deaths in this population [1]. The association between SCD and HF is predominantly mediated by ventricular arrhythmias (VA), resulting from the complex interplay between the structurally altered cardiac substrate in HF and various environmental triggers [2,3].

Guideline-directed medical therapy (GDMT) for HFrEF is founded on a cornerstone of four distinct classes of medications: beta-blockers (BB), renin-angiotensin-aldosterone system (RAAS) inhibitors, mineralocorticoid receptor antagonists (MRA), and sodium-glucose cotransporter 2 inhibitors (SGLT2i) [4]. Each of these pharmacological classes has demonstrated significant efficacy in reducing major cardiac events in HFrEF patients, including, for some, reduction in the incidence of SCD [5,6]. In this comprehensive review, we delve into the pathophysiological mechanisms underlying VA and SCD within the context of HF, and we undertake an in-depth analysis of the beneficial effects conferred by each of these medication classes in preventing SCD in this population.

2. Pathophysiology of Ventricular Arrhythmia and Sudden Cardiac Death

The pathophysiology of SCD due to VA in the context of HF is multifaceted. It involves an intricate interplay among transient factors or events that serve as triggers (e.g., ischemic episodes, metabolic disturbances, electrolyte imbalances, fluctuations in sympathetic nervous system activity), occurring in the presence of a myocardial substrate predisposed to arrhythmias [3,7].

Three primary electrophysiological mechanisms lead to VA within this context: (1) Inappropriately Increased Automaticity: This mechanism involves certain ventricular myocyte regions exhibiting increased automaticity, thereby initiating spontaneous action potentials without external stimulation, contributing to the onset of arrhythmias. (2) Triggered Activity: Triggered activity can manifest as early afterdepolarizations (occurring late in phase 2 or early in phase 3 of the action potential) or delayed afterdepolarizations (occurring after complete repolarization). These afterdepolarizations can reach the threshold potential necessary for the activation of ion channels, ultimately leading to arrhythmic events. Triggered activity typically follows a preceding impulse and is not a self-generating rhythm. (3) Reentry: This involves the circulation of electrical impulses around a barrier, often anatomical, such as scar tissue or fibrosis, perpetuating a continuous myocardial excitation, leading to sustained arrhythmias. It is noteworthy that these three mechanisms can coexist; arrhythmias may initiate through triggered activity and transition to reentrant patterns [7–9].

The pathophysiological changes in HF create an environment that favors these VA mechanisms. HF is characterized by cardiac remodeling, which includes ventricular enlargement, hypertrophy, and fibrosis [10]. Fibrosis may result from myocardial infarctions or from other structural cardiac disorders such as hypertrophic cardiomyopathy and arrhythmogenic cardiomyopathy. Factors like TGF-β1, endothelin-1, and Angiotensin II induce fibrosis, perturbing electrical excitation and repolarization [11]. Regions of fibrosis facilitate reentrant tachycardias by disrupting myocardial electrical impulses and fostering areas of slow conduction [12].

The nervous system and the RAAS, which are both markedly activated in the setting of HFrEF due to ventricular dysfunction, are significantly implicated in arrhythmogenesis. Angiotensin II and Aldosterone, acting through RAAS, induce vasoconstriction, increasing the afterload and remodeling, and stimulate fibroblasts' activity, leading to interstitial fibrosis and scar formation [10,13]. At the cellular level, angiotensin II initiates multiple signaling pathways that induce electrical remodeling, notably through alterations in the sodium current [14] and the destabilization of Kv4.3 messenger RNA [15], leading to increased Ca^{2+}/calmodulin-dependent protein kinase II (CaMKII) activity, perturbing calcium homeostasis, and predisposing to VA [16–18]. Moreover, Angiotensin II stimulates the sympathetic nervous system, contributing to VA through an increased sympathetic tone. Elevated levels of norepinephrine raise the afterload, thus increasing the myocardial oxygen demand and promoting cardiac remodeling, dilatation, and fibrosis [10]. Such structural alterations create a favorable environment for arrhythmogenesis. Additionally, sympathetic activation induces electrophysiological alterations, disrupting sodium and calcium channel currents and prolonging action's potential duration, ultimately predisposing the myocardium to early depolarizations [19]. For example, chronic adrenergic activation destabilizes Ryanodine receptors 2 (RyR2) channels, which are critical Ca^{2+} release channels located on the sarcoplasmic reticulum, playing a central role in the excitation-contraction coupling in the heart. Dysfunctional RyR2 channels lead to calcium leak and elevated cytoplasmic calcium levels via CaMKII, impairing cardiac function and exacerbating arrhythmogenesis through electrical instability, delayed afterdepolarizations, and triggered arrhythmias [18,19].

All this intricate electrical and structural remodeling in HFrEF leads to arrhythmogenesis and SCD (Figure 1). This highlights the importance of the GDMT for HFrEF in mitigating the risk of SCD in this population.

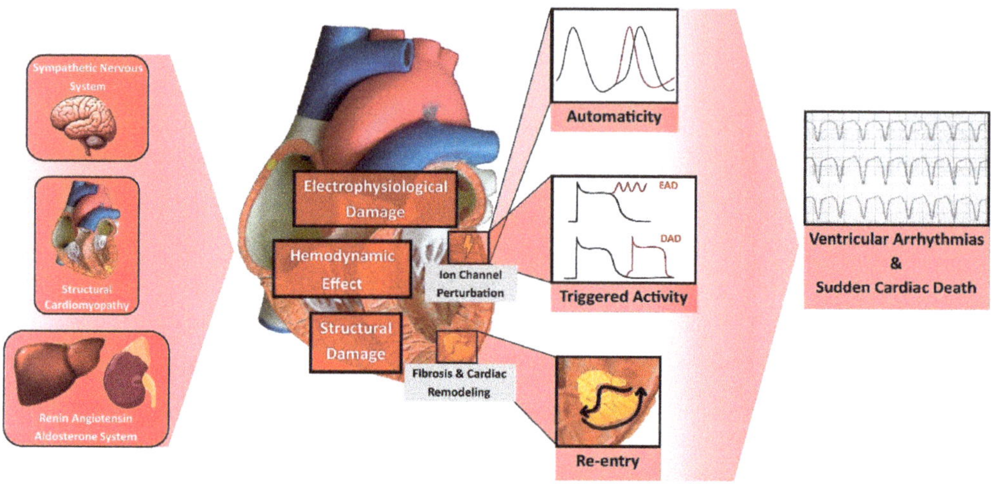

Figure 1. Pathophysiology of Ventricular Arrhythmia and Sudden Cardiac Death in Heart Failure. DAD, Delayed Afterdepolarization; EAD, Early Afterdepolarization.

3. Beta-Blockers

β-adrenergic receptors are expressed on cardiomyocytes. The activation of the cardiac sympathetic system by the binding of norepinephrine and epinephrine to these receptors initiates a cascade of intracellular reactions involving the cAMP/PKA signaling pathway [20]. This signaling pathway affects several key targets, including RyR2, L-type calcium channels, phospholamban, and others [19,20]. The net result of these signaling events is the enhancement of various aspects of cardiac function: an increased heart rate (chronotropy), an accelerated conduction velocity (dromotropy), a heightened force of contraction (inotropy), and an improved speed of relaxation (lusitropy) [21]. All these downstream effects of β-adrenergic stimulation facilitate the development of ectopic activity, including early afterdepolarizations and delayed afterdepolarizations, as well as functional reentry through action potential duration shortening, effective refractory period reduction, and conduction alterations [21]. Consequently, excessive β-adrenergic stimulation is associated with arrhythmias.

Three subtypes of β-receptors are known, with β1-receptors being predominantly localized in the cardiac tissue. The classes of BB are diverse, encompassing non-selective β-adrenergic antagonists (e.g., nadolol, propranolol), β1-selective adrenergic antagonists (e.g., acebutolol, atenolol, esmolol, metoprolol), and β-adrenergic antagonists with additional cardiovascular effects (e.g., carvedilol, labetalol, nebivolol), which may exhibit vasodilatory, anti-inflammatory, and antioxidant properties [22]. BB attenuate the sympathetic tone and sympathetically mediated triggers [22]. They mitigate automaticity by prolonging the sinus node cycle length and decelerating the atrioventricular conduction velocity by limiting calcium entry via catecholamine-dependent channels [21]. Moreover,

BB have been shown to possess antifibrotic properties, improve the left ventricular (LV) function, reduce the LV diameter, and decrease the LV mass, outcomes that are favorable in reducing SCD in HF [21].

Multiple studies have demonstrated the efficacy of BB in preventing arrhythmias and SCD in the context of HF. CIBIS II investigated the impact of Bisoprolol in HFrEF and demonstrated a significant mortality benefit, with a 42% reduction in SCD compared to the placebo group [23]. Metoprolol in HFrEF showed a similar and significant reduction in SCD in the MERIT-HF trial [24]. In the SENIORS trial, evaluating Nebivolol in an elderly HFrEF population, the SCD rate was significantly lower in the nebivolol-treated group [25]. The COPERNICUS trial in 2001, studying Carvedilol, showed a mortality benefit, although explicit data on SCD were not presented [26]. Additionally, several studies have indicated a significant reduction in shocks in patients wearing implantable cardioverter–defibrillators (ICD) when treated with BB compared to those without [27]. Meta-analyses have confirmed the benefit of BB on both mortality and SCD, without revealing statistically significant differences among the various types of BB [28–30]. Recent evidence, however, indicates a potential superiority of non-selective beta-blockers in antiarrhythmic effects. Specifically, Propranolol has been demonstrated to be superior to Metoprolol in managing electrical storms in ICD patients [31]. Carvedilol has also been associated with a substantial decrease in VA risk, compared to Metoprolol [32]. Further robust data are needed to confirm these findings.

In conclusion, BB substantially reduce proarrhythmic risk by inhibiting sympathetically mediated triggers, reducing functional reentrant substrates, and slowing the sinus node and atrioventricular nodal rates. The evidence supporting their use in HFrEF is robust and emphasizes their critical role in mitigating arrhythmias and SCD in this patient population.

4. Angiotensin-Converting Enzyme Inhibitor/Angiotensin Receptor Blocker

The RAAS exerts a critical influence on the pathophysiology of HFrEF by contributing to cardiac remodeling, interstitial fibrosis, and perturbations in various ionic currents, which collectively enhance arrhythmogenesis. The inhibition of the RAAS is principally achieved through two pharmacological classes: angiotensin-converting enzyme inhibitors (ACEi) and angiotensin II receptor blockers (ARB). ACEi act by inhibiting the conversion of angiotensin I to angiotensin II, while ARB selectively antagonize the angiotensin II type 1 receptors [33]. This blockage results in several beneficial effects, including the attenuation of ventricular remodeling, vasodilatation, a reduction in neurohormonal agents, and a decrease in the sympathetic tone and circulating catecholamines, along with favorable effects on ionic currents [10,34].

Several pivotal trials have explored the efficacy of RAAS inhibitors in the context of HFrEF. The CONSENSUS study, assessing the use of Enalapril in HFrEF, demonstrated a significant reduction in mortality, although it did not find a difference in SCD [35]. Similar results were found in the SOLVD-Prevention study [36]. In the ELITE trial, which compared Losartan to Captopril, Losartan was associated with a lower mortality, primarily driven by a lower incidence of SCD [37]. However, these results were not replicated in the ELITE II trial, where no significant differences were observed in either mortality or SCD [38]. Trials such as CHARM (exploring Candesartan) [39] and Val-HEFT (exploring Valsartan) [40] did not specifically monitor SCD as an endpoint. In patients wearing ICD, ACEi/ARB therapy has been associated with an improved freedom from shocks [41,42]. A large retrospective registry by Schupp et al. [43] indicated that ACEI/ARB treatment is associated with reduced all-cause mortality in patients who survived episodes of VA. Nonetheless, meta-analyses have shown a lack of a consistent efficacy of ACEi/ARBs in reducing the risk of SCD and VA, despite demonstrating benefits in overall mortality and hospitalization rates [30,44–46]. The exception appears to be in the context following acute myocardial infarction, where ACEi have shown a 20% reduction in SCD [47].

In conclusion, although ACEi and ARB have demonstrated favorable effects on the RAAS and have robust data supporting their beneficial impact on overall outcomes in HFrEF, their role in reducing the risk of SCD has not been definitively established, as underscored by multiple meta-analyses.

5. Angiotensin Receptor–Neprilysin Inhibitor

The Angiotensin Receptor–Neprilysin Inhibitor (ARNi) combines two active components: Valsartan, an ARB, and Sacubitril, a Neprilysin Inhibitor [48]. The molecular mechanisms underlying the anti-arrhythmic effects of ARNi are not yet fully elucidated and remain speculative to some extent. The mechanism of action encompasses effects on the RAAS via the ARB component and additional effects attributable to the Neprilysin Inhibitor, Sacubitril. At the electrophysiological level, ARNi exerts an influence on ionic currents in cardiomyocytes. Chang et al. [49] observed that ARNi had the potential to up-regulate the expression of potassium channel proteins, including KCNH2, KCNE1, and KCNE2. The consequent shortening of the action potential duration potentially ameliorates ventricular arrhythmogenicity, especially in the context of HF induced by myocardial infarction. Moreover, ARNi also appears to have a favorable effect on calcium homeostasis by downregulating the expression of CaMKII and mitigating diastolic calcium leak arising from dysfunctional RyR2 [50,51]. Additionally, neprilysin inhibition by ARNi contributes to elevated circulating levels of natriuretic peptides, which exert various cardioprotective effects countering the detrimental effects of the RAAS and sympathetic nervous system activation [52]. Natriuretic peptides increase the intracellular levels of cyclic guanosine monophosphate and its downstream effector molecule protein kinase G. This cascade leads to vasodilation, natriuresis, the inhibition of the RAAS, and sympathetic systems [52]. Furthermore, natriuretic peptides exert anti-inflammatory, anti-apoptotic, anti-hypertrophic, and anti-fibrotic effects on the myocardium [53–55]. ARNi has also been shown to significantly reduce biomarkers associated with profibrotic signaling [56].

Multiple studies and trials corroborate the beneficial effects of ARNi on VA and ICD therapy [57,58]. Post hoc analyses of the PARADIGM-HF trial, investigating ARNi in HFrEF, showed a significant reduction in VA and the risk of SCD [59,60]. Liu et al. [61] found in their meta-analyses that although ARNi did not affect the incidence of VA, it did significantly reduce the risk of SCD in heart failure patients. Another meta-analysis by Pozzi et al. [62] demonstrated a significant reduction in the burden of VA and ICD shock when comparing ARNi to ACEi/ARB therapy. Fernandes et al. [63] reported a significant reduction in SCD, VA, and appropriate ICD therapy with ARNi. Major studies and meta-analyses regarding the effect of ARNi on VA and SCD are summarized in Table 1.

Table 1. Major studies and meta-analyses regarding effect of ARNi on ventricular arrythmia and sudden cardiac death.

Authors Journal Year	Type of Study Intervention	No. of Patients in the Population	Effect on VA and SCD
Martens, et al. Clin Res Cardiol. 2019 [57].	Retrospective, cohort Pre- vs. Post-ARNi initiation	151 HFrEF with ICD	VA reduction (51 vs. 14; $p < 0.001$) ICD shock reduction (16 vs. 6; $p < 0.001$)
De Diego, et al. Heart Rhythm. 2018 [58].	Prospective, cohort ARNi vs. ACEi/ARB	240 HFrEF with ICD	VA and ICD shock reduction (0.8% vs. 6.7%; $p < 0.02$)
Russo, et al. J Clin Med. 2020 [64].	Prospective, cohort ARNi	167 HFrEF with ICD	VA reduction (15 vs. 4; $p = 0.03$) ICD shock reduction (13 vs. 3; $p = 0.02$)

Table 1. *Cont.*

Authors Journal Year	Type of Study Intervention	No. of Patients in the Population	Effect on VA and SCD
Rohde et al. JACC Heart Fail. 2020 [59].	RCT—post hoc analysis ARNi vs. ACEi	8399 HFrEF	SCD reduction in the ICD group (HR 0.49; 95% CI 0.25–0.99) and non-ICD group (HR 0.81; 95% CI 0.67–0.98)
Curtain, et al. Eur J Heart Fail. 2022 [60].	RCT—post hoc analysis ARNi vs. ACEi	8399 HFrEF	VA reduction (HR 0.76; 95% CI 0.62–0.95)
Fernandes, et al. Heart Rhythm O2. 2021 [63].	Meta-analysis ARNi vs. ACEi/ARB	11,204 HFrEF	SCD reduction (OR 0.78; 95% CI 0.63–0.96) VA reduction (OR 0.45; 95% CI 0.25–0.79) Higher BiV Pacing ($p < 0.0001$)
Liu, et al. Front Cardiovasc Med. 2022 [61].	Meta-analysis ARNi vs. ACEi/ARB/Placebo	18,500 HFrEF or HFpEF	No VA reduction (RR 0.86; 95% CI 0.68–1.10) SCD reduction (RR 0.79; 95% CI 0.70–0.90)
Mujadzic, et al. J Innoc Card Rhythm Mang. 2022 [65].	Meta-analysis ARNi vs. ACEi/ARB/Placebo	18,548 HFrEF or HFpEF	VA & SCD reduction (OR 0.71; 95% CI 0.54–0.93) ICD shock reduction (OR 0.23; 95% CI 0.11–0.47)
Pozzi, et al. Heart Fail Rev. 2023 [62].	Meta-analysis ARNi vs. ACEi/ARB	8837 HFrEF	VA reduction (OR 0.78; 95% CI 0.63–0.96 for RCT and RR 0.62; 95% CI 0.53–0.72 for observational studies) ICD shock reduction (RR 0.24; 95% CI 0.12–0.24)

ACEi, Angiotensin-Converting Enzyme Inhibitor; ARB, Angiotensin II Receptor Blocker; ARNi, Angiotensin Receptor–Neprilysin Inhibitor; BiV, Biventricular; HFpEF, Heart Failure with Preserved Ejection Fraction; HFrEF, Heart Failure with Reduced Ejection Fraction; ICD, Implantable Cardioverter–Defibrillator; RCT, Randomized Controlled Trial; SCD, Sudden Cardiac Death; VA, Ventricular Arrhythmia.

In conclusion, ARNi therapy appears to manifest favorable effects via multiple mechanisms, including vasodilation, the attenuation of sympathetic activation, the reduction in myocardial wall stretch and fibrosis, and modulatory impacts on ion channels such as potassium channels, RyR2, and the CaMKII pathway. Meta-analyses confirm ARNi's efficacy in reducing both VA and SCD, yet further investigation is needed to fully understand the precise molecular mechanisms.

6. Mineralocorticoid Receptor Antagonists

MRA provide a complementary approach to the neurohormonal suppression of the RAAS by targeting the aldosterone receptor [66]. These agents achieve a series of beneficial cardiovascular outcomes, including the prevention of the electrical remodeling of cardiac tissue [67,68], the attenuation of myocardial fibrosis and ventricular remodeling [69,70], a decrease in sympathetic activation [71], and beneficial effects on endothelial vasomotor dysfunction [72]. Through these several mechanisms, MRA have been shown to prevent SCD.

The RALES trial, which investigated the use of Spironolactone in patients with HFrEF, reported a significant reduction in both overall mortality and cardiac-specific mortality. It showed a 29% reduction in the risk of SCD [73]. Similarly, the EPHESUS trial focusing on Eplerenone demonstrated a significant reduction in all-cause mortality, cardiovascular-related death, and the risk of cardiovascular-related death or hospitalization. Notably, it also showed a significant reduction in the incidence of SCD [74]. Numerous meta-analyses have consistently shown a clear benefit for MRA in reducing SCD, reinforcing their critical role in managing patients with HFrEF [30,75–77].

7. Sodium-Glucose Cotransporter 2 Inhibitors

SGLT2i have emerged as a recent addition to the GDMT for HFrEF [4]. They primarily function by the selective inhibition of the SGLT2 receptor in the renal proximal tubules, conferring a variety of metabolic and cardiovascular benefits, including a reduction in cardiovascular mortality in patients with HFrEF [78].

The specific anti-arrhythmic mechanisms of SGLT2i are not yet completely understood, but several plausible pathways have been proposed. SGLT2i have been shown to exhibit anti-oxidative and anti-inflammatory properties by promoting multiple anti-oxidant and anti-inflammatory signaling pathways [79,80]. For instance, they activate AMP-activated protein kinase [81,82], attenuate the nucleotide-binding domain-like receptor protein 3 (NLRP3) inflammasome [83], and reduce the expression of inflammatory factors. This reduction in inflammation and oxidative stress may lead to anti-fibrotic and anti-remodeling properties, thereby decreasing the arrhythmic substrate. Data have indicated a reversal in cardiac volumes, a decrease in LV mass, and an improvement of LV function following SGLT2i treatment [84–86]. These positive changes have also been observed in the right ventricle [87]. Another anti-arrhythmic mechanism of SGLT2i is through ionic channels modulation. SGLT2i may modulate ionic channels by restoring intracellular Ca^{2+} and Na^{+} homeostasis. HF is characterized by cellular Na+ overload, often mediated by the upregulation of the Na^{+}/H^{+} exchanger 1 (NHE1), contributing to cytosolic Ca^{2+} overload, thus increasing arrhythmogenic risk [88,89]. SGLT2i can mitigate this risk by directly reducing Na^{+} overload through the inhibition of the late sodium current (INaL) and NHE1 [90,91]. Moreover, they may indirectly modulate CaMKII activity, thereby reducing calcium leakage from the sarcoplasmic reticulum and diminishing arrhythmic triggers like afterdepolarizations [92]. SGLT2i have also been shown to normalize the QT interval and QT dispersion, potentially reducing arrhythmogenic risks [93,94]. Experimental models have demonstrated that SGLT2i reduce ventricular arrhythmia vulnerability following myocardial ischemia [95].

Clinical trials, like DAPA-HF [96] and EMPEROR-Reduced [97], have shown a decrease in cardiovascular-related mortality in HFrEF with Dapagliflozin and Empagliflozin, respectively. Post-hoc analyses have indicated that Dapagliflozin reduces the risk of VA, cardiac arrest, and SCD [98]. Nonetheless, data from several meta-analyses have been inconclusive in showing a significant reduction in SCD or VAs with SGLT2i [99–101]. It is worth noting that many of these meta-analyses often included studies with SGLT2i focusing on diabetic patients without the specific consideration of HF. More recently, a meta-analysis by Oates et al. [102] focused specifically on the HF population and showed that SGLT2i therapy is associated with a reduced risk of SCD in patients with HF receiving contemporary medical therapy. The ongoing trial EMPA-ICD, assessing the effect of SGLT2i on VA in patients with type 2 diabetes (T2DM) wearing an ICD, is expected to provide additional data on the anti-arrhythmic effect of SGLT2i [103]. Major studies and meta-analyses regarding the effect of SGLT2i on VA and SCD are summarized in Table 2.

In conclusion, SGLT2i appear to exhibit anti-arrhythmic properties through various pleiotropic mechanisms, including the restoration of calcium and sodium homeostasis, the reversal of cardiac remodeling, and the exertion of antioxidant and anti-inflammatory effects. Although current data trends suggest a reduced incidence of SCD and VA, further well-designed prospective studies are imperative for the definitive validation of these anti-arrhythmic effects.

Table 2. Major studies and meta-analyses regarding the effect of SGLT2i on ventricular arrhythmia and sudden cardiac death.

Authors Journal Year	Type of Study Intervention	No. of Patients in the Population	Effect on VA and SCD
Curtain, et al. Eur Heart J. 2021 [98].	RCT—post hoc analysis Dapaglifozin vs. Placebo	4744 HFrEF	Reduction in the composite outcome of VA and SCD (HR 0.79; 95% CI 0.63–0.99)
Fernandes, et al. Heart Rhythm. 2021 [99].	Meta-analysis SGLT2i vs. Placebo	63,166 T2DM or HF	SCD reduction (HR 0.72; 95% CI 0.54–0.97) No difference in VA
Li, et al. Cardiovasc Diabetol. 2021 [104].	Meta-analysis SGLT2i vs. Placebo	52,115 T2DM or CKD or HF	VA reduction (RR 0.73; 95% CI 0.53–0.99)
Sfairopoulos et al. Europace. 2022 [100].	Meta-analysis SGLT2i vs. Placebo	55,590 T2DM or CKD or HF	No VA reduction (RR 0.84; 95% CI 0.66–1.06) No SCD reduction (RR 0.74; 95% CI 0.50–1.08)
Yin et al. Front Cardiovasc Med. 2022 [101].	Meta-analysis SGLT2i vs. Placebo	10,344 HFrEF or HFpEF	No VA reduction (VT: RR 0.90; 95% CI 0.44–1.82; VF: RR 1.40; 95% CI 0.73–2.67)
Oates, et al. J Cardiovasc Electrophysiol. 2023 [102].	Meta-analysis SGLT2i vs. Placebo	10,796 HFrEF or HFpEF	SCD reduction (RR 0.68; 95% CI 0.48–0.95) No VA reduction (RR 1.03; 95% CI 0.83–1.29)

CKD, Chronic Kidney Disease; HF, Heart Failure; HFpEF, Heart Failure with preserved ejection fraction; HFrEF, Heart Failure with reduced ejection fraction; RCT, Randomized Controlled Trial; SCD, Sudden Cardiac Death; SGLT2i, Sodium-Glucose Cotransporter 2 Inhibitor; T2DM, Type 2 Diabetes; VA, Ventricular Arrhythmia; VF, Ventricular Fibrillation; VT, Ventricular Tachycardia.

8. Implantable Cardioverter–Defibrillator in Light of New Heart Failure Treatment

ICD therapy is a cornerstone in the management of HFrEF, offering a proven benefit in reducing the risk of SCD. According to the current European Society of Cardiology (ESC) guidelines, ICD implantation is recommended with a class I indication for patients with ischemic HF and a left ventricular ejection fraction (LVEF) <35%, despite medical therapy for 3 months or more, and at a New York Heart Association (NYHA) functional class II or III. For patients with non-ischemic dilated cardiomyopathy, a Class IIa recommendation is provided [7]. Medical therapy includes the four classes of medications (BB, RAAS inhibitor, MRA, SGLT2i), each of which presents a Class I recommendation [4]. Similarly, the American Heart Association/American College of Cardiology/Heart Failure Society of America (AHA/ACC/HFSA) 2022 guidelines also endorse a Class 1 recommendation for both ischemic and non-ischemic patients [105].

These recommendations derive their basis from pivotal trials conducted over two decades ago—notably, MADIT II [106], SCD-HeFT [107], and DEFINITE [108]. In these studies, patient management included BB and RAAS inhibitors, such as ACEi and ARB, with approximately 20% of participants in the SCD-HeFT trial receiving an MRA. The more recent DANISH trial, however, did not demonstrate a significant reduction in all-cause mortality with ICD use, though a reduction in SCD was observed [109]. This outcome may be attributable to the inclusion of an older patient cohort, the extensive use of cardiac resynchronization therapy in both arms, or potentially, better medical management including the broader use of MRA and higher utilization rates of BB and ACEi/ARB compared to earlier trials. The latter highlights the importance of optimal medical therapy.

In the context of today's GDMT, including newer treatments such as ARNi and SGLT2i with a beneficial anti-arrhythmic profile, the criteria for ICD therapy may merit reconsideration. Prior data, predicated on outdated HFrEF management protocols, may no longer fully apply. Does the current GDMT have a sufficient anti-arrhythmic effect to disturb the benefit–risk balance of primary prevention ICD in HFrEF? Only proper trials could answer this question. Moreover, the timing for ICD implantation, currently recommended after 3 months of medical therapy, may also be challenged. The PROVE-HF trial indicated that within an HFrEF cohort treated with ARNi, 32% of patients exhibited an improvement in LVEF to over 35% at 6 months and 62% at 12 months [110]. Consequently, patients initially eligible for ICD therapy may no longer meet the criteria within this timeframe, suggesting that an ICD implantation at 3 months might be premature in this era of novel HF therapy. This improvement of LVEF with GDMT may play an important role in the burden reduction of VA. For example, Martens et al. [57] reported that patients treated with ARNi exhibiting more left ventricular reverse remodeling (defined by a mean improvement in LVEF of 5%) present a significantly lower burden of VA, compared to those with less reverse remodeling. Besides their direct beneficial effect on structural substrate and electrical remodeling, GDMT's improvement of LVEF may by itself decrease the arrhythmic burden, due to its hemodynamic benefit with a more favorable neurohormonal profile.

All these considerations question the exact place of ICD in this contemporary era of HF medication. In the absence of appropriate trials that incorporate the latest GDMT, adherence to existing guidelines is obligatory. However, there is a compelling need for updated research to more precisely define the indications and optimal timing for ICD implantation in the current therapeutic landscape.

9. Emerging Horizons in Heart Failure Treatment

Vericiguat and Omecamtiv Mecarbil represent newer pharmacological interventions for HFrEF. Vericiguat is a soluble guanylate cyclase (sGC) activator. By modulating the sGC-cyclic guanosine monophosphate pathway, Vericiguat induces vasodilatation, which in turn has beneficial effects on left ventricular afterload and hypertrophy [111,112]. The VICTORIA Study demonstrated that Vericiguat led to a statistically significant reduction in the primary endpoint of death from cardiovascular causes or heart failure hospitalizations. However, data specifically concerning SCD were not provided [113]. In pre-clinical mouse models, Vericiguat demonstrated the potential for anti-arrhythmic properties through favorable effects on ventricular remodeling and ionic currents, notably by inhibiting CaMKII [114]. Further investigations are warranted to validate these preliminary findings on its anti-arrhythmic properties.

Omecamtiv Mecarbil, on the other hand, was evaluated in the GALACTIC-HF trial in 2020 and showed a significant but modest lowering of the incidence of the primary composite outcome of heart failure hospitalization or death from cardiovascular causes [115]. The incidence of VA in the Omecamtiv Mecarbil cohort was analogous to that of the placebo group. Given these results, the anti-arrhythmic potential of Omecamtiv Mecarbil remains inconclusive at present.

Another drug worth mentioning is Glucagon-like peptide 1 receptor agonists (GLP-1 RA), which represent a relatively recent class of drugs introduced for the treatment of T2DM, exhibiting a range of diverse effects—notably, favorable metabolic outcomes [116]. Major trials investigating GLP-1 RA in T2DM have shown a reduction in major adverse cardiovascular events [117–119]. Regarding the HFrEF population specifically, two pivotal trials warrant mention. The FIGHT study, evaluating Liraglutide in HFrEF, reported no significant benefits, including in LVEF [120]. A post hoc analysis showed an excess risk of arrhythmias and HF events [121]. Furthermore, the LIVE study associated Liraglutide treatment with an increase in the heart rate and serious cardiac adverse events, including VT [122]. This brings concerns about the risk of VAs and SCD in HFrEF patients. Multiple meta-analyses regarding the T2DM population did not reveal an increased risk for VAs or SCD with GLP-1 RA use [123,124]. The overall impact of GLP-1 RAs on VA and SCD in the HFrEF population remains inconclusive, as does their general effect in HFrEF management. Nonetheless, their utility in heart failure with preserved ejection fraction (HFpEF) appears more promising, attributed to their broad spectrum of effects, including weight loss [116], improved diastolic function [125], and mitochondrial function enhancements [126]. This is supported by the STEP-HFpEF trial, endorsing the use of Semaglutide in HFpEF patients with an obesity phenotype [127].

All these new drugs offer innovative therapeutic approaches for HF, though the data on their anti-arrhythmic effects are limited and inconclusive (Figure 2). The outcomes of these initial trials signal the need for more targeted investigations, especially about potential anti-arrhythmic properties and their impact on SCD and VA.

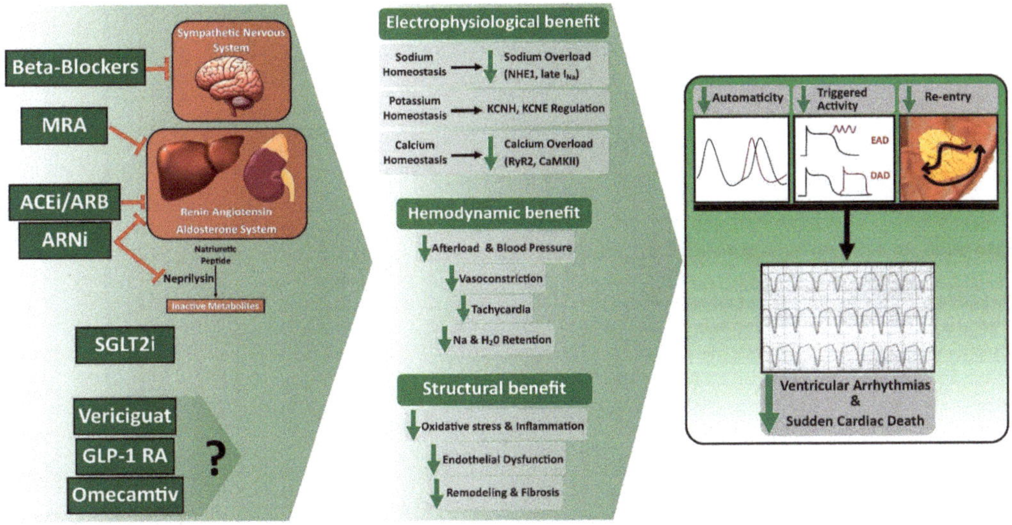

Figure 2. Effects of Guideline-directed medical therapy on Ventricular Arrhythmia and Sudden Cardiac Death. ACEi, Angiotensin-Converting Enzyme Inhibitors; ARB, Angiotensin II Receptor Blocker; ARNi, Angiotensin Receptor–Neprilysin Inhibitors; DAD, Delayed Afterdepolarization; EAD, Early Afterdepolarization; GLP-1 RA, Glucagon-like peptide 1 receptor agonists; MRA, Mineralocorticoid Receptor Antagonist; SGLT2i, Sodium-Glucose Cotransporter 2 Inhibitor.

10. Conclusions

In conclusion, SCD constitutes a critical contributor to mortality among patients with HFrEF, predominantly due to malignant VA. The optimization of GDMT serves as an effective strategy to mitigating the incidence of SCD within this population. Therapeutic interventions primarily target key systems such as the RAAS and the sympathetic nervous system, preventing both structural and electrical remodeling of the myocardium.

Despite their favorable modulatory effects on RAAS, ACEi and ARB have not been conclusively associated with a reduction in either SCD or VA. Robust evidence supports the utility of BB, ARNi, and MRA in reducing the risk of SCD. Furthermore, SGLT2i offer promising preliminary data, necessitating further well-designed prospective studies for confirmation of their anti-arrhythmic effects. Through the employment of different complementary mechanisms of action, those molecules act in synergy, highlighting the importance of optimizing GDMT to reduce arrhythmic risk in HFrEF.

Overall, the landscape of pharmacological interventions for HFrEF is progressively expanding, with novel agents undergoing evaluation. Further research is imperative for the unequivocal delineation of these agents' impact on SCD and VA, thus augmenting our arsenal in the management of HFrEF.

Author Contributions: Conceptualization, W.Z. and A.S.; literature research, W.Z.; writing—original draft, W.Z.; writing—review and editing, L.P., D.G.D.R. and A.S.; supervision and resources, S.B., C.d.A., G.-B.C. and A.S. All authors have read and agreed to the published version of the manuscript.

Funding: This research received no external funding.

Data Availability Statement: No new data were created or analyzed in this study. Data sharing is not applicable to this article.

Acknowledgments: All the figures in this manuscript were created with https://www.biorender.com/ accessed on 1 December 2023; unsplash.com accessed on 1 December 2023; and Microsoft Publisher.

Conflicts of Interest: The authors declare no conflicts of interest.

References

1. Kannel, W.B.; Plehn, J.F.; Cupples, L. Cardiac failure and sudden death in the Framingham Study. *Am. Heart J.* **1988**, *115*, 869–875. [CrossRef]
2. Zipes, D.P.; Wellens, H.J.J. Sudden Cardiac Death. *Circulation* **1998**, *98*, 2334–2351. [CrossRef]
3. Deo, R.; Albert, C.M. Epidemiology and Genetics of Sudden Cardiac Death. *Circulation* **2012**, *125*, 620–637. [CrossRef] [PubMed]
4. McDonagh, T.A.; Metra, M.; Adamo, M.; Gardner, R.S.; Baumbach, A.; Böhm, M.; Burri, H.; Butler, J.; Čelutkienė, J.; Chioncel, O.; et al. 2021 ESC guidelines for the diagnosis and treatment of acute and chronic heart failure: Developed by the Task Force for the diagnosis and treatment of acute and chronic heart failure of the European Society of Cardiology (ESC) With the special contribution of the Heart Failure Association (HFA) of the ESC. *Heart J.* **2021**, *42*, 3599–3726. [CrossRef]
5. Tromp, J.; Ouwerkerk, W.; van Veldhuisen, D.J.; Hillege, H.L.; Richards, A.M.; van der Meer, P.; Anand, I.S.; Lam, C.S.; Voors, A.A. A Systematic Review and Network Meta-Analysis of Pharmacological Treatment of Heart Failure with Reduced Ejection Fraction. *JACC Heart Fail.* **2022**, *10*, 73–84. [CrossRef] [PubMed]
6. Shen, L.; Jhund, P.S.; Petrie, M.C.; Claggett, B.L.; Barlera, S.; Cleland, J.G.F.; Dargie, H.J.; Granger, C.B.; Kjekshus, J.; Køber, L.; et al. Declining Risk of Sudden Death in Heart Failure. *N. Engl. J. Med.* **2017**, *377*, 41–51. [CrossRef] [PubMed]
7. Zeppenfeld, K.; Tfelt-Hansen, J.; de Riva, M.; Winkel, B.G.; Behr, E.R.; Blom, N.; Charron, P.; Corrado, D.; Dagres, N.; de Chillou, C.; et al. 2022 ESC Guidelines for the management of patients with ventricular arrhythmias and the prevention of sudden cardiac death. *Eur. Heart J.* **2022**, *43*, 3997–4126. [CrossRef]
8. Cherry, E.M.; Fenton, F.H.; Gilmour, R.F. Mechanisms of ventricular arrhythmias: A dynamical systems-based perspective. *Am. J. Physiol. Circ. Physiol.* **2012**, *302*, H2451–H2463. [CrossRef] [PubMed]
9. Landstrom, A.P.; Dobrev, D.; Wehrens, X.H.T. Calcium Signaling and Cardiac Arrhythmias. *Circ. Res.* **2017**, *120*, 1969–1993. [CrossRef] [PubMed]
10. Schrier, R.W.; Abraham, W.T. Hormones and Hemodynamics in Heart Failure. *N. Engl. J. Med.* **1999**, *341*, 577–585. [CrossRef]
11. Rockey, D.C.; Bell, P.D.; Hill, J.A. Fibrosis—A Common Pathway to Organ Injury and Failure. *N. Engl. J. Med.* **2015**, *372*, 1138–1149. [CrossRef]
12. Verheule, S.; Schotten, U. Electrophysiological Consequences of Cardiac Fibrosis. *Cells* **2021**, *10*, 3220. [CrossRef]
13. Weber, K.T.; Brilla, C.G. Pathological hypertrophy and cardiac interstitium. Fibrosis and renin-angiotensin-aldosterone system. *Circulation* **1991**, *83*, 1849–1865. [CrossRef]
14. Mathieu, S.; El Khoury, N.; Rivard, K.; Gélinas, R.; Goyette, P.; Paradis, P.; Nemer, M.; Fiset, C. Reduction in Na^+ current by angiotensin II is mediated by PKCα in mouse and human-induced pluripotent stem cell–derived cardiomyocytes. *Heart Rhythm.* **2016**, *13*, 1346–1354. [CrossRef]
15. Zhang, T.-T.; Takimoto, K.; Stewart, A.F.R.; Zhu, C.; Levitan, E.S. Independent Regulation of Cardiac Kv4.3 Potassium Channel Expression by Angiotensin II and Phenylephrine. *Circ. Res.* **2001**, *88*, 476–482. [CrossRef]
16. Zhao, Z.; Fefelova, N.; Shanmugam, M.; Bishara, P.; Babu, G.J.; Xie, L.-H. Angiotensin II induces afterdepolarizations via reactive oxygen species and calmodulin kinase II signaling. *J. Mol. Cell. Cardiol.* **2011**, *50*, 128–136. [CrossRef]
17. Sag, C.M.; Wadsack, D.P.; Khabbazzadeh, S.; Abesser, M.; Grefe, C.; Neumann, K.; Opiela, M.-K.; Backs, J.; Olson, E.N.; Brown, J.H.; et al. Calcium/Calmodulin-Dependent Protein Kinase II Contributes to Cardiac Arrhythmogenesis in Heart Failure. *Circ. Heart Fail.* **2009**, *2*, 664–675. [CrossRef]
18. Shannon, T.R.; Lew, W.Y. Diastolic Release of Calcium from the Sarcoplasmic Reticulum: A Potential Target for Treating Triggered Arrhythmias and Heart Failure. *J. Am. Coll. Cardiol.* **2009**, *53*, 2006–2008. [CrossRef] [PubMed]
19. Bers, D.M. Calcium Cycling and Signaling in Cardiac Myocytes. *Annu. Rev. Physiol.* **2008**, *70*, 23–49. [CrossRef] [PubMed]
20. Bers, D.M. Cardiac excitation–contraction coupling. *Nature* **2002**, *415*, 198–205. [CrossRef] [PubMed]
21. Grandi, E.; Ripplinger, C.M. Antiarrhythmic mechanisms of beta blocker therapy. *Pharmacol. Res.* **2019**, *146*, 104274. [CrossRef] [PubMed]
22. Barrese, V.; Taglialatela, M. New advances in beta-blocker therapy in heart failure. *Front. Physiol.* **2013**, *4*, 323. [CrossRef] [PubMed]
23. CIBIS-II Investigators and committees The Cardiac Insufficiency Bisoprolol Study II (CIBIS-II): A randomised trial. *Lancet* **1999**, *353*, 9–13. [CrossRef]

24. Merit-HF Study Group. Effect of metoprolol CR/XL in chronic heart failure: Metoprolol CR/XL Randomised Intervention Trial in-Congestive Heart Failure (MERIT-HF). *Lancet* **1999**, *353*, 2001–2007. [CrossRef]
25. Flather, M.D.; Shibata, M.C.; Coats, A.J.; Van Veldhuisen, D.J.; Parkhomenko, A.; Borbola, J.; Cohen-Solal, A.; Dumitrascu, D.; Ferrari, R.; Lechat, P.; et al. Randomized trial to determine the effect of nebivolol on mortality and cardiovascular hospital admission in elderly patients with heart failure (SENIORS). *Eur. Heart J.* **2005**, *26*, 215–225. [CrossRef]
26. Packer, M.; Coats, A.J.; Fowler, M.B.; Katus, H.A.; Krum, H.; Mohacsi, P.; Rouleau, J.L.; Tendera, M.; Castaigne, A.; Roecker, E.B.; et al. Effect of Carvedilol on Survival in Severe Chronic Heart Failure. *N. Engl. J. Med.* **2001**, *344*, 1651–1658. [CrossRef]
27. Connolly, S.J.; Dorian, P.; Roberts, R.S.; Gent, M.; Bailin, S.; Fain, E.S.; Thorpe, K.; Champagne, J.; Talajic, M.; Coutu, B.; et al. Comparison of β-Blockers, Amiodarone Plus β-Blockers, or Sotalol for Prevention of Shocks from Implantable Cardioverter Defibrillators: The OPTIC Study: A Randomized Trial. *JAMA* **2006**, *295*, 165–171. [CrossRef]
28. Chatterjee, S.; Biondi-Zoccai, G.; Abbate, A.; D'ascenzo, F.; Castagno, D.; Van Tassell, B.; Mukherjee, D.; Lichstein, E. Benefits of blockers in patients with heart failure and reduced ejection fraction: Network meta-analysis. *BMJ* **2013**, *346*, f55. [CrossRef]
29. Al-Gobari, M.; El Khatib, C.; Pillon, F.; Gueyffier, F. Beta-blockers for the prevention of sudden cardiac death in heart failure patients: A meta-analysis of randomized controlled trials. *BMC Cardiovasc. Disord.* **2013**, *13*, 52. [CrossRef]
30. Al-Gobari, M.; Al-Aqeel, S.; Gueyffier, F.; Burnand, B. Effectiveness of drug interventions to prevent sudden cardiac death in patients with heart failure and reduced ejection fraction: An overview of systematic reviews. *BMJ Open* **2018**, *8*, e021108. [CrossRef]
31. Chatzidou, S.; Kontogiannis, C.; Tsilimigras, D.I.; Georgiopoulos, G.; Kosmopoulos, M.; Papadopoulou, E.; Vasilopoulos, G.; Rokas, S. Propranolol Versus Metoprolol for Treatment of Electrical Storm in Patients with Implantable Cardioverter-Defibrillator. *J. Am. Coll. Cardiol.* **2018**, *71*, 1897–1906. [CrossRef]
32. Diamond, A.; Goldenberg, I.; Younis, A.; Goldenberg, I.; Sampath, R.; Kutyifa, V.; Chen, A.Y.; McNitt, S.; Polonsky, B.; Steinberg, J.S.; et al. Effect of Carvedilol vs Metoprolol on Atrial and Ventricular Arrhythmias Among Implantable Cardioverter-Defibrillator Recipients. *JACC Clin. Electrophysiol.* **2023**, *9*, 2122–2131. [CrossRef] [PubMed]
33. Goodfriend, T.L.; Elliott, M.E.; Catt, K.J. Angiotensin Receptors and Their Antagonists. *N. Engl. J. Med.* **1996**, *334*, 1649–1655. [CrossRef] [PubMed]
34. Makkar, K.M.; Sanoski, C.A.; Spinler, S.A. Role of Angiotensin-Converting Enzyme Inhibitors, Angiotensin II Receptor Blockers, and Aldosterone Antagonists in the Prevention of Atrial and Ventricular Arrhythmias. *Pharmacother. J. Hum. Pharmacol. Drug Ther.* **2009**, *29*, 31–48. [CrossRef] [PubMed]
35. CONSENSUS Trial Study Group. Effects of enalapril on mortality in severe congestive heart failure. Results of the Cooperative North Scandinavian Enalapril Survival Study (CONSENSUS). *N. Engl. J. Med.* **1987**, *316*, 1429–1435. [CrossRef] [PubMed]
36. SOLVD Investigators; Yusuf, S.; Pitt, B.; Davis, C.E.; Hood, W.B.; Cohn, J.N. Effect of Enalapril on Survival in Patients with Reduced Left Ventricular Ejection Fractions and Congestive Heart Failure. *N. Engl. J. Med.* **1991**, *325*, 293–302. [CrossRef]
37. Pitt, B.; Segal, R.; Martinez, F.A.; Meurers, G.; Cowley, A.J.; Thomas, I.; Deedwania, P.C.; Ney, D.; Snavely, D.B.; Chang, P.I. Randomised trial of losartan versus captopril in patients over 65 with heart failure (Evaluation of Losartan in the Elderly Study, ELITE). *Lancet* **1997**, *349*, 747–752. [CrossRef] [PubMed]
38. Pitt, B.; Poole-Wilson, P.A.; Segal, R.; Martinez, F.A.; Dickstein, K.; Camm, A.J.; Konstam, M.A.; Riegger, G.; Klinger, G.H.; Neaton, J.; et al. Effect of losartan compared with captopril on mortality in patients with symptomatic heart failure: Randomised trial—The Losartan Heart Failure Survival Study ELITE II. *Lancet* **2000**, *355*, 1582–1587. [CrossRef] [PubMed]
39. McMurray, J.J.; Östergren, J.; Swedberg, K.; Granger, C.B.; Held, P.; Michelson, E.L.; Olofsson, B.; Yusuf, S.; Pfeffer, M.A. Effects of candesartan in patients with chronic heart failure and reduced left-ventricular systolic function taking angiotensin-converting-enzyme inhibitors: The CHARM-Added trial. *Lancet* **2003**, *362*, 767–771. [CrossRef]
40. Cohn, J.N.; Tognoni, G. Valsartan Heart Failure Trial Investigators. A Randomized Trial of the Angiotensin-Receptor Blocker Valsartan in Chronic Heart Failure. *N. Engl. J. Med.* **2001**, *345*, 1667–1675. [CrossRef]
41. AlJaroudi, W.A.; Refaat, M.M.; Habib, R.H.; Al-Shaar, L.; Singh, M.; Gutmann, R.; Bloom, H.L.; Dudley, S.C.; Ellinor, P.T.; Saba, S.F.; et al. Effect of Angiotensin-Converting Enzyme Inhibitors and Receptor Blockers on Appropriate Implantable Cardiac Defibrillator Shock in Patients with Severe Systolic Heart Failure (from the GRADE Multicenter Study). *Am. J. Cardiol.* **2015**, *115*, 924–931. [CrossRef]
42. Schupp, T.; Behnes, M.; Weiß, C.; Nienaber, C.; Lang, S.; Reiser, L.; Bollow, A.; Taton, G.; Reichelt, T.; Ellguth, D.; et al. Prognostic Impact of Angiotensin-Converting Enzyme Inhibitors and Receptor Blockers on Recurrent Ventricular Tachyarrhythmias and Implantable Cardioverter–Defibrillator Therapies. *J. Cardiovasc. Pharmacol.* **2019**, *73*, 272–281. [CrossRef]
43. Schupp, T.; Behnes, M.; Weiß, C.; Nienaber, C.; Lang, S.; Reiser, L.; Bollow, A.; Taton, G.; Reichelt, T.; Ellguth, D.; et al. Beta-Blockers and ACE Inhibitors Are Associated with Improved Survival Secondary to Ventricular Tachyarrhythmia. *Cardiovasc. Drugs Ther.* **2018**, *32*, 353–363. [CrossRef]
44. Garg, R.; Yusuf, S.; Bussmann, W.D.; Sleight, P.; Uprichard, A.; Massie, B.; McGrath, B.; Nilsson, B.; Pitt, B.; Magnani, B.; et al. Overview of Randomized Trials of Angiotensin-Converting Enzyme Inhibitors on Mortality and Morbidity in Patients with Heart Failure. Collaborative Group on ACE Inhibitor Trials. *JAMA* **1995**, *273*, 1450–1456. [CrossRef]
45. Flather, M.D.; Yusuf, S.; Køber, L.; Pfeffer, M.; Hall, A.; Murray, G.; Torp-Pedersen, C.; Ball, S.; Pogue, J.; Moyé, L.; et al. Long-term ACE-inhibitor therapy in patients with heart failure or left-ventricular dysfunction: A systematic overview of data from individual patients. ACE-Inhibitor Myocardial Infarction Collaborative Group. *Lancet* **2000**, *355*, 1575–1581. [CrossRef]

46. Tsartsalis, D.; Korela, D.; Karlsson, L.O.; Foukarakis, E.; Svensson, A.; Anastasakis, A.; Venetsanos, D.; Aggeli, C.; Tsioufis, C.; Braunschweig, F.; et al. Risk and Protective Factors for Sudden Cardiac Death: An Umbrella Review of Meta-Analyses. *Front. Cardiovasc. Med.* **2022**, *9*, 848021. [CrossRef]
47. Domanski, M.J.; Exner, D.V.; Borkowf, C.B.; Geller, N.L.; Rosenberg, Y.; Pfeffer, M.A. Effect of angiotensin converting enzyme inhibition on sudden cardiac death in patients following acute myocardial infarction: A meta-analysis of randomized clinical trials. *J. Am. Coll. Cardiol.* **1999**, *33*, 598–604. [CrossRef]
48. Gu, J.; Noe, A.; Chandra, P.; Al-Fayoumi, S.; Ligueros-Saylan, M.; Sarangapani, R.; Maahs, S.; Ksander, G.; Rigel, D.F.; Jeng, A.Y.; et al. Pharmacokinetics and Pharmacodynamics of LCZ696, a Novel Dual-Acting Angiotensin Receptor—Neprilysin Inhibitor (ARNi). *J. Clin. Pharmacol.* **2010**, *50*, 401–414. [CrossRef]
49. Chang, P.-C.; Lin, S.-F.; Chu, Y.; Wo, H.-T.; Lee, H.-L.; Huang, Y.-C.; Wen, M.-S.; Chou, C.-C. LCZ696 Therapy Reduces Ventricular Tachyarrhythmia Inducibility in a Myocardial Infarction-Induced Heart Failure Rat Model. *Cardiovasc. Ther.* **2019**, *2019*, 6032631. [CrossRef]
50. Eiringhaus, J.; Wünsche, C.M.; Tirilomis, P.; Herting, J.; Bork, N.; Nikolaev, V.O.; Hasenfuss, G.; Sossalla, S.; Fischer, T.H. Sacubitrilat reduces pro-arrhythmogenic sarcoplasmic reticulum Ca^{2+} leak in human ventricular cardiomyocytes of patients with end-stage heart failure. *ESC Heart Fail.* **2020**, *7*, 2992–3002. [CrossRef]
51. Chang, P.-C.; Wo, H.-T.; Lee, H.-L.; Lin, S.-F.; Chu, Y.; Wen, M.-S.; Chou, C.-C. Sacubitril/Valsartan Therapy Ameliorates Ventricular Tachyarrhythmia Inducibility in a Rabbit Myocardial Infarction Model. *J. Card. Fail.* **2020**, *26*, 527–537. [CrossRef]
52. D'Elia, E.; Iacovoni, A.; Vaduganathan, M.; Lorini, F.L.; Perlini, S.; Senni, M. Neprilysin inhibition in heart failure: Mechanisms and substrates beyond modulating natriuretic peptides. *Eur. J. Heart Fail.* **2017**, *19*, 710–717. [CrossRef]
53. Pfau, D.; Thorn, S.L.; Zhang, J.; Mikush, N.; Renaud, J.M.; Klein, R.; deKemp, R.A.; Wu, X.; Hu, X.; Sinusas, A.J.; et al. Angiotensin Receptor Neprilysin Inhibitor Attenuates Myocardial Remodeling and Improves Infarct Perfusion in Experimental Heart Failure. *Sci. Rep.* **2019**, *9*, 5791. [CrossRef]
54. von Lueder, T.G.; Wang, B.H.; Kompa, A.R.; Huang, L.; Webb, R.; Jordaan, P.; Atar, D.; Krum, H. Angiotensin Receptor Neprilysin Inhibitor LCZ696 Attenuates Cardiac Remodeling and Dysfunction After Myocardial Infarction by Reducing Cardiac Fibrosis and Hypertrophy. *Circ. Heart Fail.* **2015**, *8*, 71–78. [CrossRef]
55. Sung, Y.-L.; Lin, T.-T.; Syu, J.-Y.; Hsu, H.-J.; Lin, K.-Y.; Liu, Y.-B.; Lin, S.-F. Reverse electromechanical modelling of diastolic dysfunction in spontaneous hypertensive rat after sacubitril/valsartan therapy. *ESC Heart Fail.* **2020**, *7*, 4040–4050. [CrossRef]
56. Zile, M.R.; O'Meara, E.; Claggett, B.; Prescott, M.F.; Solomon, S.D.; Swedberg, K.; Packer, M.; McMurray, J.J.; Shi, V.; Lefkowitz, M.; et al. Effects of Sacubitril/Valsartan on Biomarkers of Extracellular Matrix Regulation in Patients with HFrEF. *J. Am. Coll. Cardiol.* **2019**, *73*, 795–806. [CrossRef]
57. Martens, P.; Nuyens, D.; Rivero-Ayerza, M.; Van Herendael, H.; Vercammen, J.; Ceyssens, W.; Luwel, E.; Dupont, M.; Mullens, W. Sacubitril/valsartan reduces ventricular arrhythmias in parallel with left ventricular reverse remodeling in heart failure with reduced ejection fraction. *Clin. Res. Cardiol.* **2019**, *108*, 1074–1082. [CrossRef]
58. de Diego, C.; González-Torres, L.; Núñez, J.M.; Inda, R.C.; Martin-Langerwerf, D.A.; Sangio, A.D.; Chochowski, P.; Casasnovas, P.; Blazquéz, J.C.; Almendral, J. Effects of angiotensin-neprilysin inhibition compared to angiotensin inhibition on ventricular arrhythmias in reduced ejection fraction patients under continuous remote monitoring of implantable defibrillator devices. *Heart Rhythm.* **2018**, *15*, 395–402. [CrossRef]
59. Rohde, L.E.; Chatterjee, N.A.; Vaduganathan, M.; Claggett, B.; Packer, M.; Desai, A.S.; Zile, M.; Rouleau, J.; Swedberg, K.; Lefkowitz, M.; et al. Sacubitril/Valsartan and Sudden Cardiac Death According to Implantable Cardioverter-Defibrillator Use and Heart Failure Cause. *JACC Heart Fail.* **2020**, *8*, 844–855. [CrossRef]
60. Curtain, J.P.; Jackson, A.M.; Shen, L.; Jhund, P.S.; Docherty, K.F.; Petrie, M.C.; Castagno, D.; Desai, A.S.; Rohde, L.E.; Lefkowitz, M.P.; et al. Effect of sacubitril/valsartan on investigator-reported ventricular arrhythmias in PARADIGM-HF. *Eur. J. Heart Fail.* **2022**, *24*, 551–561. [CrossRef]
61. Liu, X.-H.; Wang, G.-L.; Xu, Q.; Zhang, L.; Liu, H.-J. Effect of sacubitril/valsartan on the occurrence of cardiac arrhythmias and the risk of sudden cardiac death in heart failure: A meta-analysis of randomized controlled trials. *Front. Cardiovasc. Med.* **2022**, *9*, 943377. [CrossRef]
62. Pozzi, A.; Abete, R.; Tavano, E.; Kristensen, S.L.; Rea, F.; Iorio, A.; Iacovoni, A.; Corrado, G.; Wong, C. Sacubitril/valsartan and arrhythmic burden in patients with heart failure and reduced ejection fraction: A systematic review and meta-analysis. *Heart Fail. Rev.* **2023**, *28*, 1395–1403. [CrossRef]
63. Fernandes, A.D.; Fernandes, G.C.; Ternes, C.M.; Cardoso, R.; Chaparro, S.V.; Goldberger, J.J. Sacubitril/valsartan versus angiotensin inhibitors and arrhythmia endpoints in heart failure with reduced ejection fraction. *Heart Rhythm. O2* **2021**, *2*, 724–732. [CrossRef]
64. Russo, V.; Bottino, R.; Rago, A.; Papa, A.A.; Liccardo, B.; Proietti, R.; Manna, V.; Golino, P.; D'Onofrio, A.; Nigro, G. The Effect of Sacubitril/Valsartan on Device Detected Arrhythmias and Electrical Parameters among Dilated Cardiomyopathy Patients with Reduced Ejection Fraction and Implantable Cardioverter Defibrillator. *J. Clin. Med.* **2020**, *9*, 1111. [CrossRef]
65. Mujadzic, H.; Prousi, G.S.; Napier, R.; Siddique, S.; Zaman, N. The Impact of Angiotensin Receptor–Neprilysin Inhibitors on Arrhythmias in Patients with Heart Failure: A Systematic Review and Meta-analysis. *J. Innov. Card. Rhythm. Manag.* **2022**, *13*, 5164–5175. [CrossRef]
66. Weber, K.T. Aldosterone in Congestive Heart Failure. *N. Engl. J. Med.* **2001**, *345*, 1689–1697. [CrossRef]

67. Perrier, E.; Kerfant, B.-G.; Lalevee, N.; Bideaux, P.; Rossier, M.F.; Richard, S.; Gómez, A.M.; Benitah, J.-P. Mineralocorticoid Receptor Antagonism Prevents the Electrical Remodeling That Precedes Cellular Hypertrophy After Myocardial Infarction. *Circ.* **2004**, *110*, 776–783. [CrossRef]
68. Ouvrard-Pascaud, A.; Sainte-Marie, Y.; Perrier, R.; Soukaseum, C.; Cat, A.N.D.; Royer, A.; Le Quang, K.; Charpentier, F.; Demolombe, S.; Mechta-Grigoriou, F.; et al. Conditional Mineralocorticoid Receptor Expression in the Heart Leads to Life-Threatening Arrhythmias. *Circulation* **2005**, *111*, 3025–3033. [CrossRef]
69. Brilla, C.G. Aldosterone and myocardial fibrosis in heart failure. *Herz* **2000**, *25*, 299–306. [CrossRef]
70. Cittadini, A.; Monti, M.G.; Isgaard, J.; Casaburi, C.; Strömer, H.; Di Gianni, A.; Serpico, R.; Saldamarco, L.; Vanasia, M.; Saccà, L. Aldosterone receptor blockade improves left ventricular remodeling and increases ventricular fibrillation threshold in experimental heart failure. *Cardiovasc. Res.* **2003**, *58*, 555–564. [CrossRef]
71. Brown, N.J. Eplerenone: Cardiovascular protection. *Circulation* **2003**, *107*, 2512–2518. [CrossRef]
72. Bauersachs, J.; Heck, M.; Fraccarollo, D.; Hildemann, S.K.; Ertl, G.; Wehling, M.; Christ, M. Addition of spironolactone to angiotensin-converting enzyme inhibition in heart failure improves endothelial vasomotor dysfunction: Role of vascular superoxide anion formation and endothelial nitric oxide synthase expression. *J. Am. Coll. Cardiol.* **2002**, *39*, 351–358. [CrossRef]
73. Pitt, B.; Zannad, F.; Remme, W.J.; Cody, R.; Castaigne, A.; Perez, A.; Palensky, J.; Wittes, J. The effect of spironolactone on morbidity and mortality in patients with severe heart failure. Randomized Aldactone Evaluation Study Investigators. *N. Engl. J. Med.* **1999**, *341*, 709–717. [CrossRef]
74. Pitt, B.; Williams, G.; Remme, W.; Martinez, F.; Lopez-Sendon, J.; Zannad, F.; Neaton, J.; Roniker, B.; Hurley, S.; Burns, D.; et al. The EPHESUS Trial: Eplerenone in Patients with Heart Failure Due to Systolic Dysfunction Complicating Acute Myocardial Infarction. Eplerenone Post-AMI Heart Failure Efficacy and Survival Study. *Cardiovasc. Drugs Ther.* **2001**, *15*, 79–87. [CrossRef]
75. Bapoje, S.R.; Bahia, A.; Hokanson, J.E.; Peterson, P.N.; Heidenreich, P.A.; Lindenfeld, J.; Allen, L.A.; Masoudi, F.A. Effects of Mineralocorticoid Receptor Antagonists on the Risk of Sudden Cardiac Death in Patients with Left Ventricular Systolic Dysfunction: A meta-analysis of randomized controlled trials. *Circ. Heart Fail.* **2013**, *6*, 166–173. [CrossRef]
76. Le, H.-H.; El-Khatib, C.; Mombled, M.; Guitarian, F.; Al-Gobari, M.; Fall, M.; Janiaud, P.; Marchant, I.; Cucherat, M.; Bejan-Angoulvant, T.; et al. Impact of Aldosterone Antagonists on Sudden Cardiac Death Prevention in Heart Failure and Post-Myocardial Infarction Patients: A Systematic Review and Meta-Analysis of Randomized Controlled Trials. *PLoS ONE* **2016**, *11*, e0145958. [CrossRef]
77. Rossello, X.; Ariti, C.; Pocock, S.J.; Ferreira, J.P.; Girerd, N.; McMurray, J.J.V.; Van Veldhuisen, D.J.; Pitt, B.; Zannad, F. Impact of mineralocorticoid receptor antagonists on the risk of sudden cardiac death in patients with heart failure and left-ventricular systolic dysfunction: An individual patient-level meta-analysis of three randomized-controlled trials. *Clin. Res. Cardiol.* **2018**, *108*, 477–486. [CrossRef]
78. Zannad, F.; Ferreira, J.P.; Pocock, S.J.; Anker, S.D.; Butler, J.; Filippatos, G.; Brueckmann, M.; Ofstad, A.P.; Pfarr, E.; Jamal, W.; et al. SGLT2 inhibitors in patients with heart failure with reduced ejection fraction: A meta-analysis of the EMPEROR-Reduced and DAPA-HF trials. *Lancet* **2020**, *396*, 819–829. [CrossRef]
79. Schönberger, E.; Mihaljević, V.; Steiner, K.; Šarić, S.; Kurevija, T.; Majnarić, L.T.; Ćurčić, I.B.; Canecki-Varžić, S. Immunomodulatory Effects of SGLT2 Inhibitors—Targeting Inflammation and Oxidative Stress in Aging. *Int. J. Environ. Res. Public Health* **2023**, *20*, 6671. [CrossRef]
80. Hasan, R.; Lasker, S.; Hasan, A.; Zerin, F.; Zamila, M.; Chowdhury, F.I.; Nayan, S.I.; Rahman, M.; Khan, F.; Subhan, N.; et al. Canagliflozin attenuates isoprenaline-induced cardiac oxidative stress by stimulating multiple antioxidant and anti-inflammatory signaling pathways. *Sci. Rep.* **2020**, *10*, 14459. [CrossRef]
81. Koyani, C.N.; Plastira, I.; Sourij, H.; Hallström, S.; Schmidt, A.; Rainer, P.P.; Bugger, H.; Frank, S.; Malle, E.; von Lewinski, D. Empagliflozin protects heart from inflammation and energy depletion via AMPK activation. *Pharmacol. Res.* **2020**, *158*, 104870. [CrossRef]
82. Fu, J.; Xu, H.; Wu, F.; Tu, Q.; Dong, X.; Xie, H.; Cao, Z. Empagliflozin inhibits macrophage inflammation through AMPK signaling pathway and plays an anti-atherosclerosis role. *Int. J. Cardiol.* **2022**, *367*, 56–62. [CrossRef]
83. Byrne, N.J.; Matsumura, N.; Maayah, Z.H.; Ferdaoussi, M.; Takahara, S.; Darwesh, A.M.; Levasseur, J.L.; Jahng, J.W.S.; Vos, D.; Parajuli, N.; et al. Empagliflozin Blunts Worsening Cardiac Dysfunction Associated with Reduced NLRP3 (Nucleotide-Binding Domain-Like Receptor Protein 3) Inflammasome Activation in Heart Failure. *Circ. Heart Fail.* **2020**, *13*, e006277. [CrossRef]
84. Santos-Gallego, C.G.; Requena-Ibanez, J.A.; Antonio, R.S.; Ishikawa, K.; Watanabe, S.; Picatoste, B.; Flores, E.; Garcia-Ropero, A.; Sanz, J.; Hajjar, R.J.; et al. Empagliflozin Ameliorates Adverse Left Ventricular Remodeling in Nondiabetic Heart Failure by Enhancing Myocardial Energetics. *J. Am. Coll. Cardiol.* **2019**, *73*, 1931–1944. [CrossRef]
85. Carluccio, E.; Biagioli, P.; Reboldi, G.; Mengoni, A.; Lauciello, R.; Zuchi, C.; D'Addario, S.; Bardelli, G.; Ambrosio, G. Left ventricular remodeling response to SGLT2 inhibitors in heart failure: An updated meta-analysis of randomized controlled studies. *Cardiovasc. Diabetol.* **2023**, *22*, 235. [CrossRef]
86. Pascual-Figal, D.A.; Zamorano, J.L.; Domingo, M.; Morillas, H.; Nuñez, J.; Marcos, M.C.; Riquelme-Pérez, A.; Teis, A.; Santas, E.; Caro-Martinez, C.; et al. Impact of dapagliflozin on cardiac remodelling in patients with chronic heart failure: The DAPA-MODA study. *Eur. J. Heart Fail.* **2023**, *25*, 1352–1360. [CrossRef]

87. Wu, J.; Liu, T.; Shi, S.; Fan, Z.; Hiram, R.; Xiong, F.; Cui, B.; Su, X.; Chang, R.; Zhang, W.; et al. Dapagliflozin reduces the vulnerability of rats with pulmonary arterial hypertension-induced right heart failure to ventricular arrhythmia by restoring calcium handling. *Cardiovasc. Diabetol.* **2022**, *21*, 197. [CrossRef]
88. Trum, M.; Riechel, J.; Wagner, S. Cardioprotection by SGLT2 Inhibitors—Does It All Come Down to Na^+? *Int. J. Mol. Sci.* **2021**, *22*, 7976. [CrossRef]
89. Despa, S.; Bers, D.M. Na+ transport in the normal and failing heart—Remember the balance. *J. Mol. Cell Cardiol.* **2013**, *61*, 2–10. [CrossRef]
90. Wichaiyo, S.; Saengklub, N. Alterations of sodium-hydrogen exchanger 1 function in response to SGLT2 inhibitors: What is the evidence? *Heart Fail. Rev.* **2022**, *27*, 1973–1990. [CrossRef]
91. Philippaert, K.; Kalyaanamoorthy, S.; Fatehi, M.; Long, W.; Soni, S.; Byrne, N.J.; Barr, A.; Singh, J.; Wong, J.; Palechuk, T.; et al. Cardiac Late Sodium Channel Current Is a Molecular Target for the Sodium/Glucose Cotransporter 2 Inhibitor Empagliflozin. *Circulation* **2021**, *143*, 2188–2204. [CrossRef]
92. Mustroph, J.; Wagemann, O.; Lücht, C.M.; Trum, M.; Hammer, K.P.; Sag, C.M.; Lebek, S.; Tarnowski, D.; Reinders, J.; Perbellini, F.; et al. Empagliflozin reduces Ca/calmodulin-dependent kinase II activity in isolated ventricular cardiomyocytes. *ESC Heart Fail.* **2018**, *5*, 642–648. [CrossRef]
93. Nakase, M.; Yahagi, K.; Horiuchi, Y.; Asami, M.; Yuzawa, H.; Komiyama, K.; Tanaka, J.; Aoki, J.; Tanabe, K. Effect of dapagliflozin on ventricular repolarization in patients with heart failure with reduced ejection fraction. *Heart Vessel.* **2023**, *38*, 1414–1421. [CrossRef]
94. Xue, G.; Yang, X.; Zhan, G.; Wang, X.; Gao, J.; Zhao, Y.; Wang, X.; Li, J.; Pan, Z.; Xia, Y. Sodium–Glucose cotransporter 2 inhibitor empagliflozin decreases ventricular arrhythmia susceptibility by alleviating electrophysiological remodeling post-myocardial-infarction in mice. *Front. Pharmacol.* **2022**, *13*, 988408. [CrossRef]
95. Azam, M.A.; Chakraborty, P.; Si, D.; Du, B.; Massé, S.; Lai, P.F.H.; Ha, A.C.T.; Nanthakumar, K. Anti-arrhythmic and inotropic effects of empagliflozin following myocardial ischemia. *Life Sci.* **2021**, *276*, 119440. [CrossRef]
96. McMurray, J.J.V.; Solomon, S.D.; Inzucchi, S.E.; Køber, L.; Kosiborod, M.N.; Martinez, F.A.; Ponikowski, P.; Sabatine, M.S.; Anand, I.S.; Bělohlávek, J.; et al. Dapagliflozin in Patients with Heart Failure and Reduced Ejection Fraction. *N. Engl. J. Med.* **2019**, *381*, 1995–2008. [CrossRef]
97. Packer, M.; Anker, S.D.; Butler, J.; Filippatos, G.; Pocock, S.J.; Carson, P.; Januzzi, J.; Verma, S.; Tsutsui, H.; Brueckmann, M.; et al. Cardiovascular and Renal Outcomes with Empagliflozin in Heart Failure. *N. Engl. J. Med.* **2020**, *383*, 1413–1424. [CrossRef]
98. Curtain, J.P.; Docherty, K.F.; Jhund, P.S.; Petrie, M.C.; Inzucchi, S.E.; Køber, L.; Kosiborod, M.N.; Martinez, F.A.; Ponikowski, P.; Sabatine, M.S.; et al. Effect of dapagliflozin on ventricular arrhythmias, resuscitated cardiac arrest, or sudden death in DAPA-HF. *Eur. Heart J.* **2021**, *42*, 3727–3738. [CrossRef]
99. Fernandes, G.C.; Fernandes, A.; Cardoso, R.; Penalver, J.; Knijnik, L.; Mitrani, R.D.; Myerburg, R.J.; Goldberger, J.J. Association of SGLT2 inhibitors with arrhythmias and sudden cardiac death in patients with type 2 diabetes or heart failure: A meta-analysis of 34 randomized controlled trials. *Heart Rhythm.* **2021**, *18*, 1098–1105. [CrossRef]
100. Sfairopoulos, D.; Zhang, N.; Wang, Y.; Chen, Z.; Letsas, K.P.; Tse, G.; Li, G.; Lip, G.Y.H.; Liu, T.; Korantzopoulos, P. Association between sodium–glucose cotransporter-2 inhibitors and risk of sudden cardiac death or ventricular arrhythmias: A meta-analysis of randomized controlled trials. *Europace* **2022**, *24*, 20–30. [CrossRef]
101. Yin, Z.; Zheng, H.; Guo, Z. Effect of Sodium-Glucose Co-transporter Protein 2 Inhibitors on Arrhythmia in Heart Failure Patients with or Without Type 2 Diabetes: A Meta-Analysis of Randomized Controlled Trials. *Front. Cardiovasc. Med.* **2022**, *9*, 902923. [CrossRef]
102. Oates, C.P.; Santos-Gallego, C.G.; Smith, A.; Basyal, B.; Moss, N.; Kawamura, I.; Musikantow, D.R.; Turagam, M.K.; Miller, M.A.; Whang, W.; et al. SGLT2 inhibitors reduce sudden cardiac death risk in heart failure: Meta-analysis of randomized clinical trials. *J. Cardiovasc. Electrophysiol.* **2023**, *34*, 1277–1285. [CrossRef]
103. Fujiki, S.; Iijima, K.; Okabe, M.; Niwano, S.; Tsujita, K.; Naito, S.; Ando, K.; Kusano, K.; Kato, R.; Nitta, J.; et al. Placebo-Controlled, Double-Blind Study of Empagliflozin (EMPA) and Implantable Cardioverter-Defibrillator (EMPA-ICD) in Patients with Type 2 Diabetes (T2DM): Rationale and Design. *Diabetes Ther.* **2020**, *11*, 2739–2755. [CrossRef]
104. Li, H.-L.; Lip, G.Y.H.; Feng, Q.; Fei, Y.; Tse, Y.-K.; Wu, M.-Z.; Ren, Q.-W.; Tse, H.-F.; Cheung, B.-M.Y.; Yiu, K.-H. Sodium-glucose cotransporter 2 inhibitors (SGLT2i) and cardiac arrhythmias: A systematic review and meta-analysis. *Cardiovasc. Diabetol.* **2021**, *20*, 100. [CrossRef]
105. Heidenreich, P.A.; Bozkurt, B.; Aguilar, D.; Allen, L.A.; Byun, J.J.; Colvin, M.M.; Deswal, A.; Drazner, M.H.; Dunlay, S.M.; Evers, L.R.; et al. 2022 AHA/ACC/HFSA Guideline for the Management of Heart Failure: Executive Summary: A Report of the American College of Cardiology/American Heart Association Joint Committee on Clinical Practice Guidelines. *Circulation* **2022**, *145*, E876–E894. [CrossRef]
106. Moss, A.J.; Zareba, W.; Hall, W.J.; Klein, H.; Wilber, D.J.; Cannom, D.S.; Daubert, J.P.; Higgins, S.L.; Brown, M.W.; Andrews, M.L. Prophylactic implantation of a defibrillator in patients with myocardial infarction and reduced ejection fraction. *N. Engl. J. Med.* **2002**, *346*, 877–883. [CrossRef]
107. Bardy, G.H.; Lee, K.L.; Mark, D.B.; Poole, J.E.; Packer, D.L.; Boineau, R.; Domanski, M.; Troutman, C.; Anderson, J.; Johnson, G.; et al. Amiodarone or an Implantable Cardioverter–Defibrillator for Congestive Heart Failure. *N. Engl. J. Med.* **2005**, *352*, 225–237. [CrossRef]

108. Kadish, A.; Dyer, A.; Daubert, J.P.; Quigg, R.; Estes, N.A.; Anderson, K.P.; Calkins, H.; Hoch, D.; Goldberger, J.; Shalaby, A.; et al. Prophylactic Defibrillator Implantation in Patients with Nonischemic Dilated Cardiomyopathy. *N. Engl. J. Med.* **2004**, *350*, 2151–2158. [CrossRef]
109. Køber, L.; Thune, J.J.; Nielsen, J.C.; Haarbo, J.; Videbæk, L.; Korup, E.; Jensen, G.; Hildebrandt, P.; Steffensen, F.H.; Bruun, N.E.; et al. Defibrillator Implantation in Patients with Nonischemic Systolic Heart Failure. *N. Engl. J. Med.* **2016**, *375*, 1221–1230. [CrossRef]
110. Felker, G.M.; Butler, J.; Ibrahim, N.E.; Piña, I.L.; Maisel, A.; Bapat, D.; Camacho, A.; Ward, J.H.; Williamson, K.M.; Solomon, S.D.; et al. Implantable Cardioverter-Defibrillator Eligibility After Initiation of Sacubitril/Valsartan in Chronic Heart Failure: Insights From PROVE-HF. *Circulation* **2021**, *144*, 180–182. [CrossRef]
111. Gheorghiade, M.; Greene, S.J.; Butler, J.; Filippatos, G.; Lam, C.S.P.; Maggioni, A.P.; Ponikowski, P.; Shah, S.J.; Solomon, S.D.; Kraigher-Krainer, E.; et al. Effect of Vericiguat, a Soluble Guanylate Cyclase Stimulator, on Natriuretic Peptide Levels in Patients with Worsening Chronic Heart Failure and Reduced Ejection Fraction: The SOCRATES-REDUCED Randomized Trial. *JAMA* **2015**, *314*, 2251–2262. [CrossRef]
112. Hulot, J.-S.; Trochu, J.-N.; Donal, E.; Galinier, M.; Logeart, D.; De Groote, P.; Juillière, Y. Vericiguat for the treatment of heart failure: Mechanism of action and pharmacological properties compared with other emerging therapeutic options. *Expert Opin. Pharmacother.* **2021**, *22*, 1847–1855. [CrossRef]
113. Armstrong, P.W.; Pieske, B.; Anstrom, K.J.; Ezekowitz, J.; Hernandez, A.F.; Butler, J.; Lam, C.S.P.; Ponikowski, P.; Voors, A.A.; Jia, G.; et al. Vericiguat in Patients with Heart Failure and Reduced Ejection Fraction. *N. Engl. J. Med.* **2020**, *382*, 1883–1893. [CrossRef]
114. Chen, T.; Kong, B.; Shuai, W.; Gong, Y.; Zhang, J.; Huang, H. Vericiguat alleviates ventricular remodeling and arrhythmias in mouse models of myocardial infarction via CaMKII signaling. *Life Sci.* **2023**, *334*, 122184. [CrossRef]
115. Teerlink, J.R.; Diaz, R.; Felker, G.M.; McMurray, J.J.V.; Metra, M.; Solomon, S.D.; Adams, K.F.; Anand, I.; Arias-Mendoza, A.; Biering-Sørensen, T.; et al. Cardiac Myosin Activation with Omecamtiv Mecarbil in Systolic Heart Failure. *N. Engl. J. Med.* **2021**, *384*, 105–116. [CrossRef]
116. Drucker, D.J. The Cardiovascular Biology of Glucagon-like Peptide-1. *Cell Metab.* **2016**, *24*, 15–30. [CrossRef]
117. Marso, S.P.; Bain, S.C.; Consoli, A.; Eliaschewitz, F.G.; Jódar, E.; Leiter, L.A.; Lingvay, I.; Rosenstock, J.; Seufert, J.; Warren, M.L.; et al. Semaglutide and Cardiovascular Outcomes in Patients with Type 2 Diabetes. *N. Engl. J. Med.* **2016**, *375*, 1834–1844. [CrossRef]
118. Hernandez, A.F.; Green, J.B.; Janmohamed, S.; D'Agostino, R.B.; Granger, C.B.; Jones, N.P.; Leiter, L.A.; Rosenberg, A.E.; Sigmon, K.N.; Somerville, M.C.; et al. Albiglutide and cardiovascular outcomes in patients with type 2 diabetes and cardiovascular disease (Harmony Outcomes): A double-blind, randomised placebo-controlled trial. *Lancet* **2018**, *392*, 1519–1529. [CrossRef]
119. Gerstein, H.C.; Colhoun, H.M.; Dagenais, G.R.; Diaz, R.; Lakshmanan, M.; Pais, P.; Probstfield, J.; Riesmeyer, J.S.; Riddle, M.C.; Rydén, L.; et al. Dulaglutide and cardiovascular outcomes in type 2 diabetes (REWIND): A double-blind, randomised placebo-controlled trial. *Lancet* **2019**, *394*, 121–130. [CrossRef]
120. Margulies, K.B.; Hernandez, A.F.; Redfield, M.M.; Givertz, M.M.; Oliveira, G.H.; Cole, R.; Mann, D.L.; Whellan, D.J.; Kiernan, M.S.; Felker, G.M.; et al. Effects of Liraglutide on Clinical Stability Among Patients with Advanced Heart Failure and Reduced Ejection Fraction: A Randomized Clinical Trial. *JAMA* **2016**, *316*, 500–508. [CrossRef]
121. Neves, J.S.; Vasques-Nóvoa, F.; Borges-Canha, M.; Leite, A.R.; Sharma, A.; Carvalho, D.; Packer, M.; Zannad, F.; Leite-Moreira, A.; Ferreira, J.P. Risk of adverse events with liraglutide in heart failure with reduced ejection fraction: A post hoc analysis of the FIGHT trial. *Diabetes Obes. Metab.* **2023**, *25*, 189–197. [CrossRef]
122. Jorsal, A.; Kistorp, C.; Holmager, P.; Tougaard, R.S.; Nielsen, R.; Hänselmann, A.; Nilsson, B.; Møller, J.E.; Hjort, J.; Rasmussen, J.; et al. Effect of liraglutide, a glucagon-like peptide-1 analogue, on left ventricular function in stable chronic heart failure patients with and without diabetes (LIVE)—A multicentre, double-blind, randomised, placebo-controlled trial. *Eur. J. Heart Fail.* **2017**, *19*, 69–77. [CrossRef]
123. Wu, S.; Lu, W.; Chen, Z.; Dai, Y.; Chen, K.; Zhang, S. Association of glucagon-like peptide-1 receptor agonists with cardiac arrhythmias in patients with type 2 diabetes or obesity: A systematic review and meta-analysis of randomized controlled trials. *Diabetol. Metab. Syndr.* **2022**, *14*, 195. [CrossRef]
124. Al-Sadawi, M.A.; Aslam, F.M.; Tao, M.; Alsaiqali, M.; Almasry, I.O.; Fan, R.; Rashba, E.J.; Singh, A. Effects of GLP-1 Agonists on mortality and arrhythmias in patients with Type II diabetes. *IJC Heart Vasc.* **2023**, *47*, 101218. [CrossRef]
125. Bizino, M.B.; Jazet, I.M.; Westenberg, J.J.M.; van Eyk, H.J.; Paiman, E.H.M.; Smit, J.W.A.; Lamb, H.J. Effect of liraglutide on cardiac function in patients with type 2 diabetes mellitus: Randomized placebo-controlled trial. *Cardiovasc. Diabetol.* **2019**, *18*, 55. [CrossRef]
126. Durak, A.; Turan, B. Liraglutide provides cardioprotection through the recovery of mitochondrial dysfunction and oxidative stress in aging hearts. *J. Physiol. Biochem.* **2023**, *79*, 297–311. [CrossRef]
127. Kosiborod, M.N.; Abildstrøm, S.Z.; Borlaug, B.A.; Butler, J.; Rasmussen, S.; Davies, M.; Hovingh, G.K.; Kitzman, D.W.; Lindegaard, M.L.; Møller, D.V.; et al. Semaglutide in Patients with Heart Failure with Preserved Ejection Fraction and Obesity. *N. Engl. J. Med.* **2023**, *389*, 1069–1084. [CrossRef]

Journal of
Clinical Medicine

MDPI

Review

High-Density and Resolution Epicardial Mapping of the Atria: Translational Research with Clinical Impact

Ziliang Ye [1,†], Yifan Jia [1,†], Mathijs S. van Schie [1], Paul Knops [1], Vehpi Yildirim [1], Yannick J. H. J. Taverne [2] and Natasja M. S. de Groot [1,3,*]

[1] Department of Cardiology, Erasmus Medical Center, 3015 GD Rotterdam, The Netherlands; z.ye@erasmusmc.nl (Z.Y.); y.jia@erasmusmc.nl (Y.J.); m.vanschie@erasmusmc.nl (M.S.v.S.); p.knops@erasmusmc.nl (P.K.); v.yildirim@erasmusmc.nl (V.Y.)
[2] Department of Cardiothoracic surgery, Erasmus Medical Center, 3015 GD Rotterdam, The Netherlands; y.j.h.j.taverne@erasmusmc.nl
[3] Department of Microelectronics, Signal Processing Systems, Faculty of Electrical Engineering, Mathematics and Computer Sciences, Delft University of Technology, 2628 CD Delft, The Netherlands
* Correspondence: n.m.s.degroot@erasmusmc.nl; Tel.: +31-10-7035018
† These authors contributed equally to this work.

Abstract: The electrical arrhythmogenic substrate underlying the most common cardiac arrhythmia atrial fibrillation (AF) may consist of conduction disorders, low-voltage areas, or fractionated potentials. High-density and resolution epicardial mapping (HDREM) approaches have been introduced to quantify and visualize electrophysiological properties of the atria. These approaches are essential for obtaining innovative insights into arrhythmogenic substrates and identifying novel targets for therapy. The aim of this review is to summarize and discuss the (1) contribution of HDREM studies to the knowledge on atrial arrhythmogenesis and (2) future applications of HDREM of atria in daily clinical practice.

Keywords: high-density and resolution epicardial mapping; atria; arrhythmogenic substrate; atrial fibrillation

1. Introduction

In the past decades, high-density and resolution epicardial mapping [1–3] (HDREM) studies of the atria have significantly contributed to our knowledge of arrhythmogenesis, particularly of the most common arrhythmia, atrial fibrillation (AF) [4,5]. To date, most HDREM studies of the atria have been performed during open chest surgery. However, the epicardium is not only accessible during open chest surgery, but nowadays also more easily during minimally invasive and video-assisted thoracoscopic surgery [6–8]. In addition to this, combined surgical percutaneous ablation strategies for AF are emerging [9,10]. Consequently, epicardial mapping becomes more "common practice" and thus increasingly important. Figure 1 summarizes the electrophysiological parameters recorded in HDREM studies and highlights their role in investigating the arrhythmogenic substrate underlying AF.

An epicardial mapping approach has several advantages over an endocardial mapping approach. First, the surgeon can see the position and orientation of the electrode array in relation to anatomical structures. Second, stable contact between the electrodes and the atrial wall is ensured by directly pressing the electrode array slightly on the epicardial surface. Third, the large opening created by median sternotomy enables introduction of relatively large mapping devices containing a large number of electrodes compared to the currently available endovascular mapping devices. This wide access also facilitates high-density recordings of contact electrograms from numerous sites simultaneously. Fourth, specific areas such as Bachmann's bundle [11] (BB), which cannot be accessed via the endocardial approach, can easily be mapped. Fifth, simultaneous mapping of the epicardium and the opposite endocardium at a high-density scale can be performed using a small incision in the atrial wall.

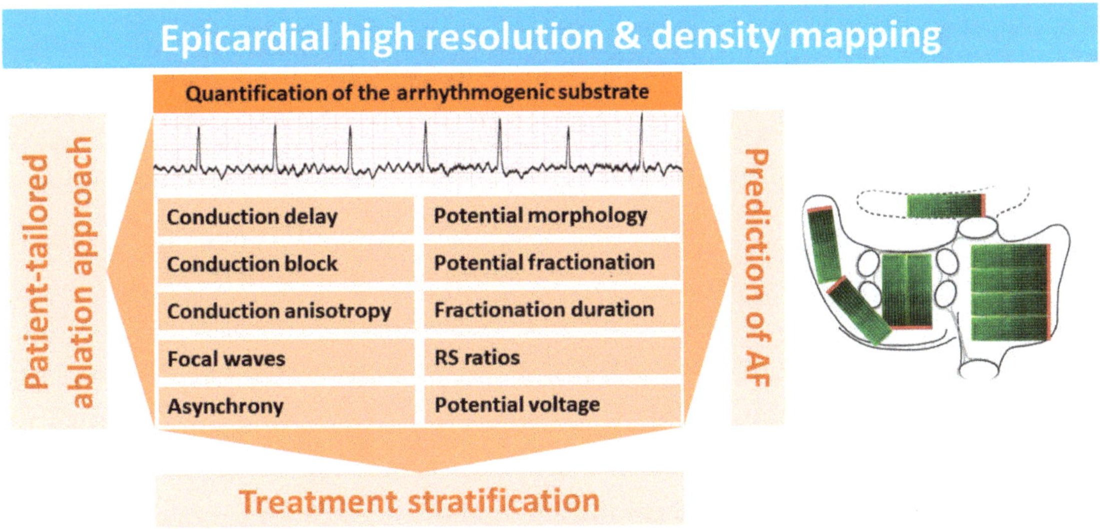

Figure 1. Summary of electrophysiological parameters used for quantification of the electrical arrhythmogenic substrate measured by using high-density and high-resolution epicardial mapping (HDREM) techniques.

In this review, we discuss the main contribution of HDREM of the atria to our knowledge of arrhythmogenesis and the impact of this technology on clinical practice.

2. History of Epicardial Mapping

2.1. Reentry as the Underlying Mechanism of AF

The first epicardial mapping of the atria was performed in dogs during sinus rhythm by Boineau et al. [12] in 1978. They used 2 electrode templates consisting of a total of 96 bipolar electrodes that were sutured to the atria (electrode diameter 0.2 mm, inter-electrode distance 1 mm, 3 mm between each bipolar pair). Later in 1991, Cox et al. [13] were the first to create an epicardial isochronal map of one sinus rhythm beat activating both the right and left atrium in a human. In addition, Cox et al. [13] performed the first epicardial mapping study of the atria during AF in patients with Wolff–Parkinson–White syndrome undergoing cardiac surgery for interruption of their accessory atrioventricular pathway. AF was induced by burst-pacing and both the right (RA) and left atria (LA) were mapped using epicardial electrode arrays (160 bipolar electrodes, inter-electrode distance 5–10 mm). Their mapping data supported reentry as the underlying mechanism of AF. Non-uniform conduction around areas of bi-directional CB resulted in multiple discrete wavefronts that were observed in all patients. Reentry mostly occurred around anatomical obstacles such as the pulmonary and caval veins, but it also occurred without the involvement of anatomical obstacles. Functional CB was observed in the atria and was sometimes associated with specific atrial structures such as the crista terminalis. In the LA, reentrant circuits were more difficult to document and seemed to occur more transiently. However, in this first epicardial mapping study of AF in humans, only *single* maps were presented, and beat-to-beat changes in patterns of activation were not analyzed.

Patterns of Activation

In 1994, HDREM of electrically *induced AF* was performed by Konings et al. [14] in 25 patients with Wolff–Parkinson–White syndrome. During cardiac surgery, the free wall of the RA was mapped with a spoon-shaped electrode array containing 244 unipolar electrodes (diameter 4 cm, inter-electrode distance 2.25 mm). The pattern of activation of the RA free wall showed a high intra- and inter-individual variation and ranged from single planar wavefronts propagating with only small areas of conduction delay to completely disorganized activation by multiple wavefronts propagating in different directions separated by long lines of CB. The degree of the organization of the activation patterns was related to the AF cycle length; long cycle lengths were associated with a higher degree of organization, whereas short cycle lengths were associated with more disorganized activation patterns.

Based on the complexity in the patterns of activation, AF was divided into three different types. During type I AF, the RA free wall was most often activated by single broad wavefronts and only small areas of slow conduction or CB occurred. These areas of conduction disorders did not affect the main course of the large fibrillation waves. During type II AF, there were either areas of local conduction delay affecting propagation of one large wavefront, or two separate wavefronts were present. During type III AF, multiple fibrillation waves were separated by functional lines of intra-atrial CB. The incidence of type I, II, and III AF in this study population of 25 patients was, respectively, 40%, 32%, and 28%. During these three distinct types of AF, there were significant differences in the average conduction velocity; type I AF was associated with the highest conduction velocity (61 ± 6 cm/s) and type III AF with the lowest conduction velocity (38 ± 10 cm/s). However, by using the "longitudinal" and "transverse" conduction velocity, Houben et al. [15] demonstrated that there was no difference in anisotropy ratio among the three types of AF. Even taking the highest degree of directional differences in conduction, the anisotropy ratio during AF still was not more than 1.80 ± 0.39. The initial mapping studies analyzing patterns of activation at the RA in patients with *(longstanding) persistent AF* were mainly performed during cardiac surgery for valvular heart disease [16,17].

Other mapping studies of chronic AF, as named at that time, focused on comparing patterns of activation in the RA and LA, which were mapped sequentially [18,19]. Surprisingly, in most patients, activation of the LA was more organized compared to RA. In three patients, organized and disorganized activation occurred alternately in the RA. However, since the mapping resolution of these studies was rather low (only 30 unipolar or 24 bipolar electrodes), conduction abnormalities occurring in small areas could easily have been missed. More recent studies performed by De Groot et al. used dedicated HDREM electrode arrays containing either 64 (8×8 electrodes, 1.10 cm^2, inter-electrode distance 1 mm) [20], 128 (8×16 electrodes, inter-electrode distance 2 mm), or 192 unipolar electrodes [21] (8×24 electrodes, electrode diameter 0.45 mm, inter-electrode distance 2 mm). Other studies of Kalman et al. [22] used custom-made electrode arrays of 128 electrodes (inter-electrode distance 2.5 mm). Electrode arrays have also more recently been used for simultaneous endo-epicardial mapping of AF [23]. Due to the emergence of "hybrid" ablation procedures, epicardial access becomes more easily achievable. Therefore, it is expected that the number of studies involving HDREM will increase considerably in the near future.

3. Historical Insights into AF Mechanisms

Konings et al. [14] observed a considerable number of focal patterns of activation at the RA epicardium during *acutely induced AF* in patients with Wolff–Parkinson–White syndrome. They described these focal waves as "new fibrillation waves" emerging in the middle of the mapping area, which could not be explained by fibrillation waves propagating in the epicardial plane. Holm et al. [17] also observed repetitive focal activation patterns in the RA during *persistent AF*, which was consistently located at the RA appendage.

Many years later, high-resolution and density epicardial fibrillation "wave" maps of the RA and LA obtained from patients with Wolff–Parkinson–White syndrome in whom

AF was acutely induced and patients with coronary artery- and valvular heart disease who had longstanding persistent AF (LSPAF) were compared [24]. A wave map shows the area activated by each individual fibrillation wave in color-code according to the moment of entrance into the mapping area. Utilizing these wave maps to count the number of fibrillation waves, it was demonstrated that persistence of AF was associated with an increase in the number of fibrillation waves (LSPAF: 4.5/cm^2 versus acutely induced AF: 2.3/cm^2, $p < 0.001$). In addition, patients with long-standing persistent AF (LSPAF) had more lines of CB (CB) (21.1 [16.6–27.5] vs. 6.1 [1.3–13.8]%, $p < 0.001$), which were also longer (total length: 21.1 [19.1–23.1] vs. 3.4 [0.3–8.8] mm/cm^2, $p < 0.001$). CB lines were defined as inter-electrode conduction times of >12 ms, representing a lower limit of 19 cm/s conduction velocity.

Recently, Van Schie et al. [25] demonstrated that increased AF complexity was associated with increased spatiotemporal variability in local conduction velocity vectors, local conduction heterogeneity, and anisotropy ratio. Interestingly, as shown by De Groot et al. [26] AF persistence was also associated with a higher frequency of epicardial breakthrough ("focal") waves, as the prevalence of focal fibrillation waves in the RA during LSPAF was almost four times higher than it was during acute AF (median, 0.46 versus 0.12 per cycle per 1 cm^2; $p < 0.0001$).

The observation that focal waves are associated with AF persistence raised the question whether focal waves can be considered as drivers of AF, and, if so, whether they can be targets for ablation therapy in patients in whom AF persists despite isolation of the pulmonary veins. However, the focal waves occurred diffusely throughout the atria, and predilection sites did not occur. Focal waves often arose as solitary events, and they rarely occurred repetitively.

Potentials recorded at the origin of the focal wave usually had clear R-waves preceding a negative deflection [26], indicating propagation of a wavefront towards the recording electrode. The coupling interval of the focal waves was <11 ms shorter than the average AF cycle length, indicating that these focal waves cannot be regarded as drivers of the fibrillatory process.

The occurrence of non-repetitive focal waves during AF was also reported by Lee et al. [27] They performed epicardial mapping (128 electrodes, inter-electrode distance of 2.5 mm) of various atrial regions—including the posterior LA wall, LA appendage, RA appendage, and right superior pulmonary vein–LA junction—in patients with LSPAF and coronary artery or valvular heart disease. None of the focal activation patterns lasted longer than two consecutive beats. Likewise, Walters et al. [3] performed in 10 patients epicardial mapping of the posterior LA wall and the RA free wall and found that the median number of consecutive focal waves was only 2 (IQR: 2–3), whereas the longest series of consecutive focal waves was 5. In a large cohort of 71 patients with different types of AF, van Staveren et al. [28] demonstrated that sites harboring focal waves were not the sites with the highest dominant frequency and highest degree of fractionated electrograms according to existing criteria for AF ablation. Hence, data from these translational mapping studies in humans did not support the concept that focal waves are the drivers of the fibrillatory process and that focal waves are suitable target sites for ablation therapy.

The Double-Layer Hypothesis

Based on the observation that focal waves were associated with AF persistence, the so-called double-layer hypothesis was introduced. In this hypothesis, the substrate of persistent AF consists of electrically dissociated muscle bundles and the mechanism of persistent AF is multiple endo-epicardial breakthroughs caused by transmural propagation of fibrillation waves from one layer to the other (right panel of Figure 2). These transmurally propagating fibrillation waves provide a constant source of new fibrillation waves for the opposite layer. However, this hypothesis requires that areas of electrical asynchrony between the endo- and epicardium are present, as otherwise, transmurally propagating waves could not excite the opposite layer.

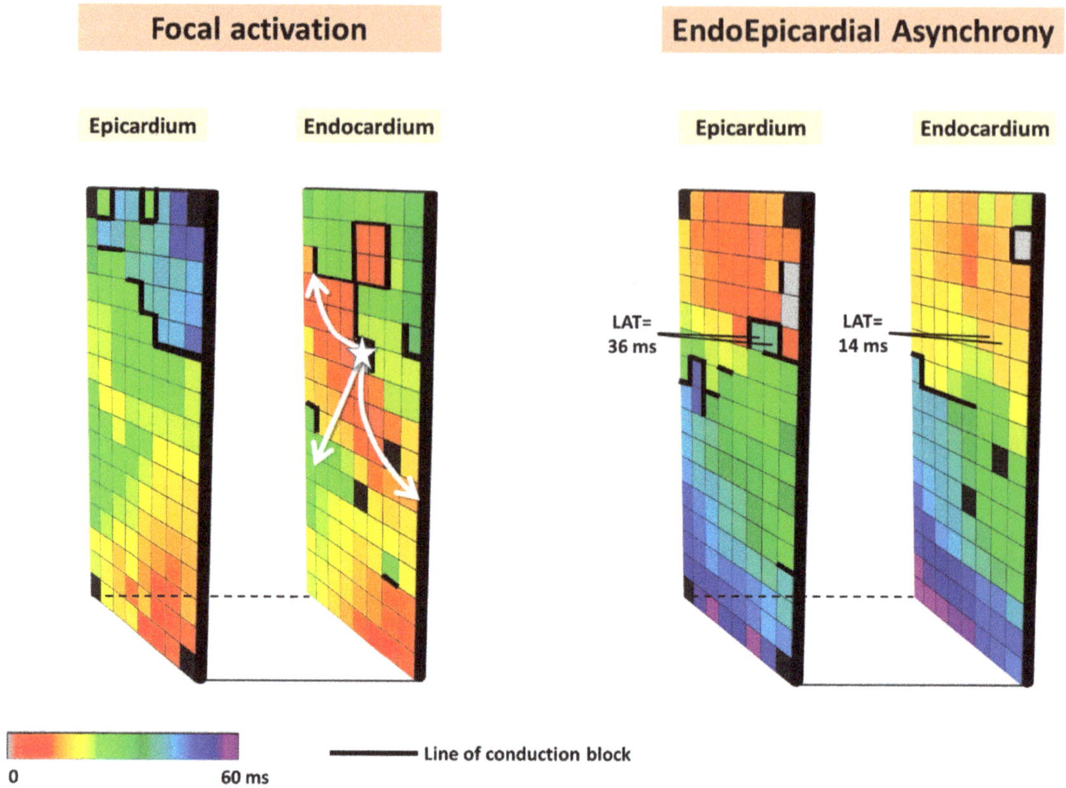

Figure 2. Simultaneously recorded epicardial and opposite endocardial activation maps. Local activation times are color-coded, and lines of CB are indicated by thick black lines. The left panel shows an example of focal activation (white star) on the endocardial layer, while the right panel shows an example of endo-epicardial asynchrony.

4. Simultaneous Endo-Epicardial Mapping during AF

In 1993, Schuessler et al. [29] performed simultaneous epicardial and endocardial mapping of isolated RA in canines during SR, electrical stimulation, and induced tachyarrhythmias. During SR, endocardial and epicardial activation occurred approximately simultaneously, as only small differences between endocardial and epicardial activation times (<1 ms) were found. Larger differences in endo- and epicardial activation times were mainly found at pectinate muscles and sites with transmural differences in fiber orientation; these differences increased during premature stimulation and induced AF. Interestingly, a focal activation pattern was observed, which was caused by a reentrant circuit in free-running muscle bundles connecting the epicardium and endocardium. The earliest activated sites giving rise to focal activation on either the endo- or epicardium were separated by 15 mm [29].

To prove that electrical asynchrony also exists in the in vivo human heart, De Groot et al. [23] performed, for the first time, simultaneous endo-epicardial mapping of the RA wall during AF in patients undergoing cardiac surgery and demonstrated frequent electrical asynchrony between the endo- and epicardial layers (up to 55.9% of the recording time). There were not only large differences in opposite local activation times but also differences in activation direction. Electrical asynchrony was more pronounced in patients with LSPAF compared to paroxysmal AF, indicating that electrical asynchrony across the atrial wall plays a key role in AF persistence. Due to the risk of air embolism, simultaneously mapping of the endo- and epicardium was limited to the RA. If extensive areas of asynchrony perpetuating the fibrillatory process are present in the atria, the *double-layer hypothesis* offers an explanation as to why patients have AF recurrences despite complete isolation of the pulmonary veins.

5. AF Potential Morphology

Konings et al. [30] were also the first to investigate the relation between unipolar potential morphology and spatial activation patterns during AF. They classified unipolar fibrillation potentials as SP, short double (SDP, two deflections, <10 ms apart), long double (LDP, two deflections, 10–50 ms apart), and fragmented potentials (FP, >2 deflections within 50 ms). Figure 3 provides typical examples of different unipolar potential morphologies. During induced AF, 77 ± 12% of potentials were SPs, 7 ± 3% SDPs, 10 ± 7% LDPs and 6 ± 4% FPs. SPs were an indicator for rapid uniform conduction (positive predictive value of 0.96). This type of conduction was present in most wavefronts (79 ± 11%); in 94 ± 4% of potentials within these wavefronts, SPs were observed. LDPs were specific for long lines of functional CB, whereas FPs were observed both during pivoting of fibrillation waves and during slowing of conduction. The complexity in patterns of activation was associated with unipolar potential morphology. Hence, the proportion of LDPs and FPs was highest during type III AF.

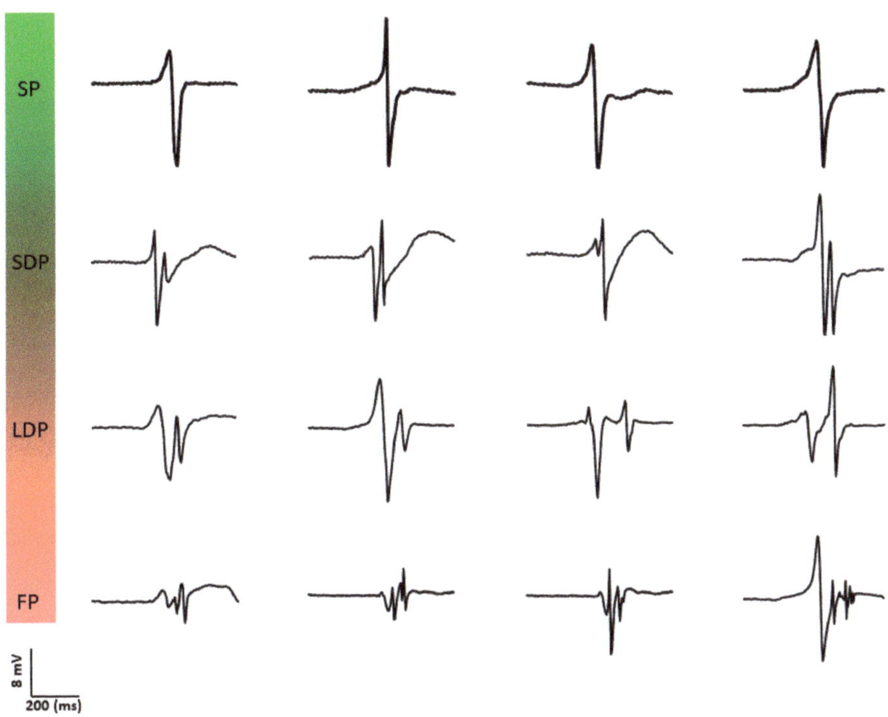

Figure 3. Examples of different types of unipolar potential morphologies. SP: single potential; SDP: short double potential; LDP: long double potential; FP: fractionated potential.

The morphology of single potentials is represented by the relative sizes of their positive (R-wave) and negative (S-wave) components (R/S ratio). Houben et al. [15] were the first to examine the morphology of SPs during acutely induced AF at the RA. In total, 413,031 unipolar fibrillation potentials were analyzed. Although there was a large intra- and inter-individual variation, a clear predominance of S-waves was found. The S-wave predominance was less pronounced during the more complex type of AF (type III) and could not be attributed to wavefront curvature or anisotropy. It was therefore hypothesized that a tilted transmural stance of the wavefront, resulting in an epicardial lead with constant epi-to-endocardial activation, could explain the S-wave predominance.

Based on the observations of Konings et al. [30], Nademanee et al. [31] developed a substrate-based AF ablation approach targeting complex fractionated atrial electrograms (CFAEs). This ablation approach has now been abandoned, which is not surprising given the significant variability in recording methodologies and definitions of CFAE used. Currently, there are at least 27 different definitions [32] used for identification of CFAEs, which leads to considerable inconsistency in treatment strategies. The CFAE approach is further complicated by the different recording techniques employed [33], including variable electrode sizes, inter-electrode distances, and filter settings. The variability in the methodology of CFAE detection explains substantial differences in ablation outcomes across different centers and operators, highlighting the need for a more standardized and reliable approach for CFAE mapping. We still believe that unipolar potentials are indicators of the AF-related arrhythmogenic substrate. However, to understand which features of potential morphologies are more closely related to AF development, thorough knowledge of the variation in these features during normal heart rhythm is essential. For this purpose, HDREM is used to quantify features of electrogram morphology, including potential voltages, degree of fractionation, duration of fractionation, and R/S ratios of single potentials.

6. Staging of AF by Quantifying Electropathology

The observation that AF persistence was associated with a larger number of fibrillation waves and more and longer lines of CB suggested that the arrhythmogenic substrate, and thus AF, can be "staged" by quantifying features of activation patterns and potential morphology. Such a diagnostic tool to stage AF could be used in clinical practice to provide patient-tailored therapy. Once an invasive "gold standard" diagnostic tool is developed and the exact AF-related electropathology has been identified, it can be used to construct less invasive and ultimately non-invasive diagnostic AF staging tools.

We hypothesize that during life, damage to atrial tissue by, e.g., cardiovascular diseases and co-morbidities causes "electropathology" manifested as pro-arrhythmogenic changes in patterns of activation and potential morphology. This tissue damage accumulates until a certain threshold of electropathology is reached and arrhythmias arise (Figure 4). From that moment on, additional electropathology contributes to perpetuation of the arrhythmia. Despite extensive research, the exact features of the AF-related arrhythmogenic substrate are unknown. To unravel the AF-related arrhythmogenic substrate, several steps are necessary, including understanding of (1) intra-atrial variation in activation patterns and potential morphology during normal heart rhythm, (2) the impact of clinical characteristics on atrial electrophysiology, and (3) differences in atrial electrophysiology between patients with and without AF. For this purpose, extensive mapping studies of the atria during sinus rhythm (SR) have been performed in a variety of patient populations.

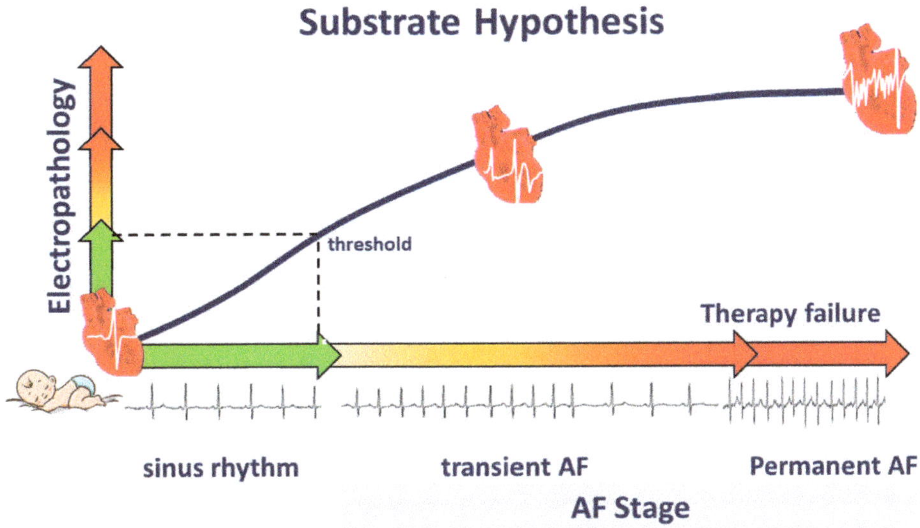

Figure 4. Substrate hypothesis. During life, electropathology progresses, and the heart rhythm changes from sinus rhythm to transient atrial fibrillation (AF), and finally to permanent AF, a condition frequently associated with therapy failure.

7. Epicardial Sinus Rhythm Mapping

The first detailed activation time mapping of the atria was performed in dogs during sinus rhythm by Boineau et al. [12] in 1978. Later, Cox et al. [13] were the first to create an epicardial isochronal map of one SR beat activating both the right and left atrium in a human. In 2018, Mouws et al. [34] were the first to investigate high-resolution atrial excitation patterns during normal SR in 253 patients with ischemic heart disease or ischemic valvular heart disease. As expected, in the vast majority (92%) of the patients, SR activations originated from the superior intercaval region of the RA. This study also highlighted the complex nature of BB activation, which exhibited various patterns, including right-to-left activation (64%), an expanding wavefront emerging from the central part (7%) of BB, by multiple wavefronts entering BB from different directions in the remaining patients. Furthermore, in 42% of the patients, the LA was activated by wavefronts propagating via BB towards the left atrioventricular groove. In a small number of patients, the SR wavefront propagated from the septum or coronary sinus across the pulmonary vein area (PVA, 3%) towards the LA appendage. However, in most patients (52%), there was a combination of both activation patterns. These findings provide insights into the variable patterns of atrial activation during normal SR. Additionally, it was found that the activation pattern of BB is particularly affected by valvular heart disease, which may explain why patients with valvular heart disease have a higher risk of developing AF.

7.1. *Influence of Prior AF Episodes on Atrial Excitation*

Mouws et al. [34] also demonstrated that patients with a history of AF were characterized by a longer total atrial excitation time during SR compared to patients without AF (136 ± 20 ms vs. 114 ± 17 ms, $p < 0.001$), which was mainly caused by longer total activation times of the right atrium and Bachmann's bundle (73 ± 13 ms vs. 67 ± 14 ms, $p = 0.018$ and 106 ± 20 ms vs. 87 ± 16 ms, $p < 0.001$, respectively). The presence of extensive conduction disorders at these areas resulted in alternative routes for activation of Bachmann's bundle and the left atrioventricular groove, as Bachmann's bundle could be activated via one wavefront from right to left, from the central part or via multiple wavefronts [35]. The left atrioventricular groove was then activated via either Bachmann's bundle, the pulmonary vein area, or via both routes, depending on which route had the shortest interatrial excitation time. However, Mouws et al. [34,36] also demonstrated that excitation of the left atrioventricular groove via only the pulmonary vein area was considerably slower than via Bachmann's bundle (90 ± 18 ms vs. 101 ± 20 ms, $p < 0.001$), and increased the risk of AF. Regional differences in local conduction velocities (CV) were investigated by Van Schie et al. [37] In 412 patients with ischemic and/or valvular heart disease, they found that CV was highest at the PVA [94.3 (83.4–101.0 cm/s)], followed by the LA [90.2 (82.2–97.0 cm/s)] and the RA [89.1 (83.3–94.3 cm/s)]; CV was lowest at BB [86.9 (77.3–96.4 cm/s)]. In patients with paroxysmal AF, local CV at BB was lower compared to those without prior AF episodes (79.1 [72.2–91.2] vs. 88.3 [79.3–97.2] cm/s, $p < 0.001$). In a subsequent case–control study, Heida et al. [38] confirmed there was a reduction in CV at Bachmann's bundle in patients with a history of AF (79 ± 12 vs. 88 ± 11 cm/s, $p = 0.02$).

The impact of underlying heart disease, including coronary artery, valvular heart, and congenital heart disease on conduction heterogeneity was explored in a study involving 447 patients who underwent epicardial mapping during SR [39]. Interestingly, the underlying heart disease had no effect on the proportion and severity of conduction disorders. However, prior AF episodes were associated with slowing of conduction in both atria and more conduction disorders at BB. In patients with AF, there are no differences in biatrial conduction characteristics between the supervulnerable period after electrical cardioversion and long-term SR in AF patients [40].

The complexity of CB even during SR is demonstrated by simultaneous endo-epicardial mapping studies of the RA, which revealed that lines of CB can be located at either the endo- or epicardium only (single-sided CB) or at both layers (transmural CB) [41]. Figure 5 illustrates different types of CBs observed during simultaneous endo-epicardial mapping.

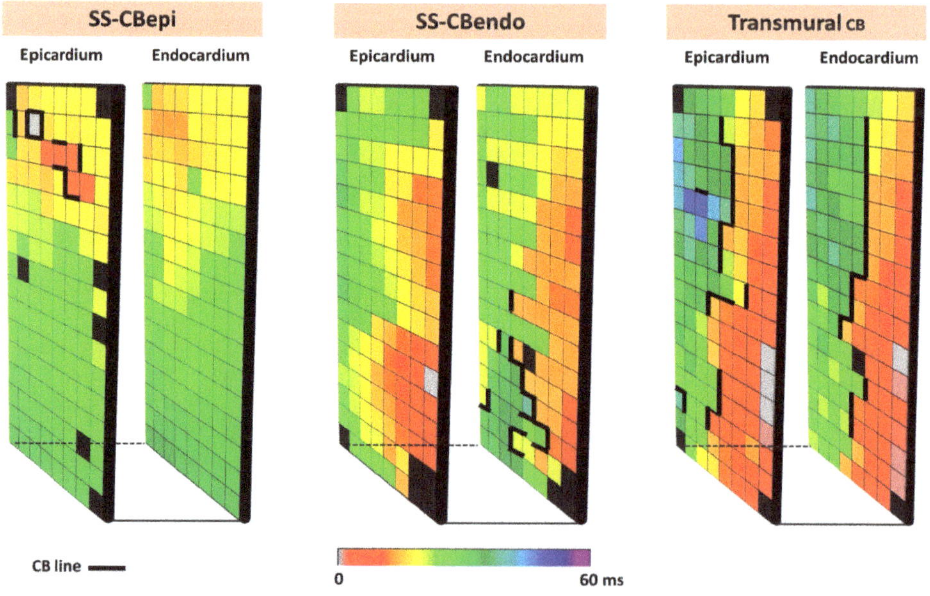

Figure 5. Different types of CB observed during endo-epicardial mapping. The left, middle, and right panels show, respectively, single-sided epicardial CB, endocardial single-sided CB, and transmural CB. SS-CB_{endo}: endocardial single-sided CB; SS-CB_{epi}: epicardial single-sided CB; Transmural CB: transmural CB.

7.2. Focal Patterns of Activation During SR

If focal waves due to transmurally propagating fibrillation waves are the result of electrically dissociated muscle bundles caused by structural changes in the atrial wall, it is most likely that focal patterns of activation may also appear during SR. In search of these focal patterns of activation during SR, Mouws et al. [42] performed epicardial mapping studies in 381 patients with ischemic or valvular heart disease. In total, 218 focal waves at various locations were found in 168 patients. These locations included mainly the RA (N = 105, 48%) but also the left atrioventricular groove (N = 67, 31%), BB (N = 27, 12%) and the PVA (N = 19, 9%). Focal waves occurred more frequently in patients with ischemic heart disease (N = 114, 49%) compared to patients with ischemic and/or valvular heart disease (N = 26, 17%). In this study [42], the morphology of SR potentials at the origin of the focal wave was also examined. These potentials were most often double or fractionated potentials (N = 137, 63%) and mainly occurred at focal patterns of activation arising from the RA and BB. In case of SPs, the majority (N = 71, 88%) contained a clear R-wave. These features of potential morphology indicate that there are indeed waves propagating from deep layers within the atrial wall towards the recording electrode.

As focal waves are present during SR, it indicates that endo-epicardial asynchrony must also be present during SR. Kharbanda et al. [43] conducted simultaneous endo-epicardial mapping of the human RA and indeed demonstrated endo-epicardial asynchrony even up to 61 ms in the thin inferior RA and up to 84 ms in the thick superior RA. Areas of endo-epicardial asynchrony are also more prevalent during SR in patients with persistent AF compared with patients without history of AF and can be more accurately detected by utilizing unipolar electrograms than bipolar electrograms.

7.3. Unipolar Potential Morphology

The value of unipolar potential morphology has been discussed for many years as a possible indicator of the electrical arrhythmogenic substrate. Potentials consisting of RS waves with high amplitudes reflect areas of fast conduction with conduction along the longitudinal axis of myocardial fibers, while in areas of slower conduction, unipolar potential amplitudes are smaller [44]. Low-voltage areas are assumed to be indicators of structurally remodeled tissue containing fibrotic areas, though study outcomes are controversial [44,45]. Asynchronous activation of (groups of) cardiomyocytes gives rise to multiple positive and negative deflections, which is known as fractionation [44,46].

7.4. Unipolar Single Potential Morphology

SPs are defined as potentials consisting of a single negative deflection, and the preceding and following wave are called, respectively, the positive R- and negative S-wave. In patients with coronary artery disease without history of arrhythmias, the majority of unipolar potentials recorded during normal SR consisted of one single deflection (81.4 [74.9–85.1]%) [40]. Even in patients with mitral valve disease and paroxysmal AF, the majority of recorded potentials still consists of SPs (81.0 [75.5–87.0]%) [47,48]. The morphology of SPs is represented by the relative positive (R-wave) and negative (S-wave) components (R/S ratio).

As described above, Houben et al. [15] were the first to examine the morphology of SPs during acutely induced AF at the RA. They proposed that the thin epicardial layer of atrial myocardium plays an important role in propagation of fibrillation waves. Simultaneous endo-epicardial mapping of the RA during SR, however, demonstrated that opposite epicardial and endocardial electrograms both have S-predominance [49], suggesting that predominant epicardial-to-endocardial activation during SR is not the cause of S-predominance.

Differences in relative R- and S-wave amplitude ratios of SPs were further studied in a cohort of 67 patients with mitral valve disease [47]. In all patients, there was a clear predominance of S-waves at BB and the RA. Comparing patients without AF and with PAF, SP morphology differences were most prominent at BB. Patients with PAF had lower amplitudes, more R-wave predominance, and slower wavefront propagation. The lower amplitude was mainly determined by a decrease in S-wave amplitude, which is observed in damaged tissue. SPs were also recorded from the origin of epicardial focal waves during SR; an R-wave was observed in 88% of all epicardial focal waves, as opposed to in only 21% of sinus node breakthrough waves [42].

7.5. Double and Fractionated Potentials

Ye et al. [50] described the distribution and the proportion of different types of atrial unipolar potential morphologies during SR. The study involved 189 patients undergoing coronary artery bypass graft surgery, preceded by epicardial mapping of the RA, BB, PVA, and LA. Various types of potential morphologies, including SPs, SDPs, LDPs, and FPs, were distributed across the different regions of the atria. The highest proportions of LDP and FP were mainly recorded at the RA and Bachmann's bundle, with fractionation at Bachmann's bundle also having the longest durations. The amount of CB was correlated with the proportion of LDPs and FPs, and duration of FPs. In a cohort of patients with mitral valve disease and paroxysmal AF, it was demonstrated that more unipolar FPs were present in the pulmonary vein area compared to patients without a history of AF [48]. However, LDPs and FPs were detected throughout the atria in patients without atrial tachyarrhythmias. This finding suggests that unipolar potential fractionation can also be physiological in nature, due to, for example, tissue discontinuities caused by anatomical structures such as capillaries. Interestingly, by performing simultaneous endo-epicardial mapping, Zhang et al. [51] demonstrated that LDPs and FPs are also indicators of areas of electrical asynchrony between the endo- and epicardial layers. The inability to discriminate physiological fractionations from pathological ones provides a possible explanation for the limited success of ablation strategies targeting CFAE.

7.6. Potential Voltages

It is generally assumed that potentials with low peak-to-peak amplitudes (voltages) are indicators of sites of structurally remodeled tissue and have therefore become targets for AF ablation [52]. For this reason, several HDREM studies have also focused on investigating potential voltages. However, the use of potential voltage as an indicator for arrhythmogenic tissue critically relies on the used voltage mapping technique. Mapping studies used several voltage mapping approaches including unipolar, bipolar, omnipolar, Laplacian, or multipolar voltage techniques, which all have their advantages and disadvantages [32]. There is no standardized definition for low-voltage areas and a clear threshold has never been histologically validated [53]. Also, low-voltage areas defined with unipolar potentials may differ considerably from low-voltage areas defined with bipolar or omnipolar voltages [54]. Simultaneous endo-epicardial mapping studies have demonstrated that low-voltage areas are not always transmural but can be present in either the endocardium or epicardium [55,56]. Interestingly, low-voltage, fractionated potentials were not only recorded in areas with slowing of conduction or CB [54,55], indicating that not all FPs are indicators of an arrhythmogenic substrate, but could simply be the result of structure of the atrial wall.

In order to fully exploit unipolar potential voltages for detecting AF vulnerability, more insights into the distribution of unipolar potential voltages during sinus rhythm were required by van Schie et al. [48]. From 67 patients with mitral valve disease, high-resolution unipolar SR voltage fingerprints to identify low-voltage areas were constructed and compared between patients with and without AF episodes. They demonstrated that there was no correlation between unipolar potential voltages and CV, although lower potential voltages were recorded in areas of conduction slowing and surrounding areas of CB.

In addition, unipolar potential voltages decreased in potentials with an increasing number of deflections. Even during SR, marked inter-individual and regional variation in potential voltages was found. However, patients with paroxysmal AF had lower unipolar potential voltages at RA, Bachmann's bundle, and PVA, and more low-voltage areas at Bachmann's bundle compared to those without AF. This difference was mainly determined by the magnitude of the S-waves, which was particularly lower at BB [47]. In 189 patients undergoing epicardial mapping of the atria during SR, Ye et al. [50] found a significant negative correlation between unipolar potential voltages and CB in the RA, BB, and the PVA. These observations suggest that unipolar potential voltages can be used to assess the severity of atrial conduction abnormalities.

8. Electrical Signal Fingerprinting

In 2021, Ye et al. [50] first introduced the concept of electrical signal fingerprinting in a large cohort of patients without atrial tachyarrhythmias. The electrical signal fingerprint uses features of unipolar potential morphology to predict the severity of atrial conduction heterogeneity in the epicardial layer. The fingerprint was then tested in 235 patients undergoing coronary artery bypass grafting; the electrical signal fingerprint score had a significant predictive value of conduction heterogeneity (entire atrium: C-index: 0.92 (0.89, 0.95)) [57]. Moreover, patients who developed postoperative AF had a markedly higher electrical signal fingerprint score compared to patients without postoperative AF. This observation suggests that the electrical signal fingerprint score could serve as a novel diagnostic tool for prediction of postoperative AF. The electrophysiological parameters of the electrical signal fingerprint and their further utilization in identifying patients at higher risk of postoperative AF are illustrated in Figure 6. Zhang et al. [41] discovered that unipolar potential morphologies were also useful in identifying areas of transmural CB, which could accurately be predicted by combining unipolar potential morphology parameters, including potential voltages, fractionation, and fractionation duration (area under the curve (AUC) = 0.91).

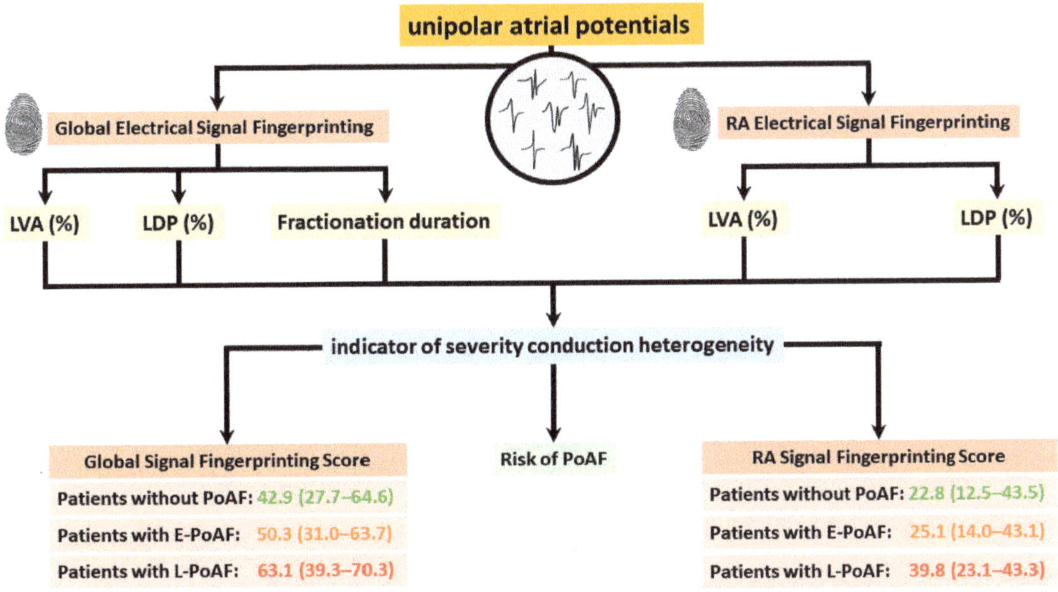

Figure 6. Electrophysiological parameters of global and right atrial electrical signal fingerprinting, along with their application in predicting postoperative atrial fibrillation, are illustrated. LVA: low-voltage area; LDP: long double potential; PoAF: postoperative atrial fibrillation.

Electrical signal fingerprints can also be used to identify areas of endo-epicardial asynchrony (EEA) during SR. Zhang et al. [51] performed simultaneous endo-epicardial mapping in a cohort of 86 participants and revealed that endocardial low-voltage areas and fractionation duration of double potentials (DPs) serve as significant predictors for the degree of EEA, achieving an AUC of 0.913. This high predictive value underscores the potential utility of these electrophysiological parameters in the assessment of EEA. Moreover, endo- and epi-asynchrony fingerprinting scores (AFS) were introduced to use either endocardial or epicardial mapping to identify EEAs. Both methods had a strong predictive value for the prediction of EEA, with AUCs of 0.901 and 0.830, respectively. These findings highlight the efficacy of AFS as a less-invasive diagnostic tool compared to simultaneous endo- and epicardial mapping to quantify the severity of EEA, which is potentially an indicator for AF vulnerability.

9. Impact of Risk Factors on Atrial Epicardial Electrophysiology

In the past decade, epicardial mapping studies have been performed in large patient cohorts undergoing cardiac surgery to study the impact of risk factors on atrial electrophysiology. These risk factors include ageing, sex, and obesity.

9.1. Ageing

The impact of age on atrial electrophysiological properties was studied in 216 patients undergoing elective coronary artery bypass surgery [58]. With aging, slowing in conduction and CB occurred during SR throughout both the RA and LA. Conduction abnormalities were particularly more prevalent at the RA and BB. Furthermore, this was the first study demonstrating that at BB, with advancing age, slowing of conduction in transverse direction occurred to a greater extent compared to the conduction slowing in longitudinal direction, reflecting enhanced lateral uncoupling.

Ye et al. [59] further explored the relationship between ageing and epicardial unipolar atrial potential morphology. Advanced age, which was defined as age $\geq$ 60 years, was associated with a decrease in SPs, an increase in SDPs, LDPs, and FPs. Even after adjusting for potential confounding factors, the impact of age on these four different types of potential morphology remained significant. Both of the above-mentioned studies were conducted during SR, and there are currently no data about the impact of age on the fibrillatory process.

9.2. Obesity

The relation between obesity and AF has been demonstrated by several clinical studies, although the pathophysiology of obesity-related AF remains largely unknown. The impact of obesity on atrial electrophysiology was investigated by Schram-Serban et al. [60], who performed epicardial mapping studies in 106 matched obese patients and non-obese patients. None of these patients had a history of AF. Compared to non-obese patients, obese patients had more areas of conduction delay, CB, and longer continuous conduction delay and CB lines. These differences were most pronounced at BB. Furthermore, in a subsequent study, Schram-Serban et al. [61] demonstrated that obese patients also had lower unipolar potential voltages, particularly at BB and the LA. Furthermore, the number of low-voltage areas positively correlated with incidences of CB, while BMI and the number of low-voltage areas were independent predictors for the incidence of early postoperative AF. This study suggests that obesity may predispose to an overall decrease in atrial potential voltages and a higher number of low-voltage areas, and that Bachmann's bundle is a predilection site for low-voltage areas within the atria of obese patients. The next step in further understanding the obesity-related electrical substrate underlying AF is to investigate the electrophysiological differences between obese and non-obese patients with a history of AF to investigate whether obesity further exacerbates atrial remodeling in AF patients.

9.3. Sex Differences

There is increasing awareness of sex-specific differences in epidemiology, pathophysiology, and therapy outcomes of AF. To fully understand these differences, knowledge on sex differences in atrial electrophysiological properties during normal heart rhythm is essential. However, data on this topic are scarce. Therefore, Veen et al. [62] used epicardial mapping to investigate the impact of sex on electrophysiological properties of the atria during SR in 53 matched post-menopausal females and males. None of these patients had a history of AF. Sex-related differences in electrophysiology were particularly found at the RA and to a lesser degree at BB. At both the RA and BB, females had significantly lower unipolar potential voltages and conduction velocities. At the RA only, females had more low-voltage areas, more CB, and continuous conduction delay and CB lines, and also longer CB and continuous conduction delay and CB lines. In future studies, it needs to be investigated whether these areas play a role in sex-based differences in vulnerability to atrial tachyarrhythmias such as AF.

10. Gaps in Current HDREM Research

At present, HDREM is used by only a small number of researchers and experience with this technology is therefore limited. As recently discussed in detail [32], differences in signal recording and particularly processing techniques may exist and it is unknown how these methodological differences affect reproducibility of study outcomes.

11. Clinical Applications of Epicardial Mapping

HDREM can also be applied to guide real-time, patient-specific therapy. Although epicardial mapping is predominantly performed during open chest surgery, it is nowadays also increasingly conducted during minimally invasive procedures. As concomitant surgical AF ablation is advised in patients with paroxysmal or persistent AF and stand-alone surgical or hybrid ablation is considered appropriate in symptomatic patients with persistent AF, the clinical applications of epicardial mapping to guide these procedures is expanding.

Comparable to endocardial pulmonary vein isolations in the electrophysiology (EP) room, HDREM can be used to evaluate continuity of epicardial lesions during arrhythmia surgery and provide feedback on exit and/or entrance block to the surgeon. Secondly, as discussed above, the *Electrical Fingerprint Scores* obtained via epicardial mapping can provide patient-tailored AF therapy. Theoretically, if the score is low, pulmonary vein isolation may be sufficient, and if this score is high, a substrate-based AF ablation approach may be more suitable. Quantification of HDRM parameters derived from epicardial mapping enables identification of the arrhythmogenic substrate with an unparalleled accuracy. Furthermore, by correlating *electrical signal fingerprinting scores* derived from epicardial mapping data with non-invasive electrocardiographic features, it may be possible to develop a more advanced non-invasive diagnostic tool to quantify the severity of conduction inhomogeneity across the entire atrium, thereby identifying individuals at higher risk of developing AF.

Epicardial mapping generates a large amount of electrophysiological data from the atria. The integration of HDREM with artificial intelligence, along with the development of less invasive and non-invasive techniques, is likely to yield novel insights into the AF-related arrhythmogenic substrate and hence unravel novel target sites for therapy. Thus, implementation of novel signal processing technologies in HDREM will be a significant advancement in the future management of AF. However, for HDREM to become implemented in daily clinical practice, a standardized approach for signal recording and processing is mandatory.

12. Conclusions

HDREM has emerged as a pivotal approach in advancing our understanding and treatment of atrial arrhythmias, particularly AF. This technology enables visualization and quantification of arrhythmogenic substrates, such as conduction disorders, low-voltage areas, or fractionated potentials. In patients with trigger-driven AF undergoing cardiac surgery, it can be used to verify the completeness of ablation lesions, whereas in patients with substrate-mediated AF, it can be used to identify target sites for ablation. In addition, HDREM can be applied to stage AF, provide patient-tailored therapy, or identify patients at high risk of developing AF. Once the exact features of the AF-related substrate have been identified using HDREM, this knowledge can be used to develop less invasive or non-invasive techniques that have broader applications in daily clinical practice.

Author Contributions: Conceptualization, Z.Y., Y.J. and N.M.S.d.G.; Critical revision, M.S.v.S., P.K., V.Y. and Y.J.H.J.T.; writing—original draft preparation, Z.Y. and Y.J.; writing—review and editing, N.M.S.d.G. and M.S.v.S.; supervision, N.M.S.d.G. All authors have read and agreed to the published version of the manuscript.

Funding: N.M.S. de Groot is supported by grants NWO-Vidi (2016-91717339) and Medical Delta NWA-ORC project CIRCULAR NWO (NWA.1389.20.157).

Data Availability Statement: Not applicable.

Conflicts of Interest: The authors have no conflicts of interest.

References

1. Jadidi, A.S.; Cochet, H.; Shah, A.J.; Kim, S.J.; Duncan, E.; Miyazaki, S.; Sermesant, M.; Lehrmann, H.; Lederlin, M.; Linton, N.; et al. Inverse relationship between fractionated electrograms and atrial fibrosis in persistent atrial fibrillation: Combined magnetic resonance imaging and high-density mapping. *J. Am. Coll. Cardiol.* **2013**, *62*, 802–812. [CrossRef] [PubMed]
2. Laţcu, D.G.; Saoudi, N. High-resolution/Density Mapping in Patients with Atrial and Ventricular Arrhythmias. *Card. Electrophysiol. Clin.* **2019**, *11*, 511–524. [CrossRef]
3. Walters, T.E.; Lee, G.; Morris, G.; Spence, S.; Larobina, M.; Atkinson, V.; Antippa, P.; Goldblatt, J.; Royse, A.; O'Keefe, M.; et al. Temporal Stability of Rotors and Atrial Activation Patterns in Persistent Human Atrial Fibrillation: A High-Density Epicardial Mapping Study of Prolonged Recordings. *JACC Clin. Electrophysiol.* **2015**, *1*, 14–24. [CrossRef] [PubMed]
4. Yamaguchi, T.; Otsubo, T.; Takahashi, Y.; Nakashima, K.; Fukui, A.; Hirota, K.; Ishii, Y.; Shinzato, K.; Osako, R.; Tahara, M.; et al. Atrial Structural Remodeling in Patients with Atrial Fibrillation Is a Diffuse Fibrotic Process: Evidence from High-Density Voltage Mapping and Atrial Biopsy. *J. Am. Heart Assoc.* **2022**, *11*, e024521. [CrossRef] [PubMed]
5. Lee, S.; Sahadevan, J.; Khrestian, C.M.; Cakulev, I.; Markowitz, A.; Waldo, A.L. Simultaneous Biatrial High-Density (510–512 Electrodes) Epicardial Mapping of Persistent and Long-Standing Persistent Atrial Fibrillation in Patients: New Insights into the Mechanism of Its Maintenance. *Circulation* **2015**, *132*, 2108–2117. [CrossRef]
6. Krul, S.P.; Pison, L.; La Meir, M.; Driessen, A.H.; Wilde, A.A.; Maessen, J.G.; De Mol, B.A.; Crijns, H.J.; de Groot, J.R. Epicardial and endocardial electrophysiological guided thoracoscopic surgery for atrial fibrillation: A multidisciplinary approach of atrial fibrillation ablation in challenging patients. *Int. J. Cardiol.* **2014**, *173*, 229–235. [CrossRef]
7. Wudel, J.H.; Chaudhuri, P.; Hiller, J.J. Video-assisted epicardial ablation and left atrial appendage exclusion for atrial fibrillation: Extended follow-up. *Ann. Thorac. Surg.* **2008**, *85*, 34–38. [CrossRef]
8. Li, H.; Li, Y.; Sun, L.; Liu, X.; Xu, C.; Han, J.; Meng, X. Minimally invasive surgical pulmonary vein isolation alone for persistent atrial fibrillation: Preliminary results of epicardial atrial electrogram analysis. *Ann. Thorac. Surg.* **2008**, *86*, 1219–1225. [CrossRef]
9. Killu, A.M.; Ebrille, E.; Asirvatham, S.J.; Munger, T.M.; McLeod, C.J.; Packer, D.L.; Friedman, P.A.; Mulpuru, S.K. Percutaneous epicardial access for mapping and ablation is feasible in patients with prior cardiac surgery, including coronary bypass surgery. *Circ. Arrhythm. Electrophysiol.* **2015**, *8*, 94–101. [CrossRef]
10. Jiang, R.; Buch, E.; Gima, J.; Upadhyay, G.A.; Nayak, H.M.; Beaser, A.D.; Aziz, Z.; Shivkumar, K.; Tung, R. Feasibility of percutaneous epicardial mapping and ablation for refractory atrial fibrillation: Insights into substrate and lesion transmurality. *Heart Rhythm.* **2019**, *16*, 1151–1159. [CrossRef]
11. van Campenhout, M.J.; Yaksh, A.; Kik, C.; de Jaegere, P.P.; Ho, S.Y.; Allessie, M.A.; de Groot, N.M. Bachmann's bundle: A key player in the development of atrial fibrillation? *Circ. Arrhythm. Electrophysiol.* **2013**, *6*, 1041–1046. [CrossRef] [PubMed]
12. Boineau, J.P.; Schuessler, R.B.; Mooney, C.R.; Wylds, A.C.; Miller, C.B.; Hudson, R.D.; Borremans, J.M.; Brockus, C.W. Multicentric origin of the atrial depolarization wave: The pacemaker complex. Relation to dynamics of atrial conduction, P-wave changes and heart rate control. *Circulation* **1978**, *58*, 1036–1048. [CrossRef]
13. Cox, J.L.; Canavan, T.E.; Schuessler, R.B.; Cain, M.E.; Lindsay, B.D.; Stone, C.; Smith, P.K.; Corr, P.B.; Boineau, J.P. The surgical treatment of atrial fibrillation. II. Intraoperative electrophysiologic mapping and description of the electrophysiologic basis of atrial flutter and atrial fibrillation. *J. Thorac. Cardiovasc. Surg.* **1991**, *101*, 406–426. [CrossRef]
14. Konings, K.T.; Kirchhof, C.J.; Smeets, J.R.; Wellens, H.J.; Penn, O.C.; Allessie, M.A. High-density mapping of electrically induced atrial fibrillation in humans. *Circulation* **1994**, *89*, 1665–1680. [CrossRef]
15. Houben, R.P.; de Groot, N.M.; Smeets, J.L.; Becker, A.E.; Lindemans, F.W.; Allessie, M.A. S-wave predominance of epicardial electrograms during atrial fibrillation in humans: Indirect evidence for a role of the thin subepicardial layer. *Heart Rhythm.* **2004**, *1*, 639–647. [CrossRef] [PubMed]

16. Holm, M.; Johansson, R.; Olsson, S.B.; Brandt, J.; Lührs, C. A new method for analysis of atrial activation during chronic atrial fibrillation in man. *IEEE Trans. Biomed. Eng.* **1996**, *43*, 198–210. [CrossRef]
17. Holm, M.; Johansson, R.; Brandt, J.; Lührs, C.; Olsson, S.B. Epicardial right atrial free wall mapping in chronic atrial fibrillation. Documentation of repetitive activation with a focal spread—A hitherto unrecognised phenomenon in man. *Eur. Heart J.* **1997**, *18*, 290–310. [CrossRef] [PubMed]
18. Harada, A.; Sasaki, K.; Fukushima, T.; Ikeshita, M.; Asano, T.; Yamauchi, S.; Tanaka, S.; Shoji, T. Atrial activation during chronic atrial fibrillation in patients with isolated mitral valve disease. *Ann. Thorac. Surg.* **1996**, *61*, 104–111, discussion 111–102. [CrossRef]
19. Sueda, T.; Nagata, H.; Shikata, H.; Orihashi, K.; Morita, S.; Sueshiro, M.; Okada, K.; Matsuura, Y. Simple left atrial procedure for chronic atrial fibrillation associated with mitral valve disease. *Ann. Thorac. Surg.* **1996**, *62*, 1796–1800. [CrossRef]
20. Yaksh, A.; Kik, C.; Knops, P.; Roos-Hesselink, J.W.; Bogers, A.J.; Zijlstra, F.; Allessie, M.; de Groot, N.M. Atrial fibrillation: To map or not to map? *Neth. Heart J.* **2014**, *22*, 259–266. [CrossRef]
21. Yaksh, A.; van der Does, L.J.; Kik, C.; Knops, P.; Oei, F.B.; van de Woestijne, P.C.; Bekkers, J.A.; Bogers, A.J.; Allessie, M.A.; de Groot, N.M. A novel intra-operative, high-resolution atrial mapping approach. *J. Interv. Card. Electrophysiol.* **2015**, *44*, 221–225. [CrossRef] [PubMed]
22. Lee, G.; Roberts-Thomson, K.; Madry, A.; Spence, S.; Teh, A.; Heck, P.M.; Kumar, S.; Kistler, P.M.; Morton, J.B.; Sanders, P.; et al. Relationship among complex signals, short cycle length activity, and dominant frequency in patients with long-lasting persistent AF: A high-density epicardial mapping study in humans. *Heart Rhythm.* **2011**, *8*, 1714–1719. [CrossRef] [PubMed]
23. de Groot, N.; van der Does, L.; Yaksh, A.; Lanters, E.; Teuwen, C.; Knops, P.; van de Woestijne, P.; Bekkers, J.; Kik, C.; Bogers, A.; et al. Direct Proof of Endo-Epicardial Asynchrony of the Atrial Wall During Atrial Fibrillation in Humans. *Circ. Arrhythm. Electrophysiol.* **2016**, *9*, e003648. [CrossRef] [PubMed]
24. Allessie, M.A.; de Groot, N.M.; Houben, R.P.; Schotten, U.; Boersma, E.; Smeets, J.L.; Crijns, H.J. Electropathological substrate of long-standing persistent atrial fibrillation in patients with structural heart disease: Longitudinal dissociation. *Circ. Arrhythm. Electrophysiol.* **2010**, *3*, 606–615. [CrossRef]
25. van Schie, M.S.; Talib, S.; Knops, P.; Taverne, Y.; de Groot, N.M.S. Conduction Velocity and Anisotropic Properties of Fibrillation Waves During Acutely Induced and Long-Standing Persistent AF. *JACC Clin. Electrophysiol.* **2024**, *10*, 1592–1604. [CrossRef]
26. de Groot, N.M.; Houben, R.P.; Smeets, J.L.; Boersma, E.; Schotten, U.; Schalij, M.J.; Crijns, H.; Allessie, M.A. Electropathological substrate of longstanding persistent atrial fibrillation in patients with structural heart disease: Epicardial breakthrough. *Circulation* **2010**, *122*, 1674–1682. [CrossRef]
27. Lee, G.; Kumar, S.; Teh, A.; Madry, A.; Spence, S.; Larobina, M.; Goldblatt, J.; Brown, R.; Atkinson, V.; Moten, S.; et al. Epicardial wave mapping in human long-lasting persistent atrial fibrillation: Transient rotational circuits, complex wavefronts, and disorganized activity. *Eur. Heart J.* **2014**, *35*, 86–97. [CrossRef]
28. van Staveren, L.N.; Hendriks, R.C.; Taverne, Y.; de Groot, N.M.S. High Dominant Frequencies and Fractionated Potentials Do Not Indicate Focal or Rotational Activation During AF. *JACC Clin. Electrophysiol.* **2023**, *9*, 1082–1096. [CrossRef]
29. Schuessler, R.B.; Kawamoto, T.; Hand, D.E.; Mitsuno, M.; Bromberg, B.I.; Cox, J.L.; Boineau, J.P. Simultaneous epicardial and endocardial activation sequence mapping in the isolated canine right atrium. *Circulation* **1993**, *88*, 250–263. [CrossRef]
30. Konings, K.T.; Smeets, J.L.; Penn, O.C.; Wellens, H.J.; Allessie, M.A. Configuration of unipolar atrial electrograms during electrically induced atrial fibrillation in humans. *Circulation* **1997**, *95*, 1231–1241. [CrossRef]
31. Nademanee, K.; McKenzie, J.; Kosar, E.; Schwab, M.; Sunsaneewitayakul, B.; Vasavakul, T.; Khunnawat, C.; Ngarmukos, T. A new approach for catheter ablation of atrial fibrillation: Mapping of the electrophysiologic substrate. *J. Am. Coll. Cardiol.* **2004**, *43*, 2044–2053. [CrossRef] [PubMed]
32. de Groot, N.M.S.; Shah, D.; Boyle, P.M.; Anter, E.; Clifford, G.D.; Deisenhofer, I.; Deneke, T.; van Dessel, P.; Doessel, O.; Dilaveris, P.; et al. Critical appraisal of technologies to assess electrical activity during atrial fibrillation: A position paper from the European Heart Rhythm Association and European Society of Cardiology Working Group on eCardiology in collaboration with the Heart Rhythm Society, Asia Pacific Heart Rhythm Society, Latin American Heart Rhythm Society and Computing in Cardiology. *Europace* **2022**, *24*, 313–330. [CrossRef] [PubMed]
33. van der Does, L.J.; de Groot, N.M. Inhomogeneity and complexity in defining fractionated electrograms. *Heart Rhythm.* **2017**, *14*, 616–624. [CrossRef] [PubMed]
34. Mouws, E.; Lanters, E.A.H.; Teuwen, C.P.; van der Does, L.; Kik, C.; Knops, P.; Yaksh, A.; Bekkers, J.A.; Bogers, A.; de Groot, N.M.S. Impact of Ischemic and Valvular Heart Disease on Atrial Excitation:A High-Resolution Epicardial Mapping Study. *J. Am. Heart Assoc.* **2018**, *7*, e008331. [CrossRef]
35. Teuwen, C.P.; Yaksh, A.; Lanters, E.A.; Kik, C.; van der Does, L.J.; Knops, P.; Taverne, Y.J.; van de Woestijne, P.C.; Oei, F.B.; Bekkers, J.A.; et al. Relevance of Conduction Disorders in Bachmann's Bundle During Sinus Rhythm in Humans. *Circ. Arrhythm. Electrophysiol.* **2016**, *9*, e003972. [CrossRef]
36. Mouws, E.; Kik, C.; van der Does, L.; Lanters, E.A.H.; Teuwen, C.P.; Knops, P.; Bogers, A.; de Groot, N.M.S. Novel Insights in the Activation Patterns at the Pulmonary Vein Area. *Circ. Arrhythm. Electrophysiol.* **2018**, *11*, e006720. [CrossRef]

37. van Schie, M.S.; Ramdat Misier, N.L.; Razavi Ebrahimi, P.; Heida, A.; Kharbanda, R.K.; Taverne, Y.; de Groot, N.M.S. Premature atrial contractions promote local directional heterogeneities in conduction velocity vectors. *Europace* **2023**, *25*, 1162–1171. [CrossRef]
38. Heida, A.; van Schie, M.S.; van der Does, W.F.B.; Taverne, Y.; Bogers, A.; de Groot, N.M.S. Reduction of Conduction Velocity in Patients with Atrial Fibrillation. *J. Clin. Med.* **2021**, *10*, 2614. [CrossRef]
39. Heida, A.; van der Does, W.F.B.; van Staveren, L.N.; Taverne, Y.; Roos-Serote, M.C.; Bogers, A.; de Groot, N.M.S. Conduction Heterogeneity: Impact of Underlying Heart Disease and Atrial Fibrillation. *JACC Clin. Electrophysiol.* **2020**, *6*, 1844–1854. [CrossRef]
40. Heida, A.; van der Does, W.F.B.; van Schie, M.S.; van Staveren, L.N.; Taverne, Y.; Bogers, A.; de Groot, N.M.S. Does conduction heterogeneity determine the supervulnerable period after atrial fibrillation? *Med. Biol. Eng. Comput.* **2023**, *61*, 897–908. [CrossRef]
41. Zhang, L.; van Schie, M.S.; Xiang, H.; Liao, R.; Zheng, J.; Knops, P.; Taverne, Y.; de Groot, N.M.S. Identification of Atrial Transmural Conduction Inhomogeneity Using Unipolar Electrogram Morphology. *J. Clin. Med.* **2024**, *13*, 1015. [CrossRef]
42. Mouws, E.; Lanters, E.A.H.; Teuwen, C.P.; van der Does, L.; Kik, C.; Knops, P.; Bekkers, J.A.; Bogers, A.; de Groot, N.M.S. Epicardial Breakthrough Waves During Sinus Rhythm: Depiction of the Arrhythmogenic Substrate? *Circ. Arrhythm. Electrophysiol.* **2017**, *10*, e005145. [CrossRef] [PubMed]
43. Kharbanda, R.K.; Knops, P.; van der Does, L.; Kik, C.; Taverne, Y.; Roos-Serote, M.C.; Heida, A.; Oei, F.B.S.; Bogers, A.; de Groot, N.M.S. Simultaneous Endo-Epicardial Mapping of the Human Right Atrium: Unraveling Atrial Excitation. *J. Am. Heart Assoc.* **2020**, *9*, e017069. [CrossRef] [PubMed]
44. Spach, M.S.; Miller, W.T., 3rd; Miller-Jones, E.; Warren, R.B.; Barr, R.C. Extracellular potentials related to intracellular action potentials during impulse conduction in anisotropic canine cardiac muscle. *Circ. Res.* **1979**, *45*, 188–204. [CrossRef] [PubMed]
45. de Groot, N.M.; Schalij, M.J.; Zeppenfeld, K.; Blom, N.A.; Van der Velde, E.T.; Van der Wall, E.E. Voltage and activation mapping: How the recording technique affects the outcome of catheter ablation procedures in patients with congenital heart disease. *Circulation* **2003**, *108*, 2099–2106. [CrossRef] [PubMed]
46. Jacquemet, V.; Virag, N.; Ihara, Z.; Dang, L.; Blanc, O.; Zozor, S.; Vesin, J.M.; Kappenberger, L.; Henriquez, C. Study of unipolar electrogram morphology in a computer model of atrial fibrillation. *J. Cardiovasc. Electrophysiol.* **2003**, *14*, S172–S179. [CrossRef]
47. van Schie, M.S.; Starreveld, R.; Roos-Serote, M.C.; Taverne, Y.; van Schaagen, F.R.N.; Bogers, A.; de Groot, N.M.S. Classification of sinus rhythm single potential morphology in patients with mitral valve disease. *Europace* **2020**, *22*, 1509–1519. [CrossRef]
48. van Schie, M.S.; Starreveld, R.; Bogers, A.; de Groot, N.M.S. Sinus rhythm voltage fingerprinting in patients with mitral valve disease using a high-density epicardial mapping approach. *Europace* **2021**, *23*, 469–478. [CrossRef]
49. van der Does, L.; Knops, P.; Teuwen, C.P.; Serban, C.; Starreveld, R.; Lanters, E.A.H.; Mouws, E.; Kik, C.; Bogers, A.; de Groot, N.M.S. Unipolar atrial electrogram morphology from an epicardial and endocardial perspective. *Heart Rhythm.* **2018**, *15*, 879–887. [CrossRef]
50. Ye, Z.; van Schie, M.S.; de Groot, N.M.S. Signal Fingerprinting as a Novel Diagnostic Tool to Identify Conduction Inhomogeneity. *Front. Physiol.* **2021**, *12*, 652128. [CrossRef] [PubMed]
51. Zhang, L.; van Schie, M.S.; Knops, P.; Taverne, Y.; de Groot, N.M.S. A novel diagnostic tool to identify atrial endo-epicardial asynchrony using signal fingerprinting. *Hell. J. Cardiol.* **2024**, *75*, 9–20. [CrossRef] [PubMed]
52. Rolf, S.; Kircher, S.; Arya, A.; Eitel, C.; Sommer, P.; Richter, S.; Gaspar, T.; Bollmann, A.; Altmann, D.; Piedra, C.; et al. Tailored atrial substrate modification based on low-voltage areas in catheter ablation of atrial fibrillation. *Circ. Arrhythm. Electrophysiol.* **2014**, *7*, 825–833. [CrossRef] [PubMed]
53. Josephson, M.E.; Anter, E. Substrate Mapping for Ventricular Tachycardia: Assumptions and Misconceptions. *JACC Clin. Electrophysiol.* **2015**, *1*, 341–352. [CrossRef]
54. van Schie, M.S.; Kharbanda, R.K.; Houck, C.A.; Lanters, E.A.H.; Taverne, Y.; Bogers, A.; de Groot, N.M.S. Identification of Low-Voltage Areas: A Unipolar, Bipolar, and Omnipolar Perspective. *Circ. Arrhythm. Electrophysiol.* **2021**, *14*, e009912. [CrossRef] [PubMed]
55. Van Schie, M.S.; Knops, P.; Zhang, L.; Van Schaagen, F.R.N.; Taverne, Y.; De Groot, N.M.S. Detection of endo-epicardial atrial low-voltage areas using unipolar and omnipolar voltage mapping. *Front. Physiol.* **2022**, *13*, 1030025. [CrossRef]
56. Piorkowski, C.; Kronborg, M.; Hourdain, J.; Piorkowski, J.; Kirstein, B.; Neudeck, S.; Wechselberger, S.; Päßler, E.; Löwen, A.; El-Armouche, A.; et al. Endo-/Epicardial Catheter Ablation of Atrial Fibrillation: Feasibility, Outcome, and Insights Into Arrhythmia Mechanisms. *Circ. Arrhythm. Electrophysiol.* **2018**, *11*, e005748. [CrossRef]
57. Ye, Z.; van Schie, M.S.; Pool, L.; Heida, A.; Knops, P.; Taverne, Y.; Brundel, B.; de Groot, N.M.S. Characterization of unipolar electrogram morphology: A novel tool for quantifying conduction inhomogeneity. *Europace* **2023**, *25*, euad324. [CrossRef]
58. van der Does, W.F.B.; Houck, C.A.; Heida, A.; van Schie, M.S.; van Schaagen, F.R.N.; Taverne, Y.; Bogers, A.; de Groot, N.M.S. Atrial electrophysiological characteristics of aging. *J. Cardiovasc. Electrophysiol.* **2021**, *32*, 903–912. [CrossRef]
59. Ye, Z.; van Schie, M.S.; Heida, A.; van Staveren, L.N.; van Schaagen, F.R.N.; Taverne, Y.; de Groot, N.M.S. Unipolar atrial electrogram morphology is affected by age: Evidence from high-resolution epicardial mapping. *Ann. Med.* **2023**, *55*, 1431–1441. [CrossRef]
60. Schram-Serban, C.; Heida, A.; Roos-Serote, M.C.; Knops, P.; Kik, C.; Brundel, B.; Bogers, A.; de Groot, N.M.S. Heterogeneity in Conduction Underlies Obesity-Related Atrial Fibrillation Vulnerability. *Circ. Arrhythm. Electrophysiol.* **2020**, *13*, e008161. [CrossRef]

61. Schram-Serban, C.; van Schie, M.S.; Knops, P.; Kik, C.; Bogers, A.; de Groot, N.M.S. Low-voltage potentials contribute to postoperative atrial fibrillation development in obese patients. *Heart Rhythm.* **2022**, *19*, 710–718. [CrossRef] [PubMed]
62. Veen, D.; Schram-Serban, C.; van Schie, M.; van Schaagen, F.; Knops, P.; Kavousi, M.; Taverne, Y.; de Groot, N.M.S. How sex affects the sinus rhythm heartbeat. *Int. J. Cardiol. Heart Vasc.* **2023**, *49*, 101314. [CrossRef] [PubMed]

Journal of
Clinical Medicine

MDPI

Review

Substrates of Sudden Cardiac Death in Hypertrophic Cardiomyopathy

Matteo Sclafani [1,2], Giulio Falasconi [3], Giacomo Tini [2], Beatrice Musumeci [2], Diego Penela [3,4], Andrea Saglietto [5], Luca Arcari [6,7], Chiara Bucciarelli-Ducci [1], Emanuele Barbato [2], Antonio Berruezo [3] and Pietro Francia [2,*]

1 Royal Brompton and Harefield Hospitals, Guy's and St Thomas' NHS Foundation Trust, London SW3 6PY, UK; matteo.sclafani@uniroma1.it (M.S.); c.bucciarelli-ducci@rbht.nhs.uk (C.B.-D.)
2 Cardiology Unit, Department of Clinical and Molecular Medicine, Sant'Andrea University Hospital, Sapienza University, 00189 Rome, Italy; giacomo.tinimelato@uniroma1.it (G.T.); beatrice.musumeci@uniroma1.it (B.M.); emanuele.barbato@uniroma1.it (E.B.)
3 Arrhythmia Department, Teknon Heart Institute, Teknon Medical Center, 08022 Barcelona, Spain; giuliofalasconi@gmail.com (G.F.); penela.maceda@gmail.com (D.P.); antonio.berruezo@quironsalud.es (A.B.)
4 IRCCS Humanitas Research Hospital, 20089 Rozzano, Italy
5 Division of Cardiology, Cardiovascular and Thoracic Department, "Citta Della Salute e Della Scienza" Hospital, 10126 Turin, Italy
6 Cardiology Unit, Madre Giuseppina Vannini Hospital, 00177 Rome, Italy; luca.arcari88@gmail.com
7 Department of Clinical Internal, Anesthesiological and Cardiovascular Sciences, Sapienza University, 00161 Rome, Italy
* Correspondence: pietro.francia@uniroma1.it

Abstract: Sudden cardiac death (SCD), the most devastating complication of hypertrophic cardiomyopathy (HCM), is primarily triggered by ventricular tachycardia or fibrillation. Despite advances in knowledge, the mechanisms driving ventricular arrhythmia in HCM remain incompletely understood, stemming from an interplay of multiple pro-arrhythmic factors. Myocyte disarray and myocardial fibrosis form a structural substrate favorable to re-entrant arrhythmias by altering myocardial electrophysiological properties, while cellular abnormalities predominate in patients without evident structural remodeling. Traditional SCD risk prediction models rely on clinical risk factors and regression-based risk estimation, often overlooking specific arrhythmic substrates. Emerging techniques now allow for the direct assessment of these substrates, providing deeper insights into the arrhythmogenic mechanisms and paving the way for more personalized SCD risk stratification. This review explores the contribution of cellular, structural, and electrophysiological substrates to arrhythmic risk in HCM, emphasizing their distinct roles. Furthermore, it highlights the potential of substrate-based approaches to refining SCD prevention strategies and improving outcomes for patients with HCM.

Keywords: hypertrophic cardiomyopathy; sudden cardiac death; ventricular tachycardia; ventricular fibrillation; substrates; cardiovascular magnetic resonance; electrophysiological study; afterdepolarizations

1. Hypertrophic Cardiomyopathy and Sudden Cardiac Death: An Overview

Hypertrophic cardiomyopathy (HCM) is a common inherited myocardial disease, affecting approximately 1 in 500 individuals in the general population [1,2]. The hallmark of HCM is left ventricular (LV) hypertrophy in the absence of other cardiac or systemic conditions that cause hemodynamic overload [3]. Hypertrophy in HCM is typically asymmetric, mainly involving the basal anterior septum and the anterolateral free wall. However, the phenotypic expression is highly variable, and hypertrophy may symmetrically involve the entire LV or be confined to the free wall or apex [4].

HCM is inherited as an autosomal dominant trait with incomplete penetrance, and around 1400 causative mutations have been identified in 11 sarcomeric genes, with pathogenic variants in the MYH7 and MYBPC3 genes accounting for the majority of cases [5,6]. These mutations are identified in up to 60% of individuals with a family history of HCM and in approximately 30–40% of sporadic cases [7]. The onset of HCM occurs in three distinct life stages: infancy, adolescence, and middle adulthood [8]. Childhood-onset HCM is predominantly linked to sarcomeric mutations, whereas non-sarcomeric HCM is most often diagnosed after age 50, with a peak incidence in the sixth decade of life [8].

Initially, HCM was considered a disease with an exceptionally poor prognosis [9]. Advancements in diagnostic techniques and findings from studies on unselected populations have significantly reshaped our understanding of the natural history of the disease [10]. HCM is now recognized as having an extremely heterogeneous clinical course, ranging from asymptomatic presentation and stable course to catastrophic outcomes such as arrhythmic sudden cardiac death (SCD) and heart failure (HF) [11,12]. While most patients with HCM have a normal life expectancy, those with a complex clinical course may experience a variety of HCM-related complications [13]. Approximately 70% of patients develop LV outflow tract obstruction at some point, which may be present at rest or induced by exertion, affecting both symptoms and prognosis [1,14–16]. About 5% of patients progress to overt LV dysfunction and refractory HF with extensive fibrosis, resulting in a hypokinetic-dilated or restrictive phenotype, and often require transplantation (end-stage phase) [17,18]. Additionally, around 5% of patients develop an apical aneurysm, associated with a high risk of arrhythmic and thromboembolic events [19,20]. A small subset, approximately 10%, experience "benign remodeling", characterized by gradual LV wall thinning with minimal changes in cavity dimension and ejection fraction, both of which remain within normal limits [21,22]. These patients generally have favorable long-term outcomes, with morbidity and mortality similar to those without LV remodeling [21]. The diverse phenotypic presentations underscore the importance of a personalized management strategy tailored to each patient's distinct clinical profile, disease progression, and associated complications.

Among the complications associated with HCM, SCD is the most unpredictable and dramatic and may occur as the first disease manifestation. Together with HF and stroke, it contributes significantly to HCM-related mortality [23]. SCD in HCM is most commonly due to sustained ventricular tachycardia (VT) or ventricular fibrillation (VF) [24]. Contrary to earlier beliefs, SCD is relatively rare in HCM, with an annual incidence of about 0.7% in unselected populations [25]. SCD predominantly affects younger individuals, reaching a cumulative incidence of approximately 8–10% over 5 years in childhood [8]. The risk of SCD decreases with age and is low in HCM patients over 60 years old [26,27]. The prevention of SCD with implantable cardioverter defibrillators (ICDs) has transformed the natural history of HCM, reducing disease-related mortality more than tenfold and becoming a cornerstone of disease management [23,28]. However, ICD therapy is not without risks [29,30]. Thus, while significant progress has been made in developing defibrillation technologies with a lower risk of long-term complications [31–34], it is essential to refine risk stratification strategies, making them more effective and personalized.

Over the past few decades, SCD risk models have been developed and integrated into clinical guidelines, providing support in identifying candidates for ICD therapy [2,35]. However, catastrophic events still occur in patients classified as "low risk" [36], while many "high-risk" patients receive ICD implants but never require appropriate therapies [37], exposing them to lifelong ICD-related complications without any survival benefit [37]. The pro-arrhythmic mechanisms underlying ventricular arrhythmias in HCM are complex and not yet fully understood. They involve cellular anomalies, macro- and microstructural abnormalities, and changes in myocardial electrophysiological properties. Current prediction models for SCD primarily focus on clinical risk factors, such as a family history of SCD, left ventricular wall thickness, non-sustained VT, an unexplained syncope, and abnormal blood pressure responses to exercise [35]. While these models effectively support clinical decision-making in refining ICD candidacy, a significant proportion of patients who experience SCD do not meet the established high-risk criteria. This underscores the need for a more individualized approach to risk assessments.

Recent advancements in molecular studies, imaging, and electrophysiological techniques have significantly deepened our understanding of the structural and functional substrates underlying arrhythmic events in HCM. Unlike traditional reviews that primarily address established clinical risk factors, this work adopts a mechanistic perspective, analyzing the electrophysiological and pathophysiological basis of ventricular arrhythmias through the integration of advanced technological insights. By leveraging modern approaches to substrate characterization, this review envisions the transition from static risk stratification models to a dynamic, physiology-driven framework for SCD prediction. This paradigmatic shift has the potential to refine risk assessment and pave the way for a more precise and personalized approach to shared decision-making in ICD implantation.

The organization of this review into distinct sections—cellular/molecular, anatomical/structural, and electrophysiological/functional—reflects a methodological approach aimed at structuring the available evidence in a systematic manner. While these domains are inherently interconnected, particularly through the influence of cellular mechanisms on structural remodeling and functional alterations, this framework allows for a more defined analysis of the current state of knowledge and its implications.

2. Cellular Substrates

HCM has traditionally been considered a disease that primarily affects the myocardium, resulting in macro- and microstructural abnormalities [22]. Therefore, research has predominantly focused on structural substrates as the main drivers of ventricular arrhythmias. Despite advances in understanding pro-arrhythmic structural substrates, fatal events continue to occur, particularly in patients without significant structural abnormalities [38–40]. Notably, the most lethal arrhythmia occurs in young patients at the early stages of the disease, when structural remodeling is minimal and replacement fibrosis may be absent. This subset of patients remains one of the greatest challenges in understanding SCD in HCM.

A primary reason for our inadequate knowledge in this area is that limited translational research exists, while most efforts have focused on clinical markers of risk derived from pathology, diagnostic tool-based evaluations, and imaging [41]. Few studies have focused on the cellular mechanisms of arrhythmogenesis, which might explain the occurrence of arrhythmias in patients without manifest structural abnormalities, though not exclusively. In this subgroup of patients, sustained arrhythmias begin with one or more premature ventricular contractions (PVCs), arising from the abnormal spontaneous depolarization of clusters of synchronized ventricular myocytes and propagating through the LV [41]. It has been hypothesized that the arrhythmogenic substrate involves early (EADs) and delayed afterdepolarizations (DADs) related to ion current dysfunctions and altered intracellular calcium (Ca^{2+}) homeostasis [42–46]. EADs occur during phases 2 or 3 of the cardiac action potential, typically when repolarization is prolonged. Patch-clamp studies on isolated HCM cardiomyocytes have shown that action potential duration (APD) is significantly prolonged compared to controls, resulting from multiple ion current abnormalities:

a reduction in potassium (K^+) currents (including inward-rectifier, transient outward, and delayed rectifier K^+ currents), an increase the L-type Ca^{2+} current (ICaL), and a heightened late sodium (Na^+) current (INaL) [43,47,48]. DADs, on the other hand, arise after the cell has fully repolarized (phase 4 of the cardiac action potential) due to intracellular Ca^{2+} overload. Calcium overload generates an inward sodium current through the Na^+/Ca^{2+} exchanger, resulting in delayed depolarization [46,49,50]. Abnormal Ca^{2+} handling has consistently been observed in both animal models and human samples of HCM [43,47,49,51–53]. Alterations in Ca^{2+} homeostasis are driven by various concurrent mechanisms, including the sustained activation of CaMKII, the increased amplitude and delayed inactivation kinetics of ICaL, a reduced SERCA/phospholamban ratio, diminished SERCA expression, the loss and disorganization of t-tubules, increased Ca^{2+} leakage from the sarcoplasmic reticulum, and an abnormal Na^+/Ca^{2+} exchanger function [42–46]. This collective cascade of mechanisms creates a vicious cycle, driving intracellular Ca^{2+} accumulation and promoting delayed depolarizations, further increasing the risk of arrhythmogenic events [43]. Adding to this complexity, an abnormal response to beta-adrenergic stimulation represents another potential cellular substrate for arrhythmogenesis in HCM, particularly during exercise or stress. A preclinical study showed that while beta-stimulation shortens APD in control cells, isoproterenol paradoxically prolongs APD in HCM cardiomyocytes, suggesting an abnormal cellular response under stress conditions [47]. Another factor to consider is the pro-arrhythmic role of myocardial wall stress mediated by the activation of stretch-activated channels (SACs). SACs are ion channels sensitive to mechanical stress that induce intracellular fluxes of calcium (Ca^{2+}) and sodium (Na^+), triggering afterdepolarizations [54]. Preclinical models have demonstrated that SAC activation can lead to electrophysiological instability and remodeling [54], with arrhythmogenic effects associated with SAC currents increasing with hypertrophy [55]. It is reasonable to hypothesize that the heightened myocardial wall stress typically observed in HCM could activate these channels, contributing to increased arrhythmic risk. However, these observations remain speculative, as no direct evidence currently supports a definitive role for SACs in the incidence of SCD in HCM.

Arrhythmogenesis due to cellular abnormalities is the hallmark of other inherited cardiac conditions associated with SCD that lack structural substrates, such as channelopathies [56]. Although concurrent mutations in both sarcomeric and ion channel genes have been observed in some patients [57], preclinical studies have identified a direct mechanistic link between mutant sarcomeric proteins (e.g., increased myofilament Ca^{2+} sensitivity) and cellular arrhythmogenicity [52,58]. Interestingly, arrhythmogenic cellular alterations were detected very early in transgenic mouse models before overt structural and functional cardiac abnormalities developed [42,59].

While these preclinical findings provide valuable pathophysiological insights, in vivo data remain limited. It has been extensively demonstrated that a family history of SCD is one of the most important risk factors, and it has been hypothesized that this is due to the transmission of proarrhythmic mutations, some of which may potentially involve cellular substrates [60–63]. Patients with sarcomere mutations are more prone to SCD and exhibit more pronounced repolarization abnormalities compared to those with a negative genetic status [64–67]. A recent prospective study showed that ventricular repolarization abnormalities are present in patients with HCM-related genetic mutations but without phenotypic expression [66]. Proarrhythmic abnormalities in the absence of scars or hypertrophy may reflect early cellular and molecular changes in response to sarcomeric mutations. These interesting findings should be interpreted with caution, keeping in mind that arrhythmogenesis in HCM is complex and involves multiple mechanisms. In fact, Diffusion Tensor Imaging (DTI) has shown that even in the absence of hypertrophy or fibrosis detectable with conventional imaging, microstructural abnormalities can be observed in the early stages of HCM and may contribute to the electrophysiological abnormalities observed [68].

While thought-provoking, the assessment of cellular substrates currently has minimal to no clinical applicability in identifying high-risk HCM patients. However, advanced ECG studies or drug challenges, similar to those used for channelopathies, may hold diagnostic and prognostic value in the near future [41]. Additionally, drugs targeting cellular pro-arrhythmic substrates could play a role in SCD prevention. Ranolazine, an INaL inhibitor, has been shown in preclinical studies to reduce APD and EADs in HCM cardiomyocytes [43,47]. It was also tested in a small multicenter, placebo-controlled, randomized trial, where it modestly reduced ventricular ectopy on a 24 h Holter ECG [69]. Similarly, disopyramide is a Na^+ channel blocker that has been used for years in obstructive HCM for its negative inotropic properties and has been found to stabilize the closed state of the RyR2 channel, thereby inhibiting Ca^{2+}-dependent arrhythmias and DADs by reducing cytosolic calcium levels [48]. Finally, novel cardiac myosin inhibitor drugs, which reversibly inhibit the myosin–actin coupling reaction, have the potential to reduce the calcium sensitivity of myocardial myosin and inhibit Ca^{2+}-dependent arrhythmias [70]. Their preventive effect on ventricular arrhythmias and SCD has not been adequately investigated, requiring longitudinal data.

Key Messages

- Cellular substrates play a critical role in the arrhythmogenic mechanisms of HCM, particularly in patients without manifest structural abnormalities.
- Ventricular arrhythmias and SCD can occur early in the disease, driven by ion current dysfunction, impaired calcium homeostasis, and abnormal beta-adrenergic responses. These proarrhythmic changes often precede overt structural remodeling and may be linked to sarcomeric mutations.
- Although cellular mechanisms currently have limited clinical applicability in identifying high-risk HCM patients, advancements in molecular diagnostics, imaging, and targeted therapies hold promise for improving SCD risk management.

3. Structural Substrates

Myocardial hypertrophy in HCM is characterized by a range of macroscopic and microscopic structural abnormalities [71]. In at least one-third of the myocardium, myocytes are hypertrophic and disorganized, displaying structural abnormalities in both shape and alignment, which is a phenomenon collectively referred to as myocardial disarray. This typically involves hypertrophic walls but may also affect areas of the ventricular wall with normal thickness [71]. In the HCM myocardium, the extracellular matrix is expanded and particularly rich in glycogen, with widespread interstitial fibrosis that can become so extensive as to cause progressive fibrotic replacement of the myocardium, leading to scar formation [72]. Furthermore, structural abnormalities of the intramyocardial coronary vessels are commonly observed, including media-layer hypertrophy, disorganized elastic fibers, and endothelial hyperplasia. These changes result in vessel wall thickening, which narrows the luminal diameter and leads to microvascular dysfunction, impairing the heart's ability to increase myocardial perfusion in response to metabolic demands. The result is myocardial ischemia, myocyte necrosis, and the replacement of these cells with additional fibrotic tissue [73–76].

The combination of myocardial disarray, increased extracellular matrix, and microvascular abnormalities results in both micro- and macroscopic structural alterations, dominated by the formation of myocardial fibrosis. This scarring, in the form of interstitial or replacement fibrosis, is a recognized hallmark of HCM and is commonly found in the necropsies of young patients with SCD [77].

Myocardial scars are essential components of re-entry circuits, the most common electrophysiological substrate of ventricular arrhythmias [78]. A re-entry circuit requires an anatomical or functional barrier, at least two distinct pathways for the electrical impulse to travel down (one of which must have different conduction properties, such as slower conduction), a unidirectional block (the impulse cannot travel in one direction but can still travel in the opposite), and sufficient excitable tissue. When these conditions are met, electrical excitation follows a slow, circular path. The time required for the excitation wave to complete the circuit exceeds the effective refractory period of the myocytes, allowing for persistent, self-sustaining re-entry. This re-entry circuit then functions as a rapid pacemaker, depolarizing the ventricular myocardium and leading to sustained ventricular tachycardia [41].

Regions of non-conductive dense scarring or anatomical structures act as anatomical obstacles that block the propagation of electrical impulses [79,80]. Conversely, myocardial disarray and interstitial fibrosis disrupt the physiological homogeneity of electrical conduction, favoring anisotropic, slow conduction [81]. Indeed, collagen strands accumulating in the spaces between cardiomyocytes can form thick insulating sheaths, impeding transversal conduction while accelerating longitudinal conduction [82,83]. Additionally, activated fibroblasts influence myocardial electrical activity directly by forming gap junctions with cardiomyocytes [84]. Ultimately, local transient ischemia due to microvascular dysfunction further contributes to arrhythmogenesis by creating regions of partial depolarization and slowed conduction, which further promotes anisotropic conduction [77,85,86].

Cardiac magnetic resonance (CMR) is the gold-standard non-invasive tool for identifying and quantifying both replacement and interstitial fibrosis [87,88]. CMR detects replacement fibrosis by exploiting the distinct kinetics of paramagnetic contrast distribution in the healthy myocardium versus scar tissue (late gadolinium enhancement technique, LGE). Fibrosis appears as hyperintense signals, varying in intensity based on the contrast accumulated in the interstitial space, which reflects the scar architecture. Scar tissue can be qualitatively assessed and quantified [87]. More recent techniques, such as T1 mapping and extracellular volume fraction (ECV) measurement, enable the detection of interstitial fibrosis by evaluating its effects on the longitudinal magnetization recovery time [89]. Finally, DTI is an emerging CMR technique that visualizes myocardial microstructure by mapping water molecule diffusion and measuring disarray [90].

Early studies assessing structural substrates as predictors of arrhythmic risk in HCM focused on total scar burden, which has proven to be a strong predictor of adverse events in several unselected prospective cohorts [79,91–93]. The largest analysis exploring LGE as a risk factor for HCM-related SCD demonstrated that events peaked in patients with a high scar mass (≥15%), while no significant increase in SCD risk was observed in patients with minimal LGE (1–5%) compared to those without any LGE [79]. Two following prospective cohort studies demonstrated that q moderate LGE extent (10–15%) predicts major arrhythmic events in patients with low-to-intermediate SCD risk [94,95]. Consequently, the American College of Cardiology/American Heart Association (ACC/AHA) incorporated a scar burden threshold of 15% as a risk factor to consider in the subgroup of patients without major clinical SCD risk factors or when ICD implantation remains uncertain [2]. However, scar burden as a sole risk factor has limited sensitivity, as demonstrated by a high rate of adverse events in patients with LGE ≤ 15% [79,94,95].

LGE in HCM patients reveals variations in presentation, signal intensity, and distribution independently of global scar extent [96]. This heterogeneity reflects the complex architecture of HCM scar tissue, which, unlike post-ischemic scars, consists of diffuse fibrosis combined with viable muscle fibers rather than dense subendocardial scarring confined to a specific vascular territory [74,97–99]. This complex architecture represents an ideal substrate for re-entry circuits. CMR studies showed that mild- or intermediate-enhanced LGE was more predictive of ventricular arrhythmias than hyper-enhanced LGE [100,101]. Furthermore, a recent study in low- and intermediate-risk patients demonstrated that a quantitative analysis of LGE dispersion is a predictor of major arrhythmic events independently of the total scar burden [96]. Visual scar heterogeneity evaluation can be challenging and is prone to significant interobserver variability. Radiomics has the potential to make this analysis more accurate and reproducible. A recent study conducted on a large unselected cohort of HCM patients demonstrated that scar heterogeneity assessed with LGE radiomics is a significant predictor of SCD risk and provides incremental risk stratification beyond the current risk models [102]. This suggests that a qualitative assessment of scar architecture through LGE signal heterogeneity may provide more detailed insights into the pro-arrhythmic substrate, enabling the risk reclassification of patients with mild-to-moderate LGE burden (<15%). The main limitation of assessing LGE heterogeneity with standard LGE images is its reliance on 2D imaging, which does not fully capture the complex three-dimensional architecture of scar tissue [96]. Recently developed post-processing software elaborated LGE images to obtain a more accurate evaluation of myocardial scar architecture [103,104]. By segmenting pixel signal intensity, these techniques enable differentiation between dense core fibrosis and diffuse border zone (BZ) fibrosis. They then reconstruct the data into 3D images and identify corridors of BZ tissue protected by dense scars or anatomical barriers that connect areas of normal myocardium between the core zones, referred to as border zone channels (BZCs) (Figure 1) [103]. From a functional point of view, BZCs are corridors of excitable myocardial tissue with slow conduction, electrically insulated by non-conductive scar tissue. By acting as slow-conducting re-entrant pathways, they can trigger and sustain ventricular tachycardia [103]. In this view, BZC may represent the imaging equivalent of the structural and functional substrate that promotes re-entrant VTs [105]. A recent CMR study demonstrated that BZCs are a strong independent predictor of ventricular arrhythmias in high-risk HCM patients and that risk assessment based on scar channels rather than total scar mass reclassified approximately 12% of patients, aiding in the identification of those at highest risk [106].

As discussed, in addition to the identification of electrically inert scars, a substrate assessment model aimed at identifying potential reentrant circuits must also be capable of detecting areas of possible impaired conduction, including those with myocardial disarray. In this regard, cardiac DTI is an innovative CMR technique that measures water diffusion in three dimensions, allowing for the characterization of the myocardial microstructure [90]. By calculating fractional anisotropy (FA), cardiac DTI quantifies the directional variability of water diffusion. FA values near zero indicate random diffusion (perfect isotropy), while values near one indicate unidirectional diffusion (perfect anisotropy). Thus, FA is expected to be high in voxels with coherently aligned myocytes and low in voxels with differing myocyte orientations due to disarray [81]. A recent study found that disarray detected by cardiac DTI (as reduced FA) correlated with ventricular arrhythmia risk independently of the presence of fibrosis and hypertrophy [81]. These findings reinforce the concept that disarray is a critical factor in arrhythmogenesis, even in the very early stages of the disease [68].

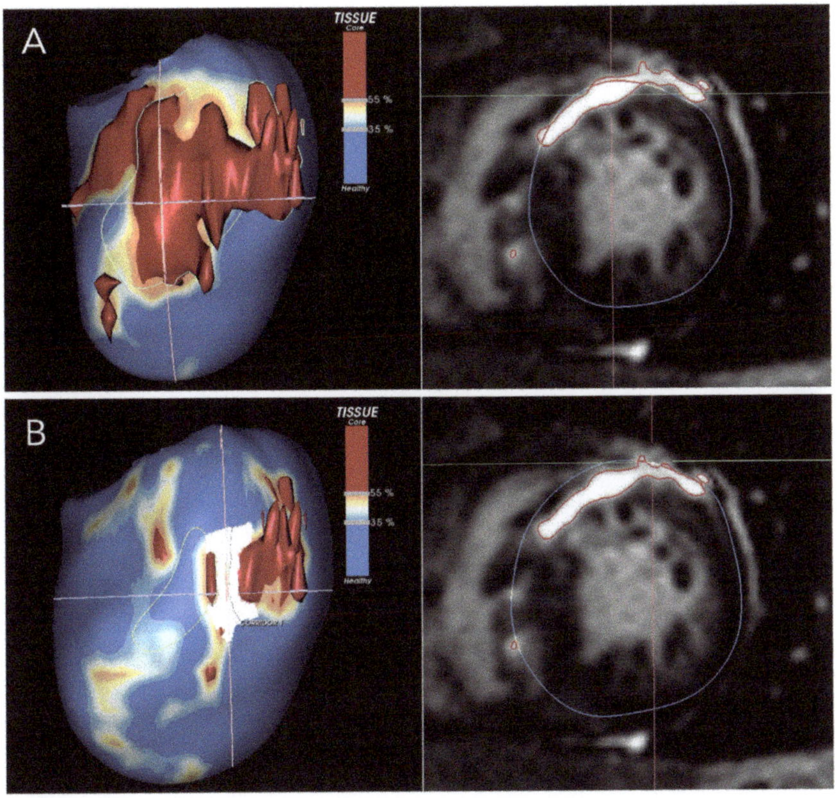

Figure 1. The figure shows a short-axis view of a CMR of a patient with HCM, highlighting an extensive scar involving the anterior wall and the interventricular septum. LGE-CMR images were post-processed using ADAS 3D (Galgo Medical, Barcelona, Spain), creating nine concentric surface layers spanning from the endocardium to the epicardium of the left ventricular wall thickness, resulting in a 3D shell for each layer. Color-coded pixel signal intensity (PSI) maps were projected onto each shell. Hyper-enhanced areas were classified as the core zone, borderline zone (BZ), or healthy tissue using thresholds of 40 ± 5% and 60 ± 5% of the maximum PSI. The scar-dense core is coded in red, BZ is coded in orange and white, and healthy myocardium is coded in blue. BZ channels are identified as continuous corridors of BZ protected by scar core tissue. In (**A**), the 50% layer is shown, representing the mid-myocardial layer. The area is entirely occupied by a dense and compact scar. In (**B**), the 3D reconstruction corresponds to the 80% epicardial layer. In the anterior wall, at the center of the crosshair, a BZ channel is visible.

Key Message

- Myocardial scars and myocyte disarray are structural substrates with recognized, significant pro-arrhythmic implications in HCM. However, the assessment of myocardial disarray is still not technically reliable and is not yet included in the definition of arrhythmic risk.
- While LGE estimation is useful as a quantitative, non-binary variable, it seems pathophysiologically inadequate to explain the structural and functional complexity of the electrical substrates.
- The heterogeneity and complexity of scar architecture and disarray in HCM necessitate a more nuanced evaluation, which is now achievable through advanced imaging techniques. This refined approach could allow for more precise identification of pro-arrhythmic substrates and lay the foundation for substrate-based risk stratification.

4. Electrophysiological Substrates

Although the etiology of SCD in HCM is arrhythmic, the study of myocardial electrophysiological properties has traditionally played a marginal and controversial prognostic role in this condition [35]. Most spontaneous non-sustained ventricular arrhythmias in HCM are monomorphic, and a significant proportion of ICD interventions are triggered by monomorphic VTs [91,107–111]. However, polymorphic VT or VF has traditionally been regarded as the most common mode of arrhythmic death and is the most frequently induced form of arrhythmia during programmed ventricular stimulation (PVS) in these patients [112,113]. Monomorphic ventricular arrhythmias are likely related primarily to scar-mediated re-entry mechanisms, whereas the anatomical and functional substrates underlying polymorphic arrhythmia in HCM remain poorly understood.

Re-entry circuits typically encompass protected isthmuses of slow-conducting tissue [78]. Of note, myocardial disarray has been associated with regions of impaired conduction [114,115], although demonstrating its effects on electrical conduction in vivo remains challenging [116]. The Paced Electrogram Fractionation Analysis (PEFA) technique is an electrophysiological method designed to assess conduction heterogeneity and electrical activity within the myocardium [117–120]. This procedure involves pacing specific sites in the right ventricle (apex, mid-septum, RVOT, and free wall) with programmed stimuli and recording the resulting electrograms. Each site is paced (S1) with a decremental sequence, and an additional premature stimulus (S2) is introduced after every third beat, with recordings made from the remaining electrodes. The electrograms are then analyzed for duration, amplitude, and fractionation—characterized by fragmented potentials at the end of the electrogram—as an indicator of slow and heterogeneous conduction. This technique exposes the electrophysiological effects of disarray, including delayed intramyocardial conduction due to slowed or tortuous pathways and a temporary conduction block [120]. Spatially heterogeneous depolarization and repolarization are known to be pro-arrhythmic by favoring the asymmetric excitability and propagation of re-entry [116]. PEFA quantifies these effects through measurements of electrogram duration and the S1-S2 coupling interval at which delays increase. Prospective studies have shown PEFA to predict major arrhythmic events with greater accuracy than non-invasive techniques [117,118,120]. Interestingly, recordings made in sinus rhythm did not show the same alterations as those observed with pacing and associated with SCD [116]. This suggests that the arrhythmogenic electrophysiological substrate is dynamic, with the myocardial perturbation that triggers arrhythmia being mimicked by pacing [116].

Scar tissue, along with disarray, is the critical structural substrate for re-entrant arrhythmias, and invasive electrophysiological studies can detect scar-induced electrophysiological alterations [79,121,122]. The extent of myocardial scarring correlates with the inducibility of ventricular arrhythmias during PVS [123]. Additionally, direct recordings from bipolar electrograms on the endocardial surface of LGE segments in HCM show low amplitude and prolonged signals, suggesting conduction delay [122]. These findings indicate the presence of the slow-conducting viable myocardium within scarred areas, creating an ideal environment for sustaining re-entrant VTs and functionally confirming what has been observed with 3D CMR imaging techniques. These regions of viable myocardial tissue within the BZ, surrounded by non-conductive scar tissue, may act as slow-conducting re-entrant pathways that sustain VT circuits. Supporting this concept, a prospective cohort study demonstrated that the presence of BZ channels correlates with the inducibility and characteristics of ventricular arrhythmias during PVS [124]. In this study, polymorphic VT or VF induced by PVS was often preceded by a short run of monomorphic VT originating from within the scar. This suggests that the arrhythmia may begin as monomorphic, utilizing re-entry circuits with BZ channels as critical components, and subsequently degenerate into disorganized arrhythmia due to the sarcomeric misalignment and non-uniform anisotropic conduction characteristic of the HCM myocardium, which favors a high degree of activation dispersion, slow conduction, and unidirectional blocks [124]. These findings derive from a single, monocentric study and require confirmation by further research; however, they offer novel insights into the pathophysiology of ventricular arrhythmias in HCM.

The role of PVS has long been controversial in HCM. For many years, PVS was considered non-specific and lacking prognostic value beyond the non-invasive risk factors, leading to its very limited use in contemporary HCM risk stratification (Figure 2) [2,35,125,126]. However, earlier studies suggested that PVS could provide prognostic information and guide therapy in specific low-risk subgroups [112]. A single-center prospective study in a cohort of unselected patients recently found that inducibility at PVS predicted SCD or appropriate device therapy in HCM, while non-inducibility correlated with prolonged event-free survival [127]. The study reported an inducibility rate of ~ 39%, with a positive predictive value of approximately 23%. This inducibility rate was notably lower than in previous studies (67–77%), likely due to differences in patient selection and the use of less aggressive stimulation protocols [126]. Indeed, the high inducibility rate due to aggressive PVS has previously led to this prognostic tool being regarded as having limited specificity [125,128]. The main limitation of PVS is that it investigates induced arrhythmias rather than spontaneous ones. As such, there is no sufficient evidence to fully rely on invasive electrophysiological studies as the sole factor for arrhythmic risk stratification in HCM. However, while further investigation is needed to confirm its prognostic accuracy, these new findings re-evaluate PVS and suggest its potential application in specific patient subgroups.

The heterogeneity of spontaneous ventricular repolarization assessed with a 12-lead ECG in HCM has been associated with CMR-detected fibrosis and has been shown to be a prognostic factor in arrhythmic risk stratification [129,130]. However, 12-lead ECG techniques quantifying depolarization and repolarization abnormalities have seen limited clinical use due to challenges related to spatial resolution, technical limitations, and bias toward more advanced disease stages [131–134]. New non-invasive techniques have been developed to map ventricular activation and repolarization with high spatial and temporal resolution [135–140]. A recent prospective study using an integrated non-invasive electrophysiological approach combined with advanced cardiovascular imaging (CMR-guided electrocardiographic imaging, ECGI) demonstrated correlations between structural substrates and functional electrophysiological alterations [66]. Moreover, the translational potential of computational modeling also offers promising paths for advancing arrhythmia management in HCM. Indeed, emerging clinical applications of digital twins [141] promise to revolutionize care by providing dynamic, personalized insights into electrophysiological behavior. If these techniques continue to evolve to become more accessible, cost-effective, and reproducible, future longitudinal studies may reassess the role of electrophysiological substrates and redefine current approaches.

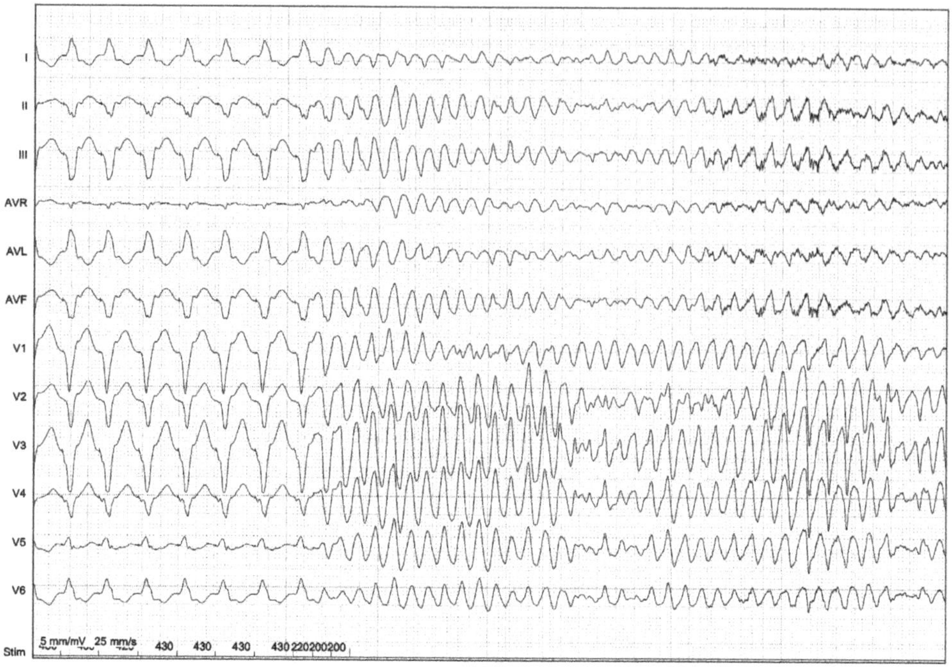

Figure 2. Induction of ventricular fibrillation by programmed ventricular stimulation (PVS) in a patient with HCM. A basic drive train cycle length of 430 ms is followed by three extra stimuli with short coupling intervals (220, 200, and 200 ms) applied in the right ventricle. The prognostic significance of polymorphic VT and VF induced with PVS in HCM is unknown. Aggressive stimulation protocols may lack specificity when identifying true arrhythmic risk.

Key Messages

- Structural substrates have functional electrophysiological counterparts that are gradually emerging as crucial in defining the mechanisms of ventricular arrhythmia in HCM patients.
- These findings open promising future perspectives for an integrated imaging–electrophysiological approach, complementing clinical risk factors for a more comprehensive and personalized risk assessment.

Table 1 summarizes the substrates of SCD in HCM.

Table 1. Substrates of sudden cardiac death in hypertrophic cardiomyopathy.

Substrate	Pathological Abnormalities	Functional Alterations	Arrhythmia	Supporting Evidence
Cellular	Ion currents dysfunction: • Reduction in K^+ currents • Increased ICaL current • Increased InaL Abnormal intracellular Ca^{2+} homeostasis	APD prolongation → EADs Ca^{2+} overload → DADs Abnormal response to beta-adrenergic stimulation	Premature ventricular contractions Polymorphic VT/VF	Coppini R. et al. Circulation 2013 [43] Olivotto I. et al. Circ Heart Fail 2018 [69]
Structural and Electrophysiological	Replacement fibrosis Interstitial fibrosis Myocardial disarray Microvascular ischemia	Conduction block Slow conduction	Reentry arrhythmia	Chan RH. et al. Circulation 2014 [79] Francia P. et al. JACC Cardiovasc Imaging 2023 [106] Saumarez RC et al. Circulation 1992 [117]

ICaL: L-type Ca^{2+} current. InaL: late sodium current. APD: action potential duration. EADs: early afterdepolarizations. DADs: delayed afterdepolarizations.

5. Conclusions

SCD is the most unpredictable and severe complication of HCM. Traditional SCD prediction models regress the clinical risk factors against events to estimate risk, with limited consideration of the underlying arrhythmic substrates. While these models have significant value in clinical practice, they also have limitations. They excel at identifying high-risk patients with advanced disease but are less effective for those in the early stages of disease, with minimal remodeling or subtle anatomical and functional substrates. The advent of new techniques could enable direct assessment of arrhythmic substrates, providing a more detailed understanding of the mechanisms involved. In the near future, these advancements may facilitate a more targeted and personalized approach to SCD risk assessment in HCM, shifting the paradigm from general clinical risk predictors to an individualized, substrate-based evaluation.

Author Contributions: M.S. and P.F. drafted the main manuscript and prepared Figures 1 and 2. All other authors reviewed the manuscript and contributed to the writing process based on their specific expertise on the subject. All authors have read and agreed to the published version of the manuscript.

Funding: This research received no external funding.

Acknowledgments: Matteo Sclafani has been supported by a research grant provided by the Digi-CardiopaTh PhD program.

Conflicts of Interest: P.F. received speaker fees from Boston Scientific and research grants from Abbott and Boston Scientific. A.B. is a stockholder of Galgo Medical.

References

1. Maron, B.J.; Ommen, S.R.; Semsarian, C.; Spirito, P.; Olivotto, I.; Maron, M.S. Hypertrophic cardiomyopathy: Present and future, with translation into contemporary cardiovascular medicine. *J. Am. Coll. Cardiol.* **2014**, *64*, 83–99. [CrossRef] [PubMed]
2. Ommen, S.R.; Mital, S.; Burke, M.A.; Day, S.M.; Deswal, A.; Elliott, P.; Evanovich, L.L.; Hung, J.; Joglar, J.A.; Kantor, P.; et al. 2020 AHA/ACC Guideline for the Diagnosis and Treatment of Patients with Hypertrophic Cardiomyopathy: A Report of the American College of Cardiology/American Heart Association Joint Committee on Clinical Practice Guidelines. *J. Am. Coll. Cardiol.* **2020**, *76*, e159–e240. [CrossRef] [PubMed]
3. Russo, D.; Sclafani, M.; Tini, G.; Musumeci, M.B.; Arcari, L.; Limite, L.R.; Francia, P.; Autore, C. Prognostic implications of different clinical profiles in hypertrophic cardiomyopathy. *Minerva Cardiol. Angiol.* **2022**, *70*, 189–206. [CrossRef]
4. Maron, M.S.; Maron, B.J.; Harrigan, C.; Buros, J.; Gibson, C.M.; Olivotto, I.; Biller, L.; Lesser, J.R.; Udelson, J.E.; Manning, W.J.; et al. Hypertrophic Cardiomyopathy Phenotype Revisited After 50 Years with Cardiovascular Magnetic Resonance. *J. Am. Coll. Cardiol.* **2009**, *54*, 220–228. [CrossRef] [PubMed]
5. Maron, B.J.; Maron, M.S. Hypertrophic cardiomyopathy. *Lancet* **2013**, *381*, 242–255. [CrossRef] [PubMed]
6. Venturiello, D.; Tiberi, P.G.; Perulli, F.; Nardoianni, G.; Guida, L.; Barsali, C.; Terrone, C.; Cianca, A.; Lustri, C.; Sclafani, M.; et al. Unveiling the Future of Cardiac Care: A Review of Gene Therapy in Cardiomyopathies. *Int. J. Mol. Sci.* **2024**, *25*, 13147. [CrossRef] [PubMed]
7. Lopes, L.R.; Ho, C.Y.; Elliott, P.M. Genetics of hypertrophic cardiomyopathy: Established and emerging implications for clinical practice. *Eur. Heart J.* **2024**, *45*, 2727–2734. [CrossRef]
8. Marston, N.A.; Han, L.; Olivotto, I.; Day, S.M.; Ashley, E.A.; Michels, M.; Pereira, A.C.; Ingles, J.; Semsarian, C.; Jacoby, D.; et al. Clinical characteristics and outcomes in childhood-onset hypertrophic cardiomyopathy. *Eur. Heart J.* **2021**, *42*, 1988–1996. [CrossRef]
9. Swan, D.A.; Bell, B.; Oakley, C.M.; Goodwin, J. Analysis of symptomatic course and prognosis and treatment of hypertrophic obstructive cardiomyopathy. *Br. Heart J.* **1971**, *33*, 671–685. [CrossRef]
10. Barry, J.; Maron, P.S. Impact of patient selection biases on the perception of hypertrophic cardiomyopathy and its natural history. *Am. J. Cardiol.* **1993**, *72*, 970–972.
11. Spirito, P.; Chiarella, F.; Carratino, L.; Berisso, M.Z.; Bellotti, P.; Vecchio, C. Clinical Course and Prognosis of Hypertrophic Cardiomyopathy in an Outpatient Population. *N. Engl. J. Med.* **1989**, *320*, 749–755. [CrossRef] [PubMed]
12. Cecchi, F.; Olivotto, I.; Montereggi, A.; Santoro, G.; Dolara, A.; Maron, B.J. Hypertrophic cardiomyopathy in tuscany: Clinical course and outcome in an unselected regional population. *J. Am. Coll. Cardiol.* **1995**, *26*, 1529–1536. [CrossRef] [PubMed]

13. Maron, B.J.; Desai, M.Y.; Nishimura, R.A.; Spirito, P.; Rakowski, H.; Towbin, J.A.; Dearani, J.A.; Rowin, E.J.; Maron, M.S.; Sherrid, M.V. Management of Hypertrophic Cardiomyopathy: JACC State-of-the-Art Review. *J. Am. Coll. Cardiol.* **2022**, *79*, 390–414. [CrossRef]
14. Maron, M.S.; Olivotto, I.; Zenovich, A.G.; Link, M.S.; Pandian, N.G.; Kuvin, J.T.; Nistri, S.; Cecchi, F.; Udelson, J.E.; Maron, B.J. Hypertrophic cardiomyopathy is predominantly a disease of left ventricular outflow tract obstruction. *Circulation* **2006**, *114*, 2232–2239. [CrossRef] [PubMed]
15. Maron, M.S.; Rowin, E.J.; Olivotto, I.; Casey, S.A.; Arretini, A.; Tomberli, B.; Garberich, R.F.; Link, M.S.; Chan, R.H.M.; Lesser, J.R. Contemporary Natural History and Management of Nonobstructive Hypertrophic Cardiomyopathy. *J. Am. Coll. Cardiol.* **2016**, *67*, 1399–1409. [CrossRef]
16. Autore, C.; Francia, P.; Tini, G.; Musumeci, B. Old and new therapeutic solutions in the treatment of hypertrophic cardiomyopathy. *Eur. Heart J.* **2023**, *25*, B12–B15. [CrossRef]
17. Harris, K.M.; Spirito, P.; Maron, M.S.; Zenovich, A.G.; Formisano, F.; Lesser, J.R.; Mackey-Bojack, S.; Manning, W.J.; Udelson, J.E.; Maron, B.J. Prevalence, clinical profile, and significance of left ventricular remodeling in the end-stage phase of hypertrophic cardiomyopathy. *Circulation* **2006**, *114*, 216–225. [CrossRef]
18. Musumeci, B.; Tini, G.; Biagini, E.; Merlo, M.; Calore, C.; Ammirati, E.; Zampieri, M.; Russo, D.; Grilli, G.; Santolamazza, C.; et al. Clinical characteristics and outcome of end stage hypertrophic cardiomyopathy: Role of age and heart failure phenotypes. *Int. J. Cardiol.* **2024**, *400*, 131784. [CrossRef] [PubMed]
19. Rowin, E.J.; Maron, B.J.; Haas, T.S.; Garberich, R.F.; Wang, W.; Link, M.S.; Maron, M.S. Hypertrophic Cardiomyopathy with Left Ventricular Apical Aneurysm: Implications for Risk Stratification and Management. *J. Am. Coll. Cardiol.* **2017**, *69*, 761–773. [CrossRef]
20. Pennacchini, E.; Musumeci, M.B.; Conte, M.R.; Stöllberger, C.; Formisano, F.; Bongioanni, S.; Francia, P.; Volpe, M.; Autore, C. Electrocardiographic evolution in patients with hypertrophic cardiomyopathy who develop a left ventricular apical aneurysm. *J. Electrocardiol.* **2015**, *48*, 818–825. [CrossRef]
21. Musumeci, M.B.; Russo, D.; Limite, L.R.; Canepa, M.; Tini, G.; Casenghi, M.; Francia, P.; Adduci, C.; Pagannone, E.; Magrì, D.; et al. Long-Term Left Ventricular Remodeling of Patients with Hypertrophic Cardiomyopathy. *Am. J. Cardiol.* **2018**, *122*, 1924–1931. [CrossRef]
22. Musumeci, B.; Tini, G.; Russo, D.; Sclafani, M.; Cava, F.; Tropea, A.; Adduci, C.; Palano, F.; Francia, P.; Autore, C. Left ventricular remodeling in hypertrophic cardiomyopathy: An overview of current knowledge. *J. Clin. Med.* **2021**, *10*, 1547. [CrossRef]
23. Maron, B.J. Clinical Course and Management of Hypertrophic Cardiomyopathy. *N. Engl. J. Med.* **2018**, *379*, 655–668. [CrossRef] [PubMed]
24. Segev, A.; Wasserstrum, Y.; Arad, M.; Larrañaga-Moreira, J.M.; Martinez-Veira, C.; Barriales-Villa, R.; Sabbag, A. Ventricular arrhythmias in patients with hypertrophic cardiomyopathy: Prevalence, distribution, predictors, and outcome. *Heart Rhythm* **2023**, *20*, 1385–1392. [CrossRef]
25. Efthimiadis, G.K.; Zegkos, T.; Meditskou, S.; Hadjimiltiades, S. Perspectives on sudden death prevention in hypertrophic cardiomyopathy. *Cardiol. Rev.* **2014**, *22*, 210–216. [CrossRef] [PubMed]
26. Maron, B.J.; Rowin, E.J.; Casey, S.A.; Haas, T.S.; Chan, R.H.M.; Udelson, J.E.; Garberich, R.F.; Lesser, J.R.; Appelbaum, E.; Manning, W.J. Risk stratification and outcome of patients with hypertrophic cardiomyopathy ≥60 years of age. *Circulation* **2013**, *127*, 585–593. [CrossRef]
27. Elliott, P.M.; Poloniecki, J.; Dickie, S.; Sharma, S.; Monserrat, L.; Varnava, A.; Mahon, N.G.; McKenna, W.J. Sudden death in hypertrophic cardiomyopathy: Identification of high risk patients. *J. Am. Coll. Cardiol.* **2000**, *36*, 2212–2218. [CrossRef] [PubMed]
28. Maron, B.J.; Casey, S.A.; Olivotto, I.; Sherrid, M.V.; Semsarian, C.; Autore, C.; Ahmed, A.; Boriani, G.; Francia, P.; Winters, S.L.; et al. Clinical Course and Quality of Life in High-Risk Patients with Hypertrophic Cardiomyopathy and Implantable Cardioverter-Defibrillators. *Circ. Arrhythm. Electrophysiol.* **2018**, *11*, e005820. [CrossRef] [PubMed]
29. Wang, N.; Xie, A.; Tjahjono, R.; Tian, D.H.; Phan, S.; Yan, T.D.; Bajona, P.; Phan, K. Implantable cardioverter defibrillator therapy in hypertrophic cardiomyopathy: An updated systematic review and meta-analysis of outcomes and complications. *Ann. Cardiothorac. Surg.* **2017**, *6*, 298–306. [CrossRef]
30. Schinkel, A.F.L.; Vriesendorp, P.A.; Sijbrands, E.J.G.; Jordaens, L.J.; ten Cate, F.J.; Michels, M. Outcome and complications after implantable cardioverter defibrillator therapy in hypertrophic cardiomyopathy: Systematic review and meta-analysis. *Circ. Heart Fail.* **2012**, *5*, 552–559. [CrossRef] [PubMed]
31. Francia, P.; Ziacchi, M.; Adduci, C.; Ammendola, E.; Pieragnoli, P.; De Filippo, P.; Rapacciuolo, A.; Rella, V.; Migliore, F.; Viani, S. Clinical course of hypertrophic cardiomyopathy patients implanted with a transvenous or subcutaneous defibrillator. *Europace* **2023**, *25*, euad270. [CrossRef] [PubMed]
32. Migliore, F.; Biffi, M.; Viani, S.; Pittorru, R.; Francia, P.; Pieragnoli, P.; De Filippo, P.; Bisignani, G.; Nigro, G.; Dello Russo, A. Modern subcutaneous implantable defibrillator therapy in patients with cardiomyopathies and channelopathies: Data from a large multicentre registry. *Europace* **2023**, *25*, euad239. [CrossRef]

33. Francia, P.; Olivotto, I.; Lambiase, P.D.; Autore, C. Implantable cardioverter-defibrillators for hypertrophic cardiomyopathy: The Times They Are a-Changin'. *Europace* **2022**, *24*, 1384–1394. [CrossRef] [PubMed]
34. Adduci, C.; Palano, F.; Francia, P. Safety, efficacy and evidence base for use of the subcutaneous implantable cardioverter defibrillator. *J. Clin. Med.* **2018**, *7*, 53. [CrossRef]
35. Elliott, P.M.; Anastasakis, A.; Borger, M.A.; Borggrefe, M.; Cecchi, F.; Charron, P.; Hagege, A.A.; Lafont, A.; Limongelli, G.; Mahrholdt, H.; et al. 2014 ESC guidelines on diagnosis and management of hypertrophic cardiomyopathy: The task force for the diagnosis and management of hypertrophic cardiomyopathy of the European Society of Cardiology (ESC). *Eur. Heart J.* **2014**, *35*, 2733–2779.
36. Spirito, P.; Autore, C.; Formisano, F.; Assenza, G.E.; Biagini, E.; Haas, T.S.; Bongioanni, S.; Semsarian, C.; Devoto, E.; Kitner, C.; et al. Abstract 12673: How Low is Low Risk in Hypertrophic Cardiomyopathy? Sudden Death in Patients Without Conventional Risk Factors. *Circulation* **2011**, *124*.
37. Maron, M.S.; Rowin, E.; Spirito, P.; Maron, B.J. Differing strategies for sudden death prevention in hypertrophic cardiomyopathy. *Heart* **2023**, *109*, 589–594. [CrossRef] [PubMed]
38. Maurizi, N.; Passantino, S.; Spaziani, G.; Girolami, F.; Arretini, A.; Targetti, M.; Pollini, I.; Tomberli, A.; Pradella, S.; Calabri, G.B.; et al. Long-term outcomes of pediatric-onset hypertrophic cardiomyopathy and age-specific risk factors for lethal arrhythmic events. *JAMA Cardiol.* **2018**, *3*, 520–525. [CrossRef]
39. Miron, A.; Lafreniere-Roula, M.; Fan, C.P.S.; Armstrong, K.R.; Dragulescu, A.; Papaz, T.; Manlhiot, C.; Kaufman, B.; Butts, R.J.; Gardin, L.; et al. A validated model for sudden cardiac death risk prediction in pediatric hypertrophic cardiomyopathy. *Circulation* **2020**, *142*, 217–229. [CrossRef]
40. Norrish, G.; Ding, T.; Field, E.; Ziólkowska, L.; Olivotto, I.; Limongelli, G.; Anastasakis, A.; Weintraub, R.; Biagini, E.; Ragni, L.; et al. Development of a Novel Risk Prediction Model for Sudden Cardiac Death in Childhood Hypertrophic Cardiomyopathy (HCM Risk-Kids). *JAMA Cardiol.* **2019**, *4*, 918–927. [CrossRef]
41. Coppini, R.; Santini, L.; Olivotto, I.; Ackerman, M.J.; Cerbai, E. Abnormalities in sodium current and calcium homoeostasis as drivers of arrhythmogenesis in hypertrophic cardiomyopathy. *Cardiovasc. Res.* **2020**, *116*, 1585–1599. [CrossRef] [PubMed]
42. Coppini, R.; Mazzoni, L.; Ferrantini, C.; Gentile, F.; Pioner, J.M.; Laurino, A.; Santini, L.; Bargelli, V.; Rotellini, M.; Bartolucci, G.; et al. Ranolazine prevents phenotype development in a mouse model of hypertrophic cardiomyopathy. *Circ. Heart Fail.* **2017**, *10*, e003565. [CrossRef] [PubMed]
43. Coppini, R.; Ferrantini, C.; Yao, L.; Fan, P.; Del Lungo, M.; Stillitano, F.; Sartiani, L.; Tosi, B.; Suffredini, S.; Tesi, C.; et al. Late sodium current inhibition reverses electromechanical dysfunction in human hypertrophic cardiomyopathy. *Circulation* **2013**, *127*, 575–584. [CrossRef]
44. Ferrantini, C.; Coppini, R.; Pioner, J.M.; Gentile, F.; Tosi, B.; Mazzoni, L.; Scellini, B.; Piroddi, N.; Laurino, A.; Santini, L.; et al. Pathogenesis of hypertrophic cardiomyopathy is mutation rather than disease specific: A comparison of the cardiac troponin T E163R and R92Q mouse models. *J. Am. Heart Assoc.* **2017**, *6*, 1–19. [CrossRef]
45. Ferrantini, C.; Pioner, J.M.; Mazzoni, L.; Gentile, F.; Tosi, B.; Rossi, A.; Belardinelli, L.; Tesi, C.; Palandri, C.; Matucci, R.; et al. Late sodium current inhibitors to treat exercise-induced obstruction in hypertrophic cardiomyopathy: An in vitro study in human myocardium. *Br. J. Pharmacol.* **2018**, *175*, 2635–2652. [CrossRef]
46. Sutanto, H.; Lyon, A.; Lumens, J.; Schotten, U.; Dobrev, D.; Heijman, J. Cardiomyocyte calcium handling in health and disease: Insights from in vitro and in silico studies. *Prog. Biophys. Mol. Biol.* **2020**, *157*, 54–75. [CrossRef]
47. Ulus, T.; Kudaiberdieva, G.; Gorenek, B. The onset mechanisms of ventricular tachycardia. *Int. J. Cardiol.* **2013**, *167*, 619–623. [CrossRef]
48. Coppini, R.; Ferrantini, C.; Pioner, J.M.; Santini, L.; Wang, Z.J.; Palandri, C.; Scardigli, M.; Vitale, G.; Sacconi, L.; Stefàno, P.; et al. Electrophysiological and Contractile Effects of Disopyramide in Patients with Obstructive Hypertrophic Cardiomyopathy: A Translational Study. *JACC Basic Transl. Sci.* **2019**, *4*, 795–813. [CrossRef] [PubMed]
49. Ashrafian, H.; McKenna, W.J.; Watkins, H. Disease pathways and novel therapeutic targets in hypertrophic cardiomyopathy. *Circ. Res.* **2011**, *109*, 86–96. [CrossRef] [PubMed]
50. Lan, F.; Lee, A.S.; Liang, P.; Sanchez-Freire, V.; Nguyen, P.K.; Wang, L.; Han, L.; Yen, M.; Wang, Y.; Sun, N.; et al. Abnormal calcium handling properties underlie familial hypertrophic cardiomyopathy pathology in patient-specific induced pluripotent stem cells. *Cell Stem Cell* **2013**, *12*, 101–113. [CrossRef] [PubMed]
51. Haim, T.E.; Dowell, C.; Diamanti, T.; Scheuer, J.; Tardiff, J.C. Independent, F.H.C-related cardiac troponin T mutations exhibit specific alterations in myocellular contractility and calcium kinetics. *J. Mol. Cell. Cardiol.* **2007**, *42*, 1098–1110. [CrossRef]
52. Knollmann, B.C.; Kirchhof, P.; Sirenko, S.G.; Degen, H.; Greene, A.E.; Schober, T.; Mackow, J.C.; Fabritz, L.; Potter, J.D.; Morad, M. Familial hypertrophic cardiomyopathy-linked mutant troponin T causes stress-induced ventricular tachycardia and Ca^{2+}-dependent action potential remodeling. *Circ. Res.* **2003**, *92*, 428–436. [CrossRef] [PubMed]

53. Fraysse, B.; Weinberger, F.; Bardswell, S.C.; Cuello, F.; Vignier, N.; Geertz, B.; Starbatty, J.; Krämer, E.; Coirault, C.; Eschenhagen, T.; et al. Increased myofilament Ca^{2+} sensitivity and diastolic dysfunction as early consequences of Mybpc3 mutation in heterozygous knock-in mice. *J. Mol. Cell. Cardiol.* **2012**, *52*, 1299–1307. [CrossRef] [PubMed]
54. Buonocunto, M.; Lyon, A.; Delhaas, T.; Heijman, J.; Lumens, J. Electrophysiological effects of stretch-activated ion channels: A systematic computational characterization. *J. Physiol.* **2023**, *18*, 4585–4604. [CrossRef] [PubMed]
55. Kamkin, A.; Kiseleva, I.; Isenberg, G. Stretch-activated currents in ventricular myocytes: Amplitude and arrhythmogenic effects increase with hypertrophy. *Cardiovasc. Res.* **2000**, *48*, 409–420. [CrossRef] [PubMed]
56. Zeppenfeld, K.; Tfelt-Hansen, J.; de Riva, M.; Winkel, B.G.; Behr, E.R.; Blom, N.A.; Charron, P.; Corrado, D.; Dagres, N.; de Chillou, C.; et al. 2022 ESC Guidelines for the management of patients with ventricular arrhythmias and the prevention of sudden cardiac death: Developed by the task force for the management of patients with ventricular arrhythmias and the prevention of sudden cardiac death. *Eur. Heart J.* **2022**, *43*, 3997–4126. [CrossRef]
57. Zhao, J.; Wang, B.; Ta, S.; Lu, X.; Zhao, X.; Liu, J.; Yuan, J.; Wang, J.; Liu, L. Association between Hypertrophic Cardiomyopathy and Variations in Sarcomere Gene and Calcium Channel Gene in Adults. *Cardiology* **2024**, *149*, 440–450. [CrossRef]
58. Baudenbacher, F.; Schober, T.; Pinto, J.R.; Sidorov, V.Y.; Hilliard, F.; Solaro, R.J.; Potter, J.D.; Knollmann, B.C. Myofilament Ca^{2+} sensitization causes susceptibility to cardiac arrhythmia in mice. *J. Clin. Investig.* **2008**, *118*, 3893–3903. [CrossRef]
59. Vakrou, S.; Fukunaga, R.; Foster, D.B.; Sorensen, L.; Liu, Y.; Guan, Y.; Woldemichael, K.; Pineda-Reyes, R.; Liu, T.; Tardiff, J.C.; et al. Allele-specific differences in transcriptome, miRNome, and mitochondrial function in two hypertrophic cardiomyopathy mouse models. *JCI Insight* **2018**, *3*, e94493. [CrossRef] [PubMed]
60. Lopes, L.R.; Syrris, P.; Guttmann, O.P.; O'Mahony, C.; Tang, H.C.; Dalageorgou, C.; Jenkins, S.; Hubank, M.; Monserrat, L.; McKenna, W.J.; et al. Novel genotype-phenotype associations demonstrated by high-throughput sequencing in patients with hypertrophic cardiomyopathy. *Heart* **2015**, *101*, 294–301. [CrossRef] [PubMed]
61. Maron, M.S. Family History of Sudden Death Should Be a Primary Indication for Implantable Cardioverter Defibrillator in Hypertrophic Cardiomyopathy. *Can. J. Cardiol.* **2015**, *31*, 1402–1406. [CrossRef] [PubMed]
62. Allegue, C.; Gil, R.; Blanco-Verea, A.; Santori, M.; Rodríguez-Calvo, M.; Concheiro, L.; Carracedo, A.; Brion, M. Prevalence of HCM and long QT syndrome mutations in young sudden cardiac death-related cases. *Int. J. Legal Med.* **2011**, *125*, 565–572. [CrossRef]
63. Bos, J.M.; Will, M.L.; Gersh, B.J.; Kruisselbrink, T.M.; Ommen, S.R.; Ackerman, M.J. Characterization of a phenotype-based genetic test prediction score for unrelated patients with hypertrophic cardiomyopathy. *Mayo Clin Proc.* **2014**, *89*, 727–737. [CrossRef] [PubMed]
64. Ho, C.Y.; Day, S.M.; Ashley, E.A.; Michels, M.; Pereira, A.C.; Jacoby, D.; Cirino, A.L.; Fox, J.C.; Lakdawala, N.K.; Ware, J.S.; et al. Genotype and lifetime burden of disease in hypertrophic cardiomyopathy insights from the sarcomeric human cardiomyopathy registry (SHaRe). *Circulation* **2018**, *138*, 1387–1398. [CrossRef]
65. Sedaghat-Hamedani, F.; Kayvanpour, E.; Tugrul, O.F.; Lai, A.; Amr, A.; Haas, J.; Proctor, T.; Ehlermann, P.; Jensen, K.; Katus, H.A.; et al. Clinical outcomes associated with sarcomere mutations in hypertrophic cardiomyopathy: A meta-analysis on 7675 individuals. *Clin. Res. Cardiol.* **2018**, *107*, 30–41. [CrossRef] [PubMed]
66. Joy, G.; Lopes, L.R.; Webber, M.; Ardissino, A.M.; Wilson, J.; Chan, F.; Pierce, I.; Hughes, R.K.; Moschonas, K.; Shiwani, H.; et al. Electrophysiological Characterization of Subclinical and Overt Hypertrophic Cardiomyopathy by Magnetic Resonance Imaging-Guided Electrocardiography. *J. Am. Coll. Cardiol.* **2024**, *83*, 1042–1055. [CrossRef] [PubMed]
67. De Ambroggi, L.; Francia, P.; De Ambroggi, G. Repolarization abnormalities and arrhythmogenesis in hypertrophic myocardium. *Anadolu Kardiyol. Derg.* **2007**, *7*, 71–72. [PubMed]
68. Joy, G.; Kelly, C.I.; Webber, M.; Pierce, I.; Teh, I.; McGrath, L.; Velazquez, P.; Hughes, R.K.; Kotwal, H.; Das, A.; et al. Microstructural and Microvascular Phenotype of Sarcomere Mutation Carriers and Overt Hypertrophic Cardiomyopathy. *Circulation* **2023**, *148*, 808–818. [CrossRef] [PubMed]
69. Olivotto, I.; Camici, P.G.; Merlini, P.A.; Rapezzi, C.; Patten, M.; Climent, V.; Sinagra, G.; Tomberli, B.; Marin, F.; Ehlermann, P.; et al. Efficacy of Ranolazine in Patients with Symptomatic Hypertrophic Cardiomyopathy: The RESTYLE-HCM Randomized, Double-Blind, Placebo-Controlled Study. *Circ. Heart Fail.* **2018**, *11*, e004124. [CrossRef] [PubMed]
70. Shen, H.; Dong, S.Y.; Ren, M.S.; Wang, R. Ventricular arrhythmia and sudden cardiac death in hypertrophic cardiomyopathy: From bench to bedside. *Front. Cardiovasc. Med.* **2022**, *9*, 949294. [CrossRef]
71. Hughes, S.E. The pathology of hypertrophic cardiomyopathy. *Histopathology* **2004**, *44*, 412–427. [CrossRef] [PubMed]
72. Olivotto, I.; Girolami, F.; Nistri, S.; Rossi, A.; Rega, L.; Garbini, F.; Grifoni, C.; Cecchi, F.; Yacoub, M.H. The many faces of hypertrophic cardiomyopathy: From developmental biology to clinical practice. *J. Cardiovasc. Transl. Res.* **2009**, *2*, 349–367. [CrossRef] [PubMed]
73. Cecchi, F.; Sgalambro, A.; Baldi, M.; Sotgia, B.; Antoniucci, D.; Camici, P.G.; Sciagrà, R.; Olivotto, I. Microvascular dysfunction, myocardial ischemia, and progression to heart failure in patients with hypertrophic cardiomyopathy. *J. Cardiovasc. Transl. Res.* **2009**, *2*, 452–461. [CrossRef] [PubMed]

74. Foà, A.; Agostini, V.; Rapezzi, C.; Olivotto, I.; Corti, B.; Potena, L.; Biagini, E.; Martin Suarez, S.; Rotellini, M.; Cecchi, F.; et al. Histopathological comparison of intramural coronary artery remodeling and myocardial fibrosis in obstructive versus end-stage hypertrophic cardiomyopathy. *Int. J. Cardiol.* **2019**, *291*, 77–82. [CrossRef] [PubMed]
75. Schwartzkopff, B.; Mundhenke, M.; Strauer, B.E. Alterations of the architecture of subendocardial arterioles in patients with hypertrophic cardiomyopathy and impaired coronary vasodilator reserve: A possible cause for myocardial ischemia. *J. Am. Coll. Cardiol.* **1998**, *31*, 1089–1096. [CrossRef]
76. Maron, B.J.; Wolfson, J.K.; Epstein, S.E.; Roberts, W.C. Intramural ("small vessel") coronary artery disease in hypertrophic cardiomyopathy. *J. Am. Coll. Cardiol.* **1986**, *8*, 545–557. [CrossRef] [PubMed]
77. Basso, C.; Thiene, G.; Corrado, D.; Buja, G.; Melacini, P.; Nava, A. Hypertrophic cardiomyopathy and sudden death in the young: Pathologic evidence of myocardial ischemia. *Hum. Pathol.* **2000**, *31*, 988–998. [CrossRef]
78. Proietti, R.; Roux, J.-F.; Verma, A.; Alturki, A.; Bernier, M.L.; Essebag, V. A Historical Perspective on the Role of Functional Lines of Block in the Re-entrant Circuit of Ventricular Tachycardia. *PACE-Pacing Clin. Electrophysiol.* **2016**, *39*, 490–496. [CrossRef]
79. Chan, R.H.; Maron, B.J.; Olivotto, I.; Pencina, M.J.; Egidy Assenza, G.; Haas, T.; Lesser, J.R.; Gruner, C.; Crean, A.M.; Rakowski, H.; et al. Prognostic value of quantitative contrast-enhanced cardiovascular magnetic resonance for the evaluation of sudden death risk in patients with hypertrophic cardiomyopathy. *Circulation* **2014**, *130*, 484–495. [CrossRef] [PubMed]
80. Galati, G.; Leone, O.; Pasquale, F.; Olivotto, I.; Biagini, E.; Grigioni, F.; Pilato, E.; Lorenzini, M.; Corti, B.; Foà, A.; et al. Histological and histometric characterization of myocardial fibrosis in end-stage hypertrophic cardiomyopathy. *Circ. Heart Fail.* **2016**, *9*, e003090. [CrossRef]
81. Ariga, R.; Tunnicliffe, E.M.; Manohar, S.G.; Mahmod, M.; Raman, B.; Piechnik, S.K.; Francis, J.M.; Robson, M.D.; Neubauer, S.; Watkins, H. Identification of Myocardial Disarray in Patients with Hypertrophic Cardiomyopathy and Ventricular Arrhythmias. *J. Am. Coll. Cardiol.* **2019**, *73*, 2493–2502. [CrossRef] [PubMed]
82. Krul, S.P.J.; Berger, W.R.; Smit, N.W.; van Amersfoorth, S.C.M.; Driessen, A.H.G.; van Boven, W.J.; Fiolet, J.W.T.; van Ginneken, A.C.G.; van der Wal, A.C.; de Bakker, J.M.T.; et al. Atrial fibrosis and conduction slowing in the left atrial appendage of patients undergoing thoracoscopic surgical pulmonary vein isolation for atrial fibrillation. *Circ. Arrhythm. Electrophysiol.* **2015**, *8*, 288–295. [CrossRef]
83. Burstein, B.; Nattel, S. Atrial Fibrosis: Mechanisms and Clinical Relevance in Atrial Fibrillation. *J. Am. Coll. Cardiol.* **2008**, *51*, 802–809. [CrossRef]
84. Camelliti, P.; Green, C.R.; LeGrice, I.; Kohl, P. Fibroblast Network in Rabbit Sinoatrial Node: Structural and Functional Identification of Homogeneous and Heterogeneous Cell Coupling. *Circ. Res.* **2004**, *94*, 828–835. [CrossRef] [PubMed]
85. Cecchi, F.; Olivotto, I.; Gistri, R.; Lorenzoni, R.; Chiriatti, G.; Camici, P.G. Coronary Microvascular Dysfunction and Prognosis in Hypertrophic Cardiomyopathy. *N. Engl. J. Med.* **2003**, *349*, 1027–1035. [CrossRef]
86. Maron, M.S.; Olivotto, I.; Maron, B.J.; Prasad, S.K.; Cecchi, F.; Udelson, J.E.; Camici, P.G. The Case for Myocardial Ischemia in Hypertrophic Cardiomyopathy. *J. Am. Coll. Cardiol.* **2009**, *54*, 866–875. [CrossRef]
87. Kellman, P.; Arai, A.E. Cardiac imaging techniques for physicians: Late enhancement. *J. Magn. Reson. Imaging* **2012**, *36*, 529–542. [CrossRef] [PubMed]
88. Sclafani, M.; Tini, G.; Musumeci, B.; Cianca, A.; Maestrini, V.; Cacciotti, L.; Arcari, L. Advanced Cardiovascular Magnetic Resonance Imaging in Takotsubo Syndrome: Update on Feature Tracking and Tissue Mapping. *Curr. Cardiovasc Imaging Rep.* **2024**, *17*, 61–71. [CrossRef]
89. Kellman, P.; Hansen, M.S. T1-mapping in the heart: Accuracy and precision. *J. Cardiovasc. Magn. Reson.* **2014**, *16*, 2. [CrossRef]
90. Nielles-Vallespin, S.; Scott, A.; Ferreira, P.; Khalique, Z.; Pennell, D.; Firmin, D. Cardiac Diffusion: Technique and Practical Applications. *J. Magn. Reson. Imaging* **2020**, *52*, 348–368. [CrossRef] [PubMed]
91. Bruder, O.; Wagner, A.; Jensen, C.J.; Schneider, S.; Ong, P.; Kispert, E.-M.; Nassenstein, K.; Schlosser, T.; Sabin, G.V.; Sechtem, U.; et al. Myocardial scar visualized by cardiovascular magnetic resonance imaging predicts major adverse events in patients with hypertrophic cardiomyopathy. *J. Am. Coll. Cardiol.* **2010**, *56*, 875–887. [CrossRef] [PubMed]
92. Kwon, D.H.; Smedira, N.G.; Rodriguez, E.R.; Tan, C.; Setser, R.; Thamilarasan, M.; Lytle, B.W.; Lever, H.M.; Desai, M.Y. Cardiac Magnetic Resonance Detection of Myocardial Scarring in Hypertrophic Cardiomyopathy. Correlation with Histopathology and Prevalence of Ventricular Tachycardia. *J. Am. Coll. Cardiol.* **2009**, *54*, 242–249. [CrossRef] [PubMed]
93. Suk, T.; Edwards, C.; Hart, H.; Christiansen, J.P. Myocardial Scar Detected by Contrast-Enhanced Cardiac Magnetic Resonance Imaging is Associated with Ventricular Tachycardia in Hypertrophic Cardiomyopathy Patients. *Heart Lung Circ.* **2008**, *17*, 370–374. [CrossRef]
94. Mentias, A.; Raeisi-Giglou, P.; Smedira, N.G.; Feng, K.; Sato, K.; Wazni, O.; Kanj, M.; Flamm, S.D.; Thamilarasan, M.; Popovic, Z.B.; et al. Late Gadolinium Enhancement in Patients with Hypertrophic Cardiomyopathy and Preserved Systolic Function. *J. Am. Coll. Cardiol.* **2018**, *72*, 857–870. [CrossRef]

95. Todiere, G.; Nugara, C.; Gentile, G.; Negri, F.; Bianco, F.; Falletta, C.; Novo, G.; Di Bella, G.; De Caterina, R.; Zachara, E.; et al. Prognostic Role of Late Gadolinium Enhancement in Patients with Hypertrophic Cardiomyopathy and Low-to-Intermediate Sudden Cardiac Death Risk Score. *Am. J. Cardiol.* **2019**, *124*, 1286–1292. [CrossRef] [PubMed]
96. Aquaro, G.D.; Grigoratos, C.; Bracco, A.; Proclemer, A.; Todiere, G.; Martini, N.; Habtemicael, Y.G.; Carerj, S.; Sinagra, G.; Di Bella, G. Late Gadolinium Enhancement-Dispersion Mapping: A New Magnetic Resonance Imaging Technique to Assess Prognosis in Patients with Hypertrophic Cardiomyopathy and Low-Intermediate 5-Year Risk of Sudden Death. *Circ. Cardiovasc. Imaging* **2020**, *13*, E010489. [CrossRef]
97. Konno, T.; Hayashi, K.; Fujino, N.; Nagata, Y.; Hodatsu, A.; Masuta, E.; Sakata, K.; Nakamura, H.; Kawashiri, M.-A.; Yamagishi, M. High sensitivity of late gadolinium enhancement for predicting microscopic myocardial scarring in biopsied specimens in hypertrophic cardiomyopathy. *PLoS ONE* **2014**, *9*, 13–16. [CrossRef]
98. Moravsky, G.; Ofek, E.; Rakowski, H.; Butany, J.; Williams, L.; Ralph-Edwards, A.; Wintersperger, B.J.; Crean, A. Myocardial fibrosis in hypertrophic cardiomyopathy: Accurate reflection of histopathological findings by, C.M.R. *JACC Cardiovasc. Imaging* **2013**, *6*, 587–596. [CrossRef]
99. De Bakker, J.M.; Van Capelle, F.J.; Janse, M.J.; Wilde, A.A.; Coronel, R.; Becker, A.E.; Dingemans, K.P.; Van Hemel, N.M.; Hauer, R.N. Reentry as a cause of ventricular tachycardia in patients with chronic ischemic heart disease: Electrophysiology and anatomic correlation. *Circulation* **1988**, *77*, 589–606. [CrossRef]
100. Appelbaum, E.; Maron, B.J.; Adabag, S.; Hauser, T.H.; Lesser, J.R.; Haas, T.S.; Riley, A.B.; Harrigan, C.J.; Delling, F.N.; Udelson, J.E.; et al. Intermediate-signal-intensity late gadolinium enhancement predicts ventricular tachyarrhythmias in patients with hypertrophic cardiomyopathy. Circ. Cardiovasc. *Imaging* **2012**, *5*, 78–85.
101. Aquaro, G.D.; Masci, P.; Formisano, F.; Barison, A.; Strata, E.; Pingitore, A.; Positano, V.; Spirito, P.; Lombardi, M. Usefulness of Delayed Enhancement by Magnetic Resonance Imaging in Hypertrophic Cardiomyopathy as a Marker of Disease and Its Severity. *Am. J. Cardiol.* **2010**, *105*, 392–397. [CrossRef] [PubMed]
102. Fahmy, A.S.; Rowin, E.J.; Jaafar, N.; Chan, R.H.; Rodriguez, J.; Nakamori, S.; Ngo, L.H.; Pradella, S.; Zocchi, C.; Olivotto, I.; et al. Radiomics of Late Gadolinium Enhancement Reveals Prognostic Value of Myocardial Scar Heterogeneity in Hypertrophic Cardiomyopathy. *JACC Cardiovasc. Imaging* **2024**, *17*, 16–27. [CrossRef] [PubMed]
103. Jáuregui, B.; Soto-Iglesias, D.; Penela, D.; Acosta, J.; Fernández-Armenta, J.; Linhart, M.; Ordóñez, A.; San Antonio, R.; Terés, C.; Chauca, A.; et al. Cardiovascular magnetic resonance determinants of ventricular arrhythmic events after myocardial infarction. *Europace* **2022**, *24*, 938–947. [CrossRef]
104. Acosta, J.; Fernández-Armenta, J.; Borràs, R.; Anguera, I.; Bisbal, F.; Martí-Almor, J.; Tolosana, J.M.; Penela, D.; Andreu, D.; Soto-Iglesias, D.; et al. Scar Characterization to Predict Life-Threatening Arrhythmic Events and Sudden Cardiac Death in Patients with Cardiac Resynchronization Therapy: The GAUDI-CRT Study. *JACC Cardiovasc. Imaging* **2018**, *11*, 561–572. [CrossRef] [PubMed]
105. De Silva, K.; Campbell, T.; Bennett, R.G.; Anderson, R.D.; Davey, C.; O'Donohue, A.K.; Schindeler, A.; Turnbull, S.; Selvakumar, D.; Bhaskaran, A.; et al. Whole-Heart Histological and Electroanatomic Assessment of Postinfarction Cardiac Magnetic Resonance Imaging Scar and Conducting Channels. *Circ. Arrhythm. Electrophysiol.* **2024**, *17*, 594–607. [CrossRef] [PubMed]
106. Francia, P.; Ocaña-Franco, P.; Cristiano, E.; Falasconi, G.; Adduci, C.; Soto-Iglesias, D.; Penela, D.; Sclafani, M.; Martì-Almor, J.; Musumeci, B.; et al. Substrates of Scar-Related Ventricular Arrhythmia in Patients with Hypertrophic Cardiomyopathy: A Cardiac Magnetic Resonance Study. *JACC Cardiovasc. Imaging* **2023**, *16*, 1359–1362. [CrossRef] [PubMed]
107. Ueda, A.; Fukamizu, S.; Soejima, K.; Tejima, T.; Nishizaki, M.; Nitta, T.; Kobayashi, Y.; Hiraoka, M.; Sakurada, H. Clinical and electrophysiological characteristics in patients with sustained monomorphic reentrant ventricular tachycardia associated with dilated-phase hypertrophic cardiomyopathy. *Europace* **2012**, *14*, 734–740. [CrossRef] [PubMed]
108. Francia, P.; Santini, D.; Musumeci, B.; Semprini, L.; Adduci, C.; Pagannone, E.; Proietti, G.; Volpe, M.; Autore, C. Clinical impact of nonsustained ventricular tachycardia recorded by the implantable cardioverter-defibrillator in patients with hypertrophic cardiomyopathy. *J. Cardiovasc. Electrophysiol.* **2014**, *25*, 1180–1187. [CrossRef] [PubMed]
109. Adduci, C.; Boldini, F.; Palano, F.; Musumeci, B.; De Lucia, C.; Russo, D.; Volpe, M.; Autore, C.; Francia, P. Prognostic implications of nonsustained ventricular tachycardia morphology in high-risk patients with hypertrophic cardiomyopathy. *J. Cardiovasc. Electrophysiol.* **2020**, *31*, 2093–2098. [CrossRef]
110. Adduci, C.; Semprini, L.; Palano, F.; Musumeci, M.B.; Volpe, M.; Autore, C.; Francia, P. Safety and efficacy of anti-tachycardia pacing in patients with hypertrophic cardiomyopathy implanted with an, I.C.D. *PACE-Pacing Clin. Electrophysiol.* **2019**, *42*, 610–616. [CrossRef]
111. Link, M.S.; Bockstall, K.; Weinstock, J.; Alsheikh-Ali, A.A.; Semsarian, C.; Estes, N.A.M., 3rd; Spirito, P.; Haas, T.S.; Rowin, E.J.; Maron, M.S.; et al. Ventricular Tachyarrhythmias in Patients with Hypertrophic Cardiomyopathy and Defibrillators: Triggers, Treatment, and Implications. *J. Cardiovasc. Electrophysiol.* **2017**, *28*, 531–537. [CrossRef]

112. Fananapazir, L.; Chang, A.C.; Epstein, S.E.; McAreavey, D. Prognostic determinants in hypertrophic cardiomyopathy: Prospective evaluation of a therapeutic strategy based on clinical, holter, hemodynamic, and electrophysiological findings. *Circulation* **1992**, *86*, 730–740. [CrossRef] [PubMed]
113. Kuck, K.H.; Kunze, K.P.; Schlüter, M.; Nienaber, C.A.; Costard, A. Programmed electrical stimulation in hypertrophic cardiomyopathy. Results in patients with and without cardiac arrest or syncope. *Eur. Heart J.* **1988**, *9*, 177–185. [CrossRef]
114. Kawai, C.; Sakurai, T.; Fujiwara, H.; Matsumori, A.; Yui, Y. Hypertrophic obstructive and non-obstructive cardiomyopathy in Japan. Diagnosis of the disease with special reference to endomyocardial catheter biopsy. *Eur. Heart J.* **1983**, *4*, 121–125. [CrossRef] [PubMed]
115. Segawa, I.; Suzuki, T.; Kato, M.; Tashiro, A.; Satodate, R. Relation between myocardial histological changes and ventricular tachycardia in cardiomyopathy: A study by 24-hour, E.C.G-monitoring and endomyocardial biopsy. *Heart Vessels* **1990**, *5*, 37–40.
116. Saumarez, R.; Silberbauer, J.; Scannell, J.; Pytkowski, M.; Behr, E.R.; Betts, T.; Della Bella, P.; Peters, N.S. Should lethal arrhythmias in hypertrophic cardiomyopathy be predicted using non-electrophysiological methods? *Europace* **2023**, *25*, euad045. [CrossRef]
117. Saumarez, R.C.; Camm, A.J.; Panagos, A.; Gill, J.S.; Stewart, J.T.; de Belder, M.A.; Simpson, I.A.; McKenna, W.J. Ventricular fibrillation in hypertrophic cardiomyopathy is associated with increased fractionation of paced right ventricular electrograms. *Circulation* **1992**, *86*, 467–474. [CrossRef]
118. Saumarez, R.C.; Grace, A.A. Paced ventricular electrogram fractionation and sudden death in hypertrophic cardiomyopathy and other non-coronary heart diseases. *Cardiovasc. Res.* **2000**, *47*, 11–22. [CrossRef]
119. Saumarez, R.C.; Chojnowska, L.; Derksen, R.; Pytkowski, M.; Sterlinski, M.; Huang, C.L.-H.; Sadoul, N.; Hauer, R.N.W.; Ruzyłło, W.; Grace, A.A. Sudden death in noncoronary heart disease is associated with delayed paced ventricular activation. *Circulation* **2003**, *107*, 2595–2600. [CrossRef]
120. Saumarez, R.C.; Slade, A.K.; Grace, A.A.; Sadoul, N.; Camm, A.J.; McKenna, W.J. The significance of paced electrogram fractionation in hypertrophic cardiomyopathy. A prospective study. *Circulation* **1995**, *91*, 2762–2768. [CrossRef] [PubMed]
121. Dias, G.M.; Lamounier Júnior, A.; Seifert, M.; Barájas-Martinez, H.; Barr, D.; Sternick, E.B.; Medina-Acosta, E.; Campos de Carvalho, A.C.; Cruz Filho, F.E. MYH7 p.Glu903Gln Is a Pathogenic Variant Associated with Hypertrophic Cardiomyopathy. *Circ. Genomic Precis. Med.* **2021**, *14*, E003476. [CrossRef]
122. Maron, B.J.; Rowin, E.J.; Maron, M.S. Evolution of risk stratification and sudden death prevention in hypertrophic cardiomyopathy: Twenty years with the implantable cardioverter-defibrillator. *Heart Rhythm* **2021**, *18*, 1012–1023. [CrossRef]
123. Fluechter, S.; Kuschyk, J.; Wolpert, C.; Doesch, C.; Veltmann, C.; Haghi, D.; Schoenberg, S.O.; Sueselbeck, T.; Germans, T.; Streitner, F.; et al. Extent of late gadolinium enhancement detected by cardiovascular magnetic resonance correlates with the inducibility of ventricular tachyarrhythmia in hypertrophic cardiomyopathy. *J. Cardiovasc. Magn. Reson.* **2010**, *12*, 30. [CrossRef] [PubMed]
124. Francia, P.; Falasconi, G.; Penela, D.; Viveros, D.; Alderete, J.; Saglietto, A.; Bellido, A.F.; Martí-Almor, J.; Franco-Ocaña, P.; Soto-Iglesias, D.; et al. Scar architecture affects the electrophysiological characteristics of induced ventricular arrhythmias in hypertrophic cardiomyopathy. *Europace* **2024**, *26*, euae050. [CrossRef]
125. Behr, E.R.; Elliott, P.; McKenna, W.J. Role of invasive, E.P. testing in the evaluation and management of hypertrophic cardiomyopathy. *Card. Electrophysiol. Rev.* **2002**, *6*, 482–486. [CrossRef] [PubMed]
126. Jansson, K.; Dahlström, U.; Karlsson, E.; Nylander, E.; Walfridsson, H.; Sonnhag, C. The Value of Exercise Test, Hotter Monitoring, and Programmed Electrical Stimulation in Detection of Ventricular Arrhythmias in Patients with Hypertrophic Cardiomyopathy. *Pacing Clin. Electrophysiol.* **1990**, *13*, 1261–1267. [CrossRef] [PubMed]
127. Gatzoulis, K.A.; Georgopoulos, S.; Antoniou, C.-K.; Anastasakis, A.; Dilaveris, P.; Arsenos, P.; Sideris, S.; Tsiachris, D.; Archontakis, S.; Sotiropoulos, E.; et al. Programmed ventricular stimulation predicts arrhythmic events and survival in hypertrophic cardiomyopathy. *Int. J. Cardiol.* **2018**, *254*, 175–181. [CrossRef]
128. Spirito, P.; Seidman, C.E.; McKenna, W.J.; Maron, B.J. The management of hypertrophic cardiomyopathy. *N. Engl. J. Med.* **1997**, *336*, 775–785. [CrossRef]
129. Magrì, D.; De Cecco, C.N.; Piccirillo, G.; Mastromarino, V.; Serdoz, A.; Muscogiuri, G.; Ricotta, A.; Gregori, M.; Marino, L.; Cauti, F.M.; et al. Myocardial repolarization dispersion and late gadolinium enhancement in patients with hypertrophic cardiomyopathy. *Circ. J.* **2014**, *78*, 1216–1223. [CrossRef]
130. Magrì, D.; Santolamazza, C.; Limite, L.; Mastromarino, V.; Casenghi, M.; Orlando, P.; Pagannone, E.; Musumeci, M.B.; Maruotti, A.; Ricotta, A.; et al. QT spatial dispersion and sudden cardiac death in hypertrophic cardiomyopathy: Time for reappraisal. *J. Cardiol.* **2017**, *70*, 310–315. [CrossRef]
131. Jalanko, M.; Väänänen, H.; Tarkiainen, M.; Sipola, P.; Jääskeläinen, P.; Lauerma, K.; Laitinen, T.; Laitinen, T.; Laine, M.; Heliö, T.; et al. Fibrosis and wall thickness affect ventricular repolarization dynamics in hypertrophic cardiomyopathy. *Ann. Noninvasive Electrocardiol.* **2018**, *23*, e12582. [CrossRef] [PubMed]
132. Maron, B.J.; Leyhe, M.J., 3rd; Casey, S.A.; Gohman, T.E.; Lawler, C.M.; Crow, R.S.; Maron, M.S.; Hodges, M. Assessment of QT dispersion as a prognostic marker for sudden death in a regional nonreferred hypertrophic cardiomyopathy cohort. *Am. J. Cardiol.* **2001**, *87*, 114–115. [CrossRef]

133. Francia, P.; Silvetti, G.; Cosentino, P.; Cristiano, E.; Adduci, C.; Tini, G.; Musumeci, M.B.; Volpe, M.; Autore, C. Relation of delayed intrinsicoid deflection of the QRS complex to sudden cardiac death in patients with hypertrophic cardiomyopathy. *Int. J. Cardiol.* **2022**, *366*, 42–47. [CrossRef]
134. Rattanawong, P.; Riangwiwat, T.; Kanitsoraphan, C.; Chongsathidkiet, P.; Kanjanahattakij, N.; Vutthikraivit, W.; Chung, E.H. Baseline fragmented QRS increases the risk of major arrhythmic events in hypertrophic cardiomyopathy: Systematic review and meta-analysis. *Ann. Noninvasive Electrocardiol.* **2018**, *23*, e12533. [CrossRef] [PubMed]
135. Orini, M.; Graham, A.J.; Martinez-Naharro, A.; Andrews, C.M.; de Marvao, A.; Statton, B.; Cook, S.A.; O'Regan, D.P.; Hawkins, P.N.; Rudy, Y.; et al. Noninvasive mapping of the electrophysiological substrate in cardiac amyloidosis and its relationship to structural abnormalities. *J. Am. Heart Assoc.* **2019**, *8*, e012097. [CrossRef] [PubMed]
136. Cuculich, P.S.; Zhang, J.; Wang, Y.; Desouza, K.A.; Vijayakumar, R.; Woodard, P.K.; Rudy, Y. The electrophysiological cardiac ventricular substrate in patients after myocardial infarction: Noninvasive characterization with electrocardiographic imaging. *J. Am. Coll. Cardiol.* **2011**, *58*, 1893–1902. [CrossRef] [PubMed]
137. Graham, A.J.; Orini, M.; Zacur, E.; Dhillon, G.; Daw, H.; Srinivasan, N.T.; Lane, J.D.; Cambridge, A.; Garcia, J.; O'Reilly, N.J.; et al. Simultaneous Comparison of Electrocardiographic Imaging and Epicardial Contact Mapping in Structural Heart Disease. *Circ. Arrhythm. Electrophysiol.* **2019**, *12*, e007120. [CrossRef] [PubMed]
138. Graham, A.J.; Orini, M.; Zacur, E.; Dhillon, G.; Daw, H.; Srinivasan, N.T.; Martin, C.; Lane, J.; Mansell, J.S.; Cambridge, A.; et al. Evaluation of, E.C.G Imaging to Map Hemodynamically Stable and Unstable Ventricular Arrhythmias. *Circ. Arrhythm. Electrophysiol.* **2020**, *13*, E007377. [CrossRef]
139. Andrews, C.M.; Srinivasan, N.T.; Rosmini, S.; Bulluck, H.; Orini, M.; Jenkins, S.; Pantazis, A.; McKenna, W.J.; Moon, J.C.; Lambiase, P.D.; et al. Electrical and Structural Substrate of Arrhythmogenic Right Ventricular Cardiomyopathy Determined Using Noninvasive Electrocardiographic Imaging and Late Gadolinium Magnetic Resonance Imaging. *Circ. Arrhythm. Electrophysiol.* **2017**, *10*, e005105. [CrossRef] [PubMed]
140. Zhang, J.; Sacher, F.; Hoffmayer, K.; O'Hara, T.; Strom, M.; Cuculich, P.; Silva, J.; Cooper, D.; Faddis, M.; Hocini, M.; et al. Cardiac electrophysiological substrate underlying the, E.C.G phenotype and electrogram abnormalities in brugada syndrome patients. *Circulation* **2015**, *131*, 1950–1959. [CrossRef]
141. Bhagirath, P.; Strocchi, M.; Bishop, M.J.; Boyle, P.M.; Plank, G. From bits to bedside: Entering the age of digital twins in cardiac electrophysiology. *Europace* **2024**, *26*, euae295. [CrossRef] [PubMed]

Journal of
Clinical Medicine

MDPI

Article

Real World Data from Catheter Ablation of Ventricular Tachycardias and Premature Ventricular Complexes in a Tertiary Care Center

Christian Schlatzer [1,†], Jan Berg [1,2,*,†], Firat Duru [1], Corinna Brunckhorst [1], Ardan M. Saguner [1] and Laurent M. Haegeli [1,2]

[1] University Hospital of Zurich, 8091 Zurich, Switzerland
[2] Department of Cardiology, Medical University Department, Kantonsspital Aarau Tellstrasse 25, 5001 Aarau, Switzerland
* Correspondence: jan.berg.hsr@gmail.com; Tel.: +41-(0)62-838-4491
† These authors contributed equally to this work.

Abstract: Background: Catheter ablation in patients with ventricular arrhythmias (VA), such as ventricular tachycardias (VT) or frequent premature ventricular complexes (PVC), is increasingly considered an effective and safe therapy when performed in experienced centers. This study sought to determine acute success rates and complication rates of ablation procedures for patients with VA in a Swiss tertiary care center. **Methods:** All patients who underwent ablation therapy for VT and PVC at the University Heart Center in Zurich, Switzerland, between March 2012 and April 2017 were included in this analysis. **Results:** A total of 120 patients underwent catheter ablation for VT and PVC (69 and 51, respectively). Seventy percent of patients were male, and the mean age was 55.3 years. The most common indication for ablation was high PVC burden (47.5%), followed by paroxysmal VT (38.3%), ICD shocks (23.3%), incessant VT (12.5%), electrical storm (7.5%), and syncope (3.3%). Acute success rates for VT and PVC ablations were 94.2% and 92.2%, respectively. Rates for complications (including major and minor) for VT and PVC were 10.1% and 7.8%, respectively. Complications occurred only in patients with structural heart disease; no complications were noted in structurally normal hearts. **Conclusions:** Our results suggest that catheter ablation for VT and PVC has high acute success rates with a reasonable risk for complications in the setting of tertiary care centers, comparable to those reported in other studies.

Keywords: ventricular tachycardia; premature ventricular complex; catheter ablation; acute success; clinical outcome

1. Introduction

The catheter ablation of ventricular arrhythmias is increasingly considered a treatment option for patients with and without structural heart disease. Symptoms, risk of sudden cardiac death (SCD) and recurrence of ventricular arrhythmias determine the treatment choice. The importance of catheter ablation for the treatment of ventricular tachycardia (VT) and premature ventricular complexes (PVC) increased significantly over the last decades [1–3]. Often, catheter ablation is performed as a sole therapy in patients with an idiopathic VT or with idiopathic PVCs [4]. This is different for patients with an underlying structural heart disease, where the implantation of an implantable cardioverter defibrillator (ICD) is the mainstay for SCD prevention [5]. These are life-saving devices; however, they are associated with significant morbidity, including posttraumatic stress disorder [6] or depression [7], due to ICD shocks. Antiarrhythmic drugs are then usually prescribed to reduce the recurrence of VTs and consecutive ICD therapies. However, the efficacy of these drugs is limited, and moreover, significant side effects as well as proarrhythmias may occur [8].

Catheter ablation can be an effective and safe alternative or adjunct to pharmacological therapy to reduce the recurrence of VT in these patients when performed in experienced centers. It is the only treatment option that can change the arrhythmogenic substrate. In recent years, significant progress has been made in identifying and ablating the right targets due to improved techniques and increased experience.

The purpose of this retrospective analysis of consecutive ablation procedures for VTs and PVCs was to report on acute success rates and procedural complication rates in an experienced tertiary care center in Switzerland.

2. Methods

All patients who underwent ablation therapy for VT or PVC at the University Heart Center in Zurich, Switzerland, between March 2012 and April 2017 were included in this study.

Prior to ablation in the left ventricle, transthoracic echocardiography (TTE) was performed in all patients to exclude intracardiac thrombi. If feasible, cardiac computed tomography (CT) or cardiac magnetic resonance imaging (MRI) scans were also performed. The data were then merged into the electroanatomic mapping system (CARTO, Biosense Webster, Diamond Bar, CA, USA).

Acute complete success of VT ablation was defined as abolition of all sustained VTs. Acute partial success was defined by abolition of the clinical VT. At the end of the procedure, the initial induction protocol was repeated to demonstrate non-inducibility of the VT in all patients when the clinical VT was hemodynamically stable. The non-inducibility protocol included 3 extrastimuli and was performed at two different sites of the right ventricle, RV apex and RV outflow tract. In those patients with hemodynamically unstable VT who underwent substrate mapping and substrate-based ablation, success was defined as abolition of all local late potentials and fragmented electrograms in the scar area.

In PVC ablation, complete abolition of the clinical PVC was labeled an acute success. Ability to induce single PVCs at the end of the procedure but to a significantly reduced degree or with a different morphology not resembling the spontaneous clinical PVC was labeled a partial success.

2.1. Catheter Ablation

Anterograde and/or retrograde access routes were chosen at the operator's discretion, often according to cardiac anatomy and the targeted arrhythmia. Decision for epicardial access could be made by the responsible operator when the substrate was deemed to be epicardial based on etiology of the VT (non-ischemic cardiomyopathies) or in patients after failed endocardial ablations.

Various techniques were used prior to ablation in all patients to map the ventricle for localization of specific targets. In activation mapping, endocardial electrograms were sampled by a mapping catheter and then compared with the timing of the QRS complex on the surface electrocardiogram (ECG). A site that was activated 20 to 40 ms before the onset of the surface QRS complex was considered close to the origin of the VT/PVC. In pace mapping, different sites of the ventricle were stimulated until a QRS pattern was induced that matched the QRS pattern of the spontaneous VT. Pace mapping was used when the relevant VT could not be induced, and a surface ECG of the spontaneous VT was obtained prior to ablation. Entrainment mapping was also used in patients with scar-based VT and involved pacing during a VT at a slightly faster rate than the VT rate. An isolated mid-diastolic potential with a low amplitude from within the critical isthmus of the VT, where entrainment with concealed fusion could be demonstrated, was considered a good site for ablation. Some patients, especially those with structural heart disease, would not have tolerated activation mapping and entrainment due to hemodynamic instability. Inability to induce sustained VT during a procedure was another situation where different techniques came into consideration, categorized as substrate mapping. In substrate mapping, areas of low electrical voltage or delayed potentials were recorded during sinus rhythm (examples shown in Figures 1 and 2).

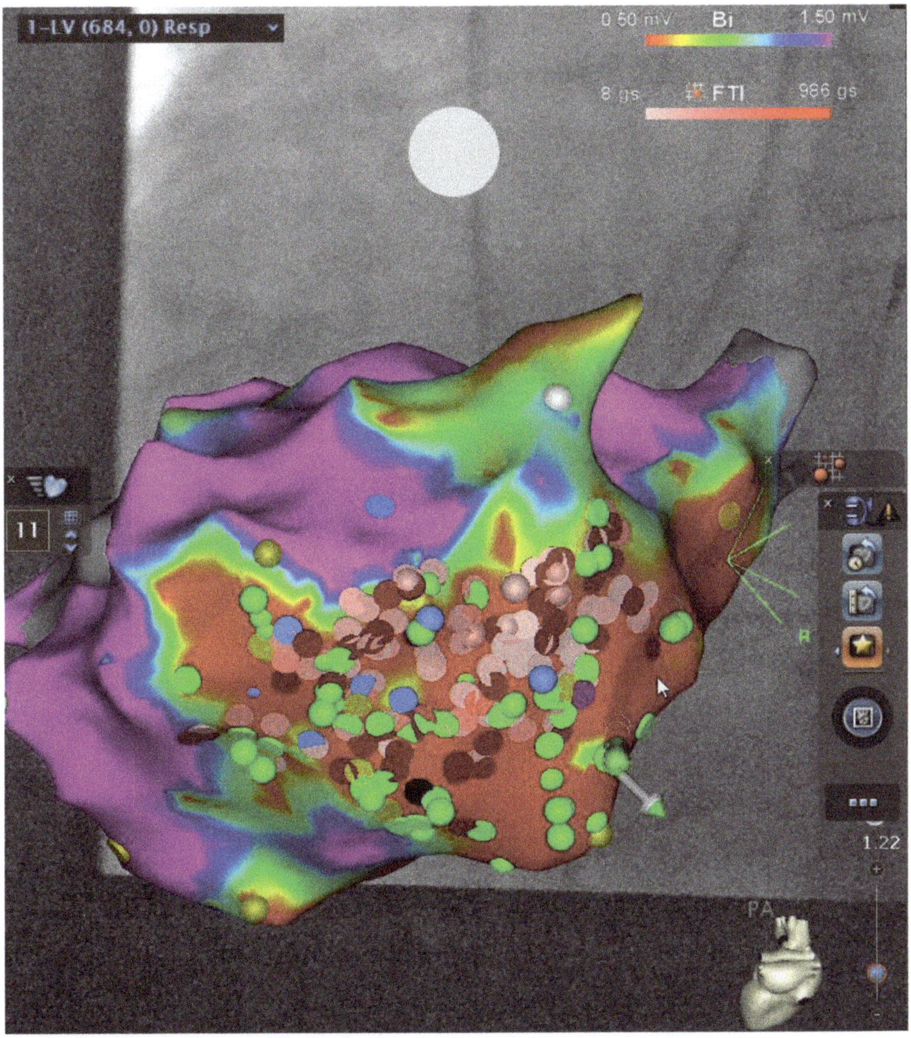

Figure 1. An example of substrate mapping in a patient with hemodynamically unstable VT. A large region of areas with low voltage (red) in the inferior left ventricle is shown. Postero-anterior (PA) view.

2.2. Statistical Analysis

Continuous variables were summarized as mean (SD), and categorical values were summarized as n/total or % of total. Descriptive analyses were performed with Microsoft Excel. To detect differences between groups for acute success and acute complication rates, Fisher's exact test was performed with GraphPad Prism version 10. A p-value < 0.05 was considered statistically significant.

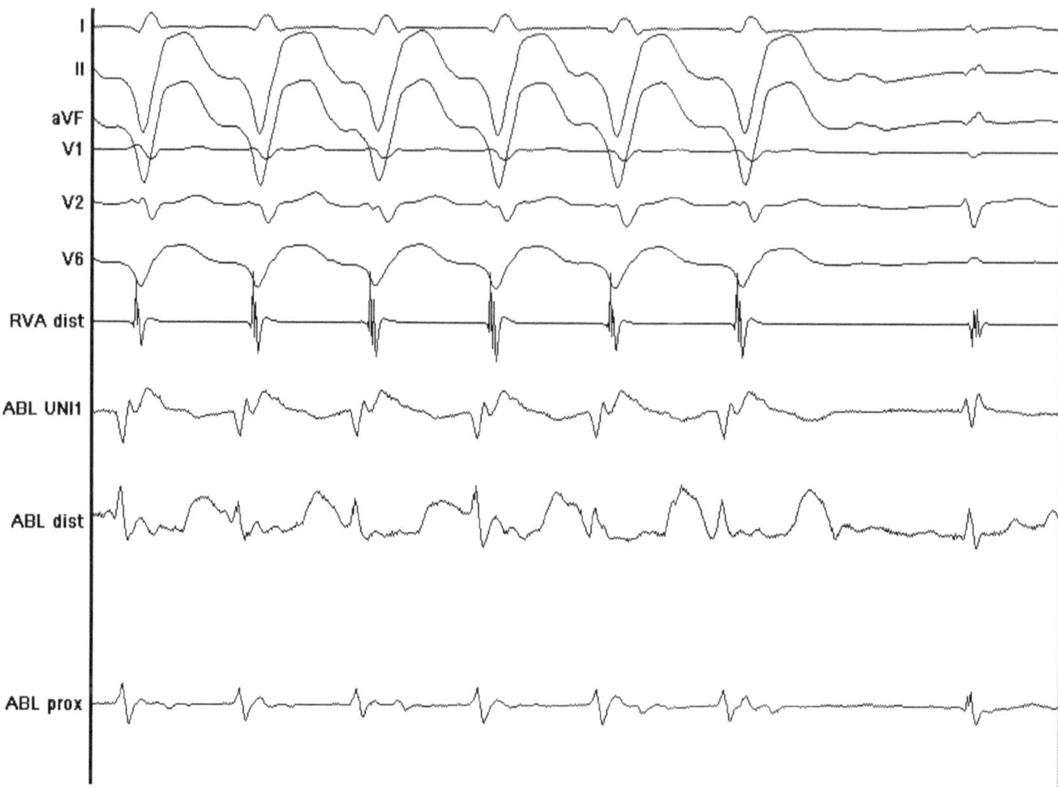

Figure 2. Ventricular tachycardia termination during RF ablation application at the site of late potentials.

3. Results

3.1. Baseline Characteristics

The demographic and clinical baseline characteristics are summarized in Table 1. Patients were predominantly male (84 out of 120 patients; 70%), and the mean age was 55 ± 15 years. Out of 120 patients who were included, 69 (57.5%) were ablated for VT and 51 (42.5%) for PVC. The etiology of arrhythmias was due to structural heart disease in 70 patients (58%), mainly ischemic cardiomyopathy (Table 1). The remaining 50 patients (42%) were diagnosed with idiopathic arrhythmias.

Table 1. Baseline characteristics.

Baseline Characteristics	All Patients (n = 120)	VT (n = 69)	PVC (n = 51)
Age, years (SD)	55.3 (15)	59 (13.8)	50.3 (15.1)
Male gender, n (%)	84 (70)	57 (82.6)	27 (52.9)
BMI (SD)	27 (4.6)	27.6 (4.8)	26.3 (4.2)
Diabetes mellitus, n (%)	20 (16.7)	17 (24.6)	3 (5.9)
Arterial hypertension, n (%)	50 (41.7)	34 (49.3)	16 (31.4)
Atrial fibrillation, n (%)	13 (10.8)	12 (17.4)	1 (2)
Prior myocardial infarction, n (%)	33 (27.5)	30 (43.5)	3 (5.9)

Table 1. *Cont.*

Baseline Characteristics	All Patients (n = 120)	VT (n = 69)	PVC (n = 51)
Prior SCD or ICD shock, n (%)	38 (31.7)	38 (55.1)	0 (0)
Prior VT/PVC ablation, n (%)	20 (16.7)	14 (20.3)	6 (11.8)
Structural cardiomyopathy, n (%)	70 (58.3)	53 (76.8)	17 (33.3)
Idiopathic VT/PVC, n (%)	50 (41.7)	16 (23.2)	34 (66.7)
Acetylsalicylate, n (%)	40 (33.3)	27 (39.1)	13 (25.5)
Oral anticoagulation, n (%)	20 (16.7)	18 (26.1)	2 (3.92)
ACE-I/ARB/ARNI, n (%)	56 (46.7)	42 (60.9)	14 (27.5)
Beta blocker, n (%)	70 (58.3)	55 (79.7)	15 (29.4)
Amiodarone, n (%)	28 (23.3)	27 (39.1)	1 (2)
Mexiletine, n (%)	8 (6.7)	8 (11.6)	0 (0)
Sotalol, n (%)	2 (1.7)	2 (2.9)	0 (0)
Verapamil/Diltiazem, n (%)	11 (9.2)	5 (7.2)	6 (11.8)
Class Ic, n (%)	2 (1.7)	1 (1.4)	1 (2)
ICD/CRT-D, n (%)	47 (39.2)	4 (66.7)	1 (2)

SCD: sudden cardiac death. ICD: implantable cardioverter defibrillator. VT: ventricular tachycardia. PVC: premature ventricular complex. ACE-I: Acetylcholine esterase inhibitor. ARB: Angiotensin receptor blocker. ARNI: Angiotensin receptor neprilysin inhibitor. CRT-D: cardiac resynchronization therapy defibrillator.

Indications for ablation treatment are summarized in Table 2. Several indications were possible (33 patients had two indications, and 3 patients had three indications). Antiarrhythmic drugs prior to ablation were used in a majority of patients (86 patients; 72%), mostly patients undergoing VT ablation. Details concerning the use of antiarrhythmic drugs are summarized in Table 1.

Table 2. Indication for ablation (multiple indications possible).

Paroxysmal VT	ICD Shocks	Incessant VT	Electrical Storm	High PVC Burden	Syncope
46 (38.33%)	28 (23.33%)	15 (12.5%)	9 (7.5%)	57 (47.5%)	4 (3.33%)

VT: ventricular tachycardia. PVC: premature ventricular complexes. ICD: implantable cardioverter defibrillator.

Left ventricular ejection fraction (LVEF) was assessed with TTE in all patients undergoing VT ablation and in 48 out of 51 patients (94%) undergoing PVC ablation. Mean LVEF was 44 percent and 56 percent, respectively. This gap is understandable when different rates of structural vs. idiopathic origins of arrhythmias are being taken into account.

3.2. Catheter Ablation Procedure

In all 120 but one patient, radiofrequency was the energy source used for ablation. In one patient, cryo ablation was used for the ablation of PVC after failure with radiofrequency ablation. Most procedures were performed with local anesthesia or mild deep sedation; however, 26 out of 120 procedures (21%), mostly VT ablations, were performed with general anesthesia. Regarding the entire patient cohort, 66/120 patients (55%) underwent left-sided ablation only. Right-sided only ablation was performed in 43/120 (35.8%) patients. Four patients (3.3%) underwent ablation both in the left and in the right ventricle. In six cases (5%), additional epicardial ablation was performed, and in one patient (8.3%), ablation was performed in the left coronary cusp.

Most of the VT ablations were performed in the LV only (48 out of 69 patients, 69.6%). In 15 out of 69 patients (21.7%), VT ablation was performed in the RV only. In 8 out of 69 patients undergoing VT ablation (11.6% of all VT patients), where an epicardial substrate was expected due to history or ECG morphology, subxiphoidal epicardial access was chosen, and in 6 out of 69 VT patients (8.7%), epicardial ablation was performed (in four cases, ablation was in the LV plus epicardial; in two cases, ablation was in the RV plus epicardial).

In PVC patients, ablation only in the LV was performed in 18/51 patients (35.3%). In 28 out of 51 patients (54.9%), PVC ablation was performed in the RV only. However, in 4/51 patients (7.8%), PVC ablation was performed both in the left and in the right ventricle. In 1 out of 51 patients (2%), PVC ablation was performed in the left coronary cusp.

In 27 out of 120 procedures (23%) in this study, substrate mapping was the preferred mapping method because of hemodynamic instability during VT. We used a multielectrode mapping catheter (Pentaray, Biosense Webster, Inc., Irvine, CA, USA) from 2015 onward in 31/120 procedures (26%).

3.3. Acute Procedural Success

In the entire patient cohort, ablation procedures were successful in 112 out of 120 patients (93.3%).

In VT ablation, acute success rate was 94.2%. Complete success was achieved in 52 out of 69 patients (75.4%), whereas partial success was achieved in 13 out of 69 patients (18.8%). Success rates in VT ablation were numerically higher for patients with ischemic cardiomyopathy as compared with non-ischemic cardiomyopathy, with complete success in 26 out of 31 patients (83.9%) vs. 26 out of 38 patients (68%) and partial success in 5 out of 31 patients (16.1%) in ischemic vs. 8 out of 38 patients (21.1%). However, the differences in success rates between ischemic and non-ischemic cardiomyopathy were not statistically different (p = ns, Appendix A Figure A1). In 24 out of 69 VT ablations (35%), at least one external defibrillation was necessary to treat hemodynamically unstable VT not responding to overstimulation. This was necessary in just one patient (2%) undergoing PVC ablation.

In PVC ablation, acute success rate was 92.2%. Complete success was achieved in 36 out of 51 patients (70.6%), whereas partial success was achieved in 11 out of 51 patients (21.6%). Success rates in PVC ablation were numerically higher for patients without structural heart disease as compared with patients with structural heart disease, with complete success in 26 out of 34 patients (76.5%) vs. 10 out of 17 patients (58.8%) and partial success in 6 out of 34 patients (17.7%) vs. 5 out of 17 patients (29.4%). The differences in success rates between normal hearts and structural heart disease in PVC ablation were not statistically different (p = ns, Appendix A Figure A2).

In most patients, one single target was ablated. However, in 36 out of 120 procedures (30%), two targets were ablated; in 18 procedures (15%), three targets were ablated and in 7 procedures (6%), four or more targets were ablated. In 32 out of 120 patients (27%), one or more antiarrhythmic drug could be discontinued after successful ablation.

3.4. Acute Complications

In 11 out of 120 patients (9%), minor or major procedural complications occurred (Table 3). The most frequent complication was pericardial tamponade, which occurred in 6 patients (5%). Five cases of pericardial tamponade (83%) were resolved by means of percutaneous puncture, whereas one case (17%) had to be resolved by thoracotomy. Vascular complications occurred in two patients (2%). Third-degree AV block occurred in one patient (1%) and left bundle branch block in one patient (1%). In one patient (1%), periprocedural stroke was suspected, as assessed by cerebral MRI. There was no procedural complication leading to death.

Table 3. Procedural complications, number, and percentages.

Procedural Complications; n (%)	All Patients (n = 120)	VT (n = 69)	PVC (n = 51)
AV block	1 (0.8)	1 (1.4)	0 (0)
Pericardial tamponade	6 (5.0)	4 (5.8)	2 (3.9)
Aneurysma spurium and/or fistula	2 (1.7)	1 (1.4)	1 (2.0)
Stroke	1 (0.8)	0 (0)	1 (2)
Left bundle branch block	1 (0.8)	1 (1.4)	0 (0)
Death	0 (0)	0 (0)	0 (0)

AV: atrio-ventricular. VT: ventricular tachycardia. PVC: premature ventricular complexes.

3.5. Procedural Safety according to Ablation Site and Approach

In general, there was a trend towards a higher complication rate in patients undergoing left-sided ablation (8 out of 66, 12.1%) when compared with right-sided ablation (1 out of 43, 2.3%). However, this did not reach statistical significance ($p = 0.085$). In patients with ablation in the LV and RV (n = 4) and aortic cusp (n = 1), no complications were reported.

In patients undergoing epicardial ablation (n = 6), the complication rate was 33% (two out of six patients) with one tamponade and one left bundle branch block (epicardial plus endocardial ablation was performed in this case). Thus, we report a numerically higher rate for these patients in comparison to the remaining VT ablation group, where complications occurred in 5 out of 63 patients (7.9%). However, this did not reach statistical significance (p = ns).

3.6. Procedural Safety according to Arrhythmia Type VT vs. PVC

There were numerically higher procedural complications during VT ablations when compared with PVC ablations (7/69; 10% and 4/51; 8%, respectively). Also, the rate of pericardial tamponade was numerically higher in patients undergoing VT ablations (four patients, 6%) when compared with patients undergoing PVC ablations (two patients, 4%), but both differences were not statistically significant (p = ns).

3.7. Procedural Safety according to Presence or Absence of Structural Heart Disease

Of note, all 11 complications in our study cohort occurred in patients with structural heart disease in comparison to no complications in patients with the absence of structural heart disease. This difference was statistically significant ($p = 0.0025$).

In the VT subgroup, 76.8% of individuals had structural heart disease, whereas within the PVC group, 33.3% had structural heart disease. Seven complications in VT ablation (100%) occurred in patients with structural heart disease, whereas no complication occurred in patients without structural heart disease, but this difference was statistically not significant (p = ns). However, in PVC ablation, where all four complications (100%) occurred in patients with structural heart disease and none in patients without heart disease, the difference was statistically significant ($p = 0.0095$).

4. Discussion

4.1. Acute Success Rates of Catheter Ablation

Acute procedural success rates were reassuringly higher than 90% both in VT and PVC ablations. Comparing the acute success rates in our study with those of other studies is difficult due to large heterogeneity in patient selection, definition of clinical endpoints, ablation techniques, and other factors. The Cooled RF Ablation System clinical trial was a multicenter, prospective, nonrandomized study, enrolling patients with ischemic cardiomyopathy (ICM) with previous ICD implantation and reported acute success rates of 75 percent [9]. It needs to be noted, however, that acute success was defined as the elimination of all mappable VTs. The Multicenter THERMOCOOL VT Ablation Trial [10] enrolled high-risk patients with hemodynamically unstable and unmappable VTs, thus explaining the lower acute success rates of 49 percent [10]. Another observational study [11] reported an 81 percent rate of acute procedural success in patients with ICM.

In a study from Germany [12], acute procedural success rates for ablation of PVC were reported to be 67% and 73% in patients <65 and >65 years of age, respectively. The authors of the German Ablation Registry [13] reported acute success rates for PVC ablations of 82% in the overall patient group. In patients without structural heart disease, acute procedural success was significantly higher when compared with patients with structural heart disease (86 vs. 74%, $p = 0.002$). Another study from the United States [14] described acute procedural success rates of 76% in a series of 194 consecutively enrolled patients undergoing catheter ablation for PVC.

4.2. Procedural Complications

Procedural complication rates are in part driven by the degree of structural heart disease as well as by comorbidities. In the Multicenter THERMOCOOL VT Ablation Trial [10], high-risk patients with hemodynamically unstable and unmappable VTs were enrolled. This helps explain the reported procedural mortality of 3% in the latter study. At the other end of the spectrum, some authors report no major procedural complications in low-risk patients after the ablation of PVC originating from the right ventricular outflow tract (RVOT) [15].

In our study, two major complications occurred: one pericardial tamponade had to be resolved by means of cardiac surgery, and in one patient, periprocedural stroke was suspected as assessed by cranial MRI. Balancing between interventional success and complications is very important. Our study contains a heterogeneous patient cohort, including patients with structural heart disease (majority of patients undergoing VT ablation) and patients without structural heart disease (majority of patients undergoing PVC ablation). It is important to emphasize that all of the 11 complications in our study occurred in patients with structural heart disease. None of the patients without structural heart disease suffered from complications. We also observed a trend towards a higher number of complications in patients undergoing left-sided ablation in comparison with right-sided ablation; however, the difference did not result in statistical significance. Of note, the complication in our patient cohort that occurred in the group of right-sided ablation was a stroke. But this occurred after retrograde access of the LVOT, and thus, left-sided ablation was finally not performed.

4.3. Catheter Ablation vs. Pharmacological Treatment

A multicenter randomized controlled trial (VANISH) [8] compared catheter ablation with escalation of antiarrhythmic drug therapy (AAD) in patients with ICM and implanted ICD who experienced VT despite treatment with AAD. The primary endpoint in the VANISH trial was a composite endpoint of all-cause mortality, appropriate ICD shock after 30 days of treatment or VT storm. There was a 28 percent relative risk reduction, reaching statistical significance, in experiencing the composite endpoint in the 132 patients randomized to the catheter ablation group. Very recently, Della Bella et al. showed in the PARTITA trial that VT ablation after the first ICD shock is associated with a reduced risk of heart failure hospitalization, mortality and recurrent ICD shocks as compared with standard therapy [16]. Arenal et al. found reassuring results in their multicenter randomized SURVIVE-VT trial: patients with ischemic cardiomyopathy and ICD had reduced cardiovascular death, ICD shock, heart failure hospitalization or severe treatment-related complications in comparison to antiarrhythmic drug therapy [17]. These encouraging findings may shift the field more towards catheter ablation in this patient group.

5. Conclusions

Our results confirm that catheter ablation for VT and PVC is an effective and safe therapy when performed by experienced professionals in experienced centers. Recognition of this development in the community led to increasing numbers of ablation procedures during the last years, and that will likely further increase. Patients should be considered for catheter ablation for VT at an earlier stage, given that this treatment option can change the arrhythmogenic substrate and, thereby, prevent progression over time. This argument weighs even more in young patients with idiopathic PVC, where a one-time ablation procedure is often considered curative and can prevent patients from taking AAD for long periods and, thus, from significant long-term complications.

In summary, the data in our study suggest that catheter ablation of ventricular arrhythmia in structurally normal hearts is safe, whereas periprocedural complications have to be taken into account when dealing with structural heart disease.

Limitations

We reported on acute success and complications in the catheter ablation of VT and PVC in 120 consecutive patients over 5 years. However, the population and the results concern very different patients. Moreover, we reported on acute success rates, which can be high after ablation but different a few days after. It is well known that recurrences of VT and PVC are frequent. Mortality after ablation can be delayed. Immediate good results do not mean that the patient will always improve. Our results are limited to acute success since long-term follow-up data are missing in our patient cohort.

Author Contributions: Validation, C.B.; Formal analysis, C.S. and J.B.; Investigation, L.M.H.; Data curation, C.S. and A.M.S.; Writing—original draft, C.S. and J.B.; Writing—review & editing, J.B., F.D., A.M.S. and L.M.H.; Visualization, J.B.; Supervision, F.D. and C.B. All authors have read and agreed to the published version of the manuscript.

Funding: This research received no external funding.

Institutional Review Board Statement: The study was conducted in accordance with the Declaration of Helsinki, and approved by the Kantonale Ethikkommission of the Canton of Zurich, 2016-00116 on 11 April 2016.

Informed Consent Statement: Patient consent was waived due to the retrospective and anonymized nature of the analysis.

Data Availability Statement: The data presented in this study are available on request from the corresponding author.

Conflicts of Interest: A.M.S. has received educational grants through his institution from Abbott, Bayer Healthcare, Biosense Webster, Biotronik, Boston Scientific, BMS/Pfizer, and Medtronic; and speaker/advisory board/consulting fees from Bayer Healthcare, Biotronik, Daiichi-Sankyo, Medtronic, Novartis, Pfizer, Stride Bio Inc. and Zoll. L.M.H. has received institutional grants from Abbott, Abiomed, Amgen, Astra Zeneca, Bayer, Biosense Webster, Biotronik, Boston Scientific, Bracco, B. Braun, Daiichi-Sankyo, Edwards, Medtronic, MicroPort, Novartis, Vascular Medical and Zoll. The other authors declare no conflict of interest.

Appendix A

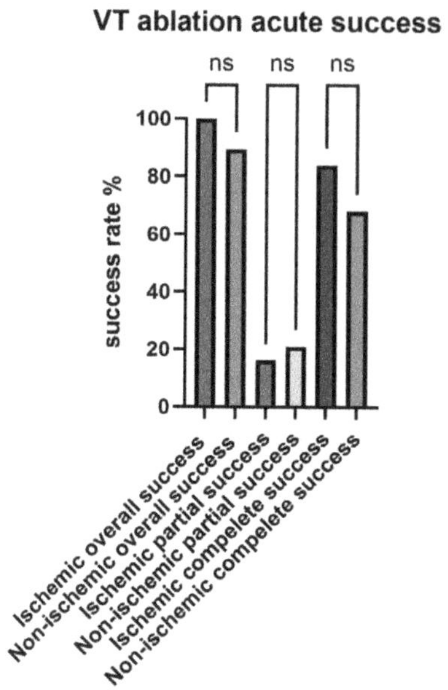

Figure A1. Differences in acute success rates in VT ablation (ischemic vs. non-ischemic); ns = not significant.

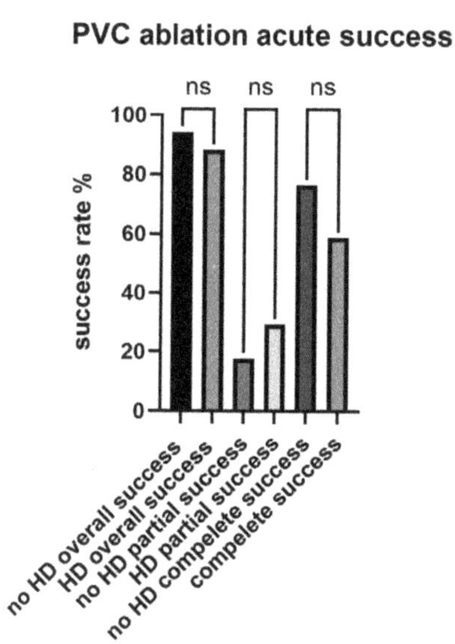

Figure A2. Differences in acute success rates in PVC ablation (no structural heart disease vs. structural heart disease); ns = not significant; HD = heart disease.

References

1. Brunckhorst, C.B.; Delacretaz, E.; Soejima, K.; Maisel, W.H.; Friedman, P.L.; Stevenson, W.G. Identification of the Ventricular Tachycardia Isthmus After Infarction by Pace Mapping. *Circulation* **2004**, *110*, 652–659. [CrossRef] [PubMed]
2. Palaniswamy, C.; Kolte, D.; Harikrishnan, P.; Khera, S.; Aronow, W.S.; Mujib, M.; Mellana, W.M.; Eugenio, P.; Lessner, S.; Ferrick, A.; et al. Catheter ablation of postinfarction ventricular tachycardia: Ten-year trends in utilization, in-hospital complications, and in-hospital mortality in the United States. *Hear. Rhythm.* **2014**, *11*, 2056–2063. [CrossRef] [PubMed]
3. Gasperetti, A.; Sicuso, R.; Russo, A.D.; Zucchelli, G.; Saguner, A.M.; Notarstefano, P.; Soldati, E.; Bongiorni, M.G.; Della Rocca, D.G.; Mohanty, S.; et al. Prospective use of ablation index for the ablation of right ventricle outflow tract premature ventricular contractions: A proof of concept study. *Europace* **2021**, *23*, 91–98. [CrossRef] [PubMed]
4. Yamada, T.; Doppalapudi, H.; McELDERRY, H.T.; Okada, T.; Murakami, Y.; Inden, Y.; Yoshida, Y.; Kaneko, S.; Yoshida, N.; Murohara, T.; et al. Idiopathic Ventricular Arrhythmias Originating from the Papillary Muscles in the Left Ventricle: Prevalence, Electrocardiographic and Electrophysiological Characteristics, and Results of the Radiofrequency Catheter Ablation. *J. Cardiovasc. Electrophysiol.* **2010**, *21*, 62–69. [CrossRef] [PubMed]
5. Zeppenfeld, K.; Tfelt-Hansen, J.; de Riva, M.; Winkel, B.G.; Behr, E.R.; A Blom, N.; Charron, P.; Corrado, D.; Dagres, N.; de Chillou, C.; et al. 2022 ESC Guidelines for the management of patients with ventricular arrhythmias and the prevention of sudden cardiac death. *Eur. Hear. J.* **2022**, *43*, 3997–4126. [CrossRef] [PubMed]
6. Sears, S.F.; Hauf, J.D.; Kirian, K.; Hazelton, G.; Conti, J.B. Posttraumatic stress and the implantable cardioverter-defibrillator patient what the electrophysiologist needs to know. *Circ. Arrhythm. Electrophysiol.* **2011**, *4*, 242–250. [CrossRef] [PubMed]
7. Ensslin, C.; Berg, J.; Hermes-Laufer, J.; Keller, L.S.; Niederseer, D.; Pazhenkottil, A.; von Känel, R.; Schmied, C. Depressive symptoms in patients after primary and secondary prophylactic ICD implantation. *Clin. Res. Cardiol.* **2022**, *111*, 1210–1218. [CrossRef] [PubMed]
8. Sapp, J.L.; Wells, G.A.; Parkash, R.; Stevenson, W.G.; Blier, L.; Sarrazin, J.-F.; Thibault, B.; Rivard, L.; Gula, L.; Leong-Sit, P.; et al. Ventricular Tachycardia Ablation versus Escalation of Antiarrhythmic Drugs. *N. Engl. J. Med.* **2016**, *375*, 111–121. [CrossRef] [PubMed]
9. Calkins, H.; Epstein, A.; Packer, D.; Arria, A.M.; Hummel, J.; Gilligan, D.M. Catheter Ablation of Ventricular Tachycardia in Patients with Structural Heart Disease Using Cooled Ra-diofrequency Energy Results of a Prospective Multicenter Study. *J. Am. Coll. Cardiol.* **2000**, *35*, 1905–1914. [CrossRef] [PubMed]
10. Stevenson, W.G.; Wilber, D.J.; Natale, A.; Jackman, W.M.; Marchlinski, F.E.; Talbert, T.; Nakagawa, H. Irrigated radiofrequency catheter ablation guided by electroanatomic mapping for recurrent ventricular tachycardia after myocardial infarction the multicenter thermocool ventricular tachycardia ablation trial. *Circulation* **2008**, *118*, 2773–2782. [CrossRef] [PubMed]
11. Tanner, H.; Hindricks, G.; Volkmer, M.; Furniss, S.; Kühlkamp, V.; Lacroix, D.; DE Chillou, C.; Almendral, J.; Caponi, D.; Kuck, K.; et al. Catheter Ablation of Recurrent Scar-Related Ventricular Tachycardia Using Electroanatomical Mapping and Irrigated Ablation Technology: Results of the Prospective Multicenter Euro-VT-Study. *J. Cardiovasc. Electrophysiol.* **2010**, *21*, 47–53. [CrossRef] [PubMed]
12. Attanasio, P.; Jungmann, J.; Huemer, M.; Parwani, A.S.; Boldt, L.-H.; Haverkamp, W.; Wutzler, A. Catheter ablation of premature ventricular contractions in elderly patients: Feasibility and success. *Aging Clin. Exp. Res.* **2016**, *28*, 527–531. [CrossRef] [PubMed]
13. Fichtner, S.; Registry, F.T.G.A.; Senges, J.; Hochadel, M.; Tilz, R.; Willems, S.; Eckardt, L.; Deneke, T.; Lewalter, T.; Dorwarth, U.; et al. Safety and efficacy in ablation of premature ventricular contraction: Data from the German ablation registry. *Clin. Res. Cardiol.* **2017**, *106*, 49–57. [CrossRef] [PubMed]
14. Baser, K.; Bas, H.D.; Yokokawa, M.; Latchamsetty, R.; Morady, F.; Bogun, F. Infrequent Intraprocedural Premature Ventricular Complexes: Implications for Ablation Outcome. *J. Cardiovasc. Electrophysiol.* **2014**, *25*, 1088–1092. [CrossRef] [PubMed]
15. Darrieux, F.C.; Scanavacca, M.I.; Hachul, D.T.; Melo, S.L.; D'Ávilla, A.B.; Gruppi, C.J.; Sosa, E.A. Radiofrequency Catheter Ablation of Premature Ventricular Contractions Originating in the Right Ventricular Outflow Tract. *Arq. Bras. Cardiol.* **2007**, *88*, 265–272. [CrossRef] [PubMed]
16. Della Bella, P.; Baratto, F.; Vergara, P.; Bertocchi, P.; Santamaria, M.; Notarstefano, P.; Radinovic, A. Does Timing of Ventricular Tachycardia Ablation Affect Prognosis in Patients with an Implantable Car-dioverter Defibrillator? Results from the Multicenter Randomized PARTITA Trial. *Circulation* **2022**, *145*, 1829–1838. [CrossRef] [PubMed]
17. Arenal, Á.; Ávila, P.; Jiménez-Candil, J.; Tercedor, L.; Calvo, D.; Arribas, F.; Fernández-Portales, J.; Merino, J.L.; Hernández-Madrid, A.; Fernández-Avilés, F.J.; et al. Substrate Ablation vs Antiarrhythmic Drug Therapy for Symptomatic Ventricular Tachycardia. *J. Am. Coll. Cardiol.* **2022**, *79*, 1441–1453. [CrossRef] [PubMed]

Journal of
Clinical Medicine

MDPI

Article

Anatomical and Electrophysiological Characteristics of Dual-Loop Re-Entry in Atypical Atrial Flutter: Implications for Mapping and Catheter Ablation

Nicolas Johner, Mehdi Namdar and Dipen C. Shah *

Cardiology Division, Geneva University Hospitals, Rue Gabrielle-Perret-Gentil 4, 1205 Geneva, Switzerland; nicolas.johner@hug.ch (N.J.); mehdi.namdar@hug.ch (M.N.)
* Correspondence: dipen.shah@hug.ch; Tel.: +41-22-372-7202; Fax: +41-22-372-7229

Abstract: Background: Atypical atrial flutter (AFL) can be challenging to ablate, especially when involving dual-loop re-entry. We sought to assess the electroanatomical characteristics of single- and dual-loop AFLs in patients undergoing catheter ablation. **Methods:** We analyzed 25 non-cavotricuspid isthmus-dependent macro-re-entrant AFL in 19 consecutive patients. Three-dimensional high-density activation mapping was performed, and active re-entry loops were confirmed by entrainment mapping. **Results:** Of 25 AFLs (24 left, 1 right atrial), 13 (52%) exhibited dual-loop re-entry. The most common circuits included, in 6/13 (46% of dual loops), a perimitral re-entry with a second loop around the right/left pulmonary veins (PV) and, in 6/13 (46%), involved a right PV ostium with a second loop around either a functional conduction block or another PV. Ablation at the common isthmus of dual-loop AFLs and at the critical isthmus of single-loop AFLs terminated the arrhythmia more frequently than ablation at a secondary isthmus of dual-loop AFLs (5/6 (83%) and 8/11 (73%) versus 1/8 (13%), respectively, $p = 0.013$). **Conclusions:** More than half of AFLs exhibited a dual-loop re-entrant mechanism. Most critical isthmuses were found at the mitral isthmus, the left atrial roof or right PV ostia. Ablation targeting the common isthmus resulted in a higher termination rate.

Keywords: atrial flutter; atrial tachycardia; dual-loop; re-entry; macro-re-entry; catheter ablation; isthmus; mapping; substrate

1. Introduction

Atypical atrial flutter (AFL) represents a heterogeneous set of complex arrhythmias defined as non-cavotricuspid isthmus (CTI)-dependent macro-re-entrant atrial tachycardia. The arrhythmogenic substrate generally consists of combination(s) of anatomical obstacles (valves and other orifices) and left or right atrial myocardial scars, the latter often resulting from catheter ablation [1–3] (e.g., atrial fibrillation [AF] ablation) or cardiac surgery [2,4,5], but may also occur without prior interventions in the setting of advanced atrial cardiomyopathy [6]. AFL is often difficult to manage medically and catheter ablation is an established treatment. Because AFL has highly variable anatomy, the selection of appropriate ablation targets relies on the individualized identification of critical isthmuses within the re-entry circuit. Three-dimensional (3D) high-density electroanatomical mapping allows delineation of the complete re-entry circuit and facilitates the identification of narrow slow-conducting critical isthmuses [7]. Despite modern tools, however, AFL can be challenging to map and ablate, owing in part to its sometimes complex and frequently variable anatomy, and long-term rates of freedom from arrhythmia after catheter ablation have been modest. In one of the largest studies on complex atrial tachycardias, Derval et al. reported recurrence in 45 of 101 (45%) patients after ablation of re-entrant atrial tachycardia during a follow-up of 13 $\pm$ 9 months [2]. Dual-loop re-entry (or figure-of-8 re-entry) can be defined by the presence of two synchronous active loops without delay compared to other loops and confirmed by entrainment mapping. Dual-loop AFLs pose specific challenges due to circuit complexity and the multiplicity of potential ablation targets. While dual-loop atrial macro-re-entry was first reported more than two decades ago [5], data remains scarce regarding its prevalence, electroanatomical characteristics and optimal ablation strategy. In the largest study on multiple-loop AFL ablation, Takigawa et al. reported recurrence of atrial tachycardia in 19 of 42 (45%) patients 1 year after ablation [1], highlighting the challenge that these arrhythmias represent.

We sought to assess the prevalence of dual-loop re-entry and to describe its electroanatomical characteristics in patients undergoing catheter ablation of AFL using high-density 3D electroanatomical mapping.

2. Methods

2.1. Design

We retrospectively studied 19 consecutive patients who underwent catheter ablation of AFL at our institution. AFL was defined as non-CTI-dependent atrial tachycardia with regular monomorphic atrial activity and a re-entrant mechanism confirmed by electrophysiology study. CTI-dependent atrial flutters were excluded from the analysis. Inclusion criteria were: (1) clinically-indicated catheter ablation of AFL and (2) availability of at least one complete electroanatomical map (see Section 2.2. Electrophysiology Study) confirming a non-CTI-dependent re-entrant mechanism. The exclusion criterion was the absence of any documented non-CTI-dependent re-entrant AFL at electrophysiology study. Written informed consent was obtained for the procedures and the study was approved by the institutional review board.

2.2. Electrophysiology Study

Antiarrhythmic drugs were discontinued 5 half-lives before ablation, except amiodarone, which was discontinued for >3–10 days. A 10-electrode mapping catheter (5 mm electrodes, 2–5–2 mm spacing, Abbott, Abbott Park, IL, USA) was placed in the coronary sinus (CS) with the catheter tip in the distal CS or great cardiac vein and all electrodes inside the CS. Another identical catheter was placed on the right atrium (RA) free wall with the catheter tip close to the lateral CTI. Left atrial (LA) access was routinely obtained up-front by transseptal puncture under fluoroscopic guidance. Entrainment mapping was performed and, in case of a post-pacing interval (PPI) to tachycardia cycle length (TCL) difference (PPI-TCL) $\geq$ 40 ms at the CTI and at $\geq$ 2 sites on the RA free wall, ruling out RA AFL, LA mapping was performed.

High-density 3D electroanatomical maps were acquired sequentially (Rhythmia mapping system, Boston Scientific, Marlborough, MA, USA) during ongoing arrhythmia using a 64-electrode basket catheter (IntellaMap Orion, Boston Scientific). A re-entrant mechanism was confirmed based on documentation of >90% of TCL with early-meets-late circular activation. Entrainment mapping was performed at several candidate sites to confirm active re-entry loops. Entrainment was obtained at a pacing cycle length 15–20 ms shorter than TCL at a 25 mA output from the distal bipole of the ablation catheter (TactiCath Quartz Contact Force Ablation Catheter, Abbott). Entrainment was defined based on conventional criteria and a PPI-TCL < 20 ms was considered indicative of a site within an active component of the re-entry circuit. Entrainment locations and the corresponding PPI measures were routinely annotated on the electroanatomical maps for subsequent analysis.

Radiofrequency ablation was performed by targeting the narrowest accessible critical isthmus, aiming for both arrhythmia termination and anatomically complete ablation across the targeted isthmus. On an individual basis, the potential impact of ablation lesions on sinus rhythm atrial activation was considered at operator's discretion when selecting ablation targets (e.g., to avoid the risk of left atrial appendage isolation in case of extensive LA scarring). After flutter termination, lesions were assessed based on abolition of local electrograms or the presence of double potentials. When applicable, differential pacing or activation mapping in sinus or paced rhythm was performed to confirm conduction block across ablation lines. When applicable, in patients with a history of AF or pulmonary vein isolation, PVs were mapped in sinus rhythm and re-isolated in case of reconnection. Following ablation, arrhythmia inducibility was assessed by atrial burst pacing in 10 ms decrements from 300 to 200 ms and incremented back to 300 ms. In case of induced arrhythmia sustained for >5 min, mapping and ablation were pursued at operator's discretion based on estimated clinical benefit. Procedure endpoints were arrhythmia termination, non-inducibility of sustained arrhythmias by atrial burst pacing, and, when applicable, conduction block confirmation across ablation lines and PV isolation.

Bipolar electrograms were filtered (band-pass 30–500 Hz) and digitally recorded at a sampling frequency of 1000 Hz (LabSystem Pro, Boston Scientific) along with surface ECG.

2.3. Electroanatomical Map Analysis

The leading tachycardia wavefront was identified from activation maps based on the tip of consecutive isochrones indicative of the shortest active re-entry loop. Multi-loop re-entry was defined by the presence of ≥2 synchronous active loops without delay compared to other leading wavefronts and confirmed by entrainment mapping (PPI-TCLs < 20 ms). Isthmuses were defined as relative narrowing < 30 mm along the path of the leading re-entry wavefront(s) and delimited on both sides by the presence of anatomical obstacles (e.g., valve annulus or thoracic veins), electrical scars (bipolar electrogram voltage < 0.05 mV) or lines of conduction block (identified based on activation mapping). In case of dual-loop re-entry, a common isthmus was defined as an isthmus < 30 mm located along the common segment between both re-entry loops, while a secondary isthmus was defined as an isthmus < 30 mm at any other location along the active re-entry wavefronts. Isthmus width was measured using Rhythmia's distance tool. Isthmus conduction velocity was calculated as the time interval between wavefront entry and exit to and from the isthmus divided by isthmus length. Entry and exit locations were identified as the sites with an abrupt change in width and/or in the direction of wavefront propagation, representative of the extremities of a protected channel. In the absence of a protected channel, i.e., isthmuses < 5 mm in length (localized narrowing), isthmus conduction velocity was measured by selecting two representative sites around the center of the isthmus, with an axis parallel to wavefront propagation and a distance of 5–15 mm (depending on map density at that site). Bipolar electrogram voltage was measured from representative electrograms (corresponding to the most common amplitude) within the isthmus. When available, PPI measures within the isthmus were verified offline (to exclude incorrect annotation or TCL variability) and PPI-TCL was calculated.

2.4. Acute Ablation Outcome

The effect of ablation at the targeted isthmus was defined based on the following categories: (1) AFL termination to sinus rhythm, (2) sustained increase in TCL by >15 ms, (3) manifest modification of the atrial activation sequence, and (4) absence of manifest effect on the arrhythmia.

2.5. Statistical Analysis

Unless otherwise specified, continuous variables are expressed as mean (±standard deviation) if normally distributed and as median (interquartile range) if not. Categorical variables are expressed as number (percentage). The distribution of continuous variables was assessed by visual examination of histograms and the Kolmogoroff-Smirnov test. Normally distributed continuous variables were compared using paired and unpaired two-tailed t-test (Welch approximation) as appropriate. Continuous variables with non-normal distribution were compared using the Mann-Whitney U-test, or the Kruskal-Wallis rank test for comparisons involving ≥ 3 groups. For categorical variables, Pearson's Chi-squared test was used when expected frequencies were >5 across all categories and the Fischer exact test was used in case of expected frequencies ≤ 5. Statistical significance was defined at a bilateral alpha < 0.05.

3. Results

3.1. Clinical Characteristics

Baseline clinical characteristics are summarized in Table 1. Nineteen patients (age 66 ± 15 years, 79% male) who underwent 20 catheter ablation procedures were included and a total of 25 AFLs were analyzed, for which complete high-density electroanatomical activation maps were acquired and entrainment mapping at several candidate sites was performed. A presumed etiology of AFL was identified in 17 (89%) patients: 14 (74%) patients had undergone previous AF ablation (of which 13 had a history of prior AF ablation and 1 exhibited AFL during de novo AF ablation), 2 (11%) patients had undergone previous cardiac surgery (mitral and aortic valve replacement along with Maze procedure in one, and mitral valve repair along with Maze, patent foramen ovale closure and coronary artery bypass graft in one) and 1 (5%) patient had a history of bipulmonary transplant (and exhibited re-entry around the right pulmonary veins [PVs] suture). AFL had no clear etiology in 2 (11%) patients: one patient only had a history of medically managed moderate-to-severe (grade 3/4) tricuspid regurgitation (but exhibited left atrial flutter) and one patient had no significant past medical history except for arterial hypertension and no evidence of structural heart disease (except for tachycardiomyopathy, which recovered fully after catheter ablation of AFL).

Table 1. Baseline characteristics.

	All Patients (N = 19)
Age (years)	66 (±15)
Male gender	15 (79%)
BMI (kg/m^2)	25.9 (±4.6)
Associated conditions	
Arterial hypertension	8 (42%)
Diabetes mellitus	1 (5.3%)
Dyslipidemia	5 (26%)
Structural heart disease	5 (26%)
Prior stroke or transient ischemic attack	3 (15.8%)
CHA_2DS_2-VASc score	
0–1	8 (42%)
≥2	11 (58%)
LA surface (cm^2)	24.9 (±5.1)
RA surface (cm^2)	20.3 (±5.2)
LVEF ≤ 50%	4 (21%)

Data presented as mean (±standard deviation) for continuous variables and number (percentage) for categorical variables. BMI denotes body mass index; LA, left atrium; LVEF, left ventricular ejection fraction; RA, right atrium.

3.2. Electroanatomical Mapping

Out of 25 AFL, 13 (52%) exhibited a dual-loop re-entrant mechanism and 12 (48%) consisted of a single-loop re-entry. Re-entry was located entirely in the LA in 24 (96%) and in the RA in 1 AFL (4%). Average TCL was 261 ± 35 ms. Activation maps contained an average 18,522 points (range 8216–33,368).

Table 2 and Figure 1 summarize the anatomy of single- and dual-loop AFLs. Single-loop circuits (N = 12) were distributed as follows: 6 perimitral (50% of single-loop AFLs), 2 around the right PVs, 2 coronary sinus (CS)-dependent flutters with an endo-epicardial component, 1 around a scar on the interatrial septum, and 1 around a scar on the RA free wall. Dual-loop circuits (N = 13) had the following paths: 4 perimitral with a second loop around the left PVs, 4 around the right PVs with a second loop around a line of conduction block, 2 perimitral with a second loop around the right PVs, 1 with a loop around each right PV, 1 around the right PVs with a second loop around the left PVs, and 1 around the left PVs with a second loop around a line of conduction block. The most common configuration of dual-loop re-entry was therefore a perimitral loop with a second roof-dependent loop (around either the right of left PVs), which accounted for 6 of 13 (46%) dual-loop AFLs.

Table 2. Anatomy of single- and dual-loop atypical atrial flutters.

	Single-Loop Re-Entry (N = 12)	Dual-Loop Re-Entry (N = 13)	
Perimitral	6 (50%)	6 (46%)	4 with second loop around left PVs 2 with second loop around right PVs
Around right PVs	2 (17%)	6 (46%)	4 with second loop around a line of block 1 with one loop around each right PV 1 with second loop around left PVs
Coronary sinus-dependent	2 (17%)		
Around a septal scar	1 (8%)		
Around a right atrial free wall scar	1 (8%)		
Around left PVs		1 (8%)	Second loop around a functional block

Data described as number (percentage). PV denotes pulmonary vein.

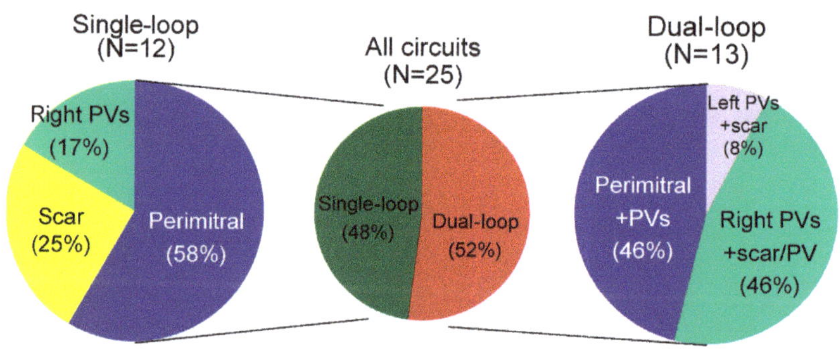

Figure 1. Circuit anatomy in single- and dual-loop macro-re-entrant atrial tachycardias, identified by the central obstacle defining each re-entrant loop. PV denotes pulmonary vein.

Isthmuses < 30 mm (not limited to the common isthmus in case of dual-loop re-entry) were identified at the following locations, and summarized in Table 3 and Figure 2: 9 at the posterior mitral isthmus (defined as the region between the left inferior PV and the posterior mitral annulus), 6 at the LA roof, 5 at a right PV ostium or carina, 3 at the posterior LA wall, 3 at the anterior mitral isthmus (defined as the region between the left superior PV/left atrial appendage and the anterior mitral annulus), 3 at the interatrial septum near the mitral annulus, 2 within the CS (epicardial), 2 at the interatrial septum near the right PVs, 1 at a left PV ostium, and 1 at the superior vena cava-RA free wall junction.

Table 3. Anatomical location of isthmuses.

	All Isthmuses	Common Isthmuses of Dual-Loop Reentries
Posterior mitral isthmus	9 (26%)	3 (27%)
Pulmonary vein ostium	6 (17%)	3 (27%)
Left atrial roof	6 (17%)	2 (18%)
Posterior left atrial wall	3 (9%)	2 (18%)
Anterior mitral isthmus	3 (9%)	1 (9%)
Inferior interatrial septum	3 (9%)	
Coronary sinus (epicardial)	2 (6%)	
Superior interatrial septum	2 (6%)	
Superior vena cava—right atrial free wall junction	1 (3%)	

Data described as number (percentage). PV denotes pulmonary vein.

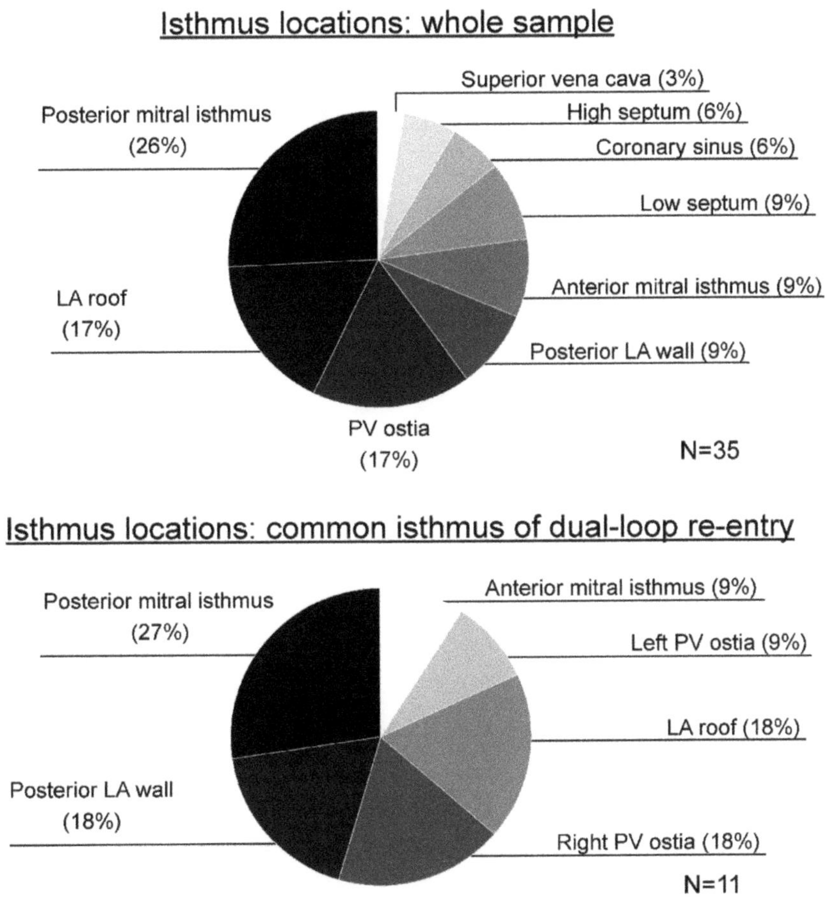

Figure 2. Location of narrow isthmuses (<30 mm). Top panel includes all identified narrow isthmuses in single- and dual-loop atypical atrial flutters. Bottom panel includes only narrow isthmuses located on the segment common to both loops in dual-loop re-entry. LA denotes left atrium; PV, pulmonary vein.

Compared to single-loop re-entry, dual-loop AFLs exhibited isthmuses characterized by greater isthmus width (17.1 ± 5.9 versus 11.4 ± 2.8 mm in dual-loop versus single-loop, respectively, $p = 0.001$), faster local conduction velocity (0.56 ± 0.42 versus 0.29 ± 0.16 m/s, respectively, $p = 0.014$), and greater bipolar electrogram voltage (0.53 ± 0.40 versus 0.27 ± 0.26 mV, respectively, $p = 0.0499$). PPI-TCL at isthmuses of dual- versus single-loop AFLs did not differ significantly (−6.6 ± 10.0 versus −12.8 ± 14.2 ms, respectively, $p = 0.29$). TCL did not differ significantly between dual- and single-loop AFLs (250 ± 28 versus 271 ± 38 ms, respectively, $p = 0.14$).

Among dual-loop AFLs, 11 (85%) exhibited a common isthmus < 30 mm along the common path of both re-entry loops, the location of which were as follows: 3 at the posterior mitral isthmus, 2 at the LA roof, 2 at a right PV ostium, 2 at the posterior LA wall, 1 at the anterior mitral isthmus, and 1 at a left PV ostium.

Among dual-loop AFLs, common isthmuses (N = 11) and secondary isthmuses (N = 12) did not differ significantly with respect to isthmus width (15.8 ± 5.9 versus 18.3 ± 5.7 mm, respectively, $p = 0.33$), local conduction velocity (0.45 ± 0.33 versus 0.68 ± 0.47 m/s, respectively, $p = 0.23$), bipolar electrogram voltage (0.52 ± 0.47 versus

0.55 ± 0.32 mV, respectively, $p = 0.88$), or local PPI-TCL (−11.1 ± 6.3 versus −2.6 ± 10.9 ms, respectively, $p = 0.08$).

3.3. Effect of Ablation

In dual-loop AFLs, ablation more frequently resulted in AFL termination to sinus rhythm when targeting a common isthmus compared to a secondary isthmus (Figure 3): 5 of 6 (83%) common isthmus ablations versus 1 of 8 (13%) secondary isthmus ablations resulted in arrhythmia termination to sinus rhythm, $p = 0.026$. Ablation of a secondary isthmus resulted in sustained TCL increase > 15 ms in 5 of 8 (71%) and in a change in activation sequence in 2 of 8 (29%).

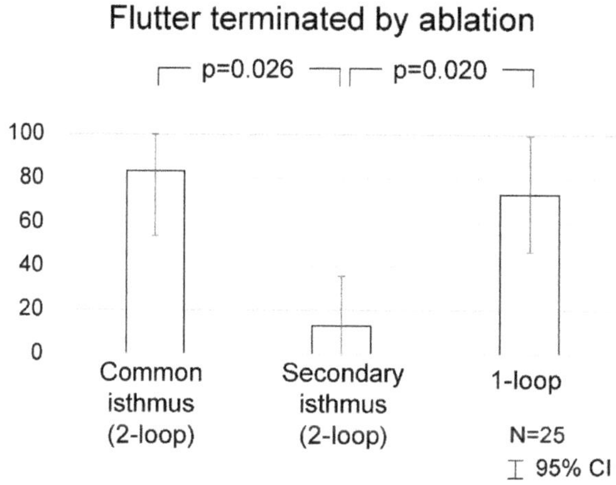

Figure 3. Rate of arrhythmia termination to sinus rhythm during radiofrequency ablation, by flutter type (single- or dual-loop) and isthmus type (common path or side loop).

Ablation of the narrowest accessible isthmus of single-loop AFLs resulted in termination to sinus rhythm in 8 of 11 (73%), a rate similar to that of dual-loop common isthmus ablation (83%, $p = 1.0$) and higher than that of dual-loop secondary isthmus ablation (13%, $p = 0.020$).

3.4. Procedure Outcome

When accounting for all arrhythmias targeted for ablation during the 20 procedures (including those that were not fully mapped), ablation targets/lesions were: a posterior mitral line in 8, a pulmonary vein ostium or carina in 6, an LA roof line in 5, the interatrial septum in 3, an anterolateral mitral line in 3, the CS in 2, an anteroseptal line in 2 and the superior vena cava-RA free wall junction in 1. Procedure endpoint was tachycardia termination to sinus rhythm followed by non-inducibility in 14 of 20 (70%), ablation in sinus rhythm followed by non-inducibility in 2 of 20 (10%), transformation of AFL into AF during ablation followed by non-inducibility in 2 of 20 (10%) and some residual inducible sustained AFL in 2 of 20 (10%) which were not ablated due to multiple inducible atrial tachycardias that could not be readily mapped and/or ablated. Complete block across ablation lines was confirmed in 11 of 20 (55%) procedures, including 4 of 8 posterior mitral lines, 5 of 5 LA roof lines, 2 of 3 anterolateral mitral lines, 2 of 2 anteroseptal mitral lines and 1 of 1 superior vena cava-RA free wall line.

Follow-up data was available for 13 patients with a median follow-up of 429 (IQR 114–461) days. Of those, 5 (38%) exhibited arrhythmia recurrence after a median of 142 (IQR 114–429) days. Three of the patients with arrhythmia recurrence had exhibited at least one dual-loop AFL at the index procedure. Two patients with arrhythmia recurrence underwent repeat procedures, which showed recurrence of perimitral AFL in both cases: one patient previously had dual-loop perimitral and roof-dependent AFL (activation map of index procedure is shown in Figure 4) which was ablated by a roof line and anterolateral mitral line (with confirmed conduction block) and exhibited recurrence in the form of single-loop perimitral AFL due to conduction recovery across the anterolateral mitral line through an epicardial CS connection; the second patient previously had single-loop perimitral AFL which was ablated by a posterior mitral line (requiring CS lesions, and with confirmed conduction block) and exhibited recurrence in the form of single-loop perimitral AFL due to conduction recovery across the posterior mitral line.

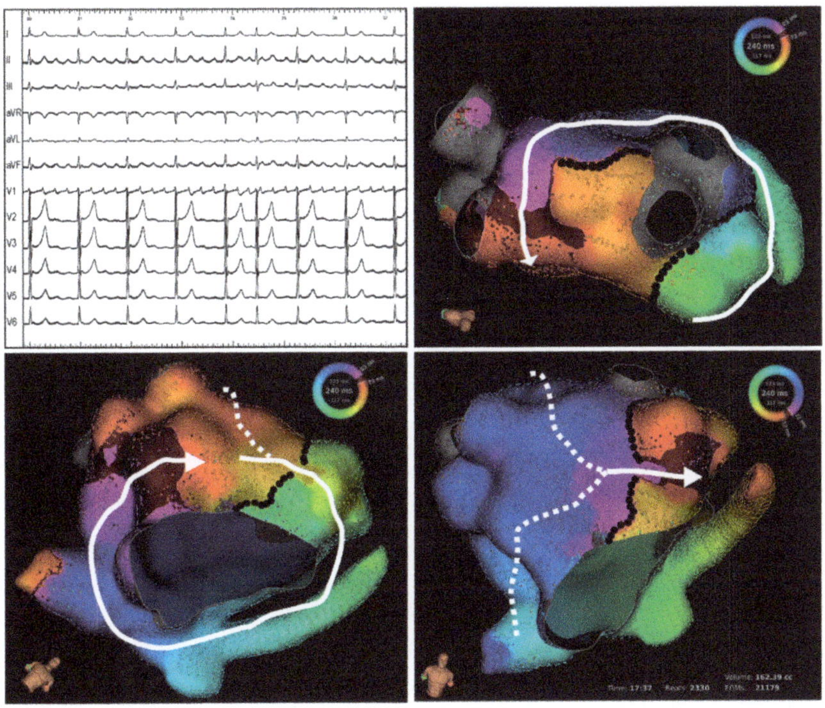

Figure 4. Example of a dual-loop atypical atrial flutter in a patient with a history of atrial fibrillation ablation. Top left panel shows 12-lead ECG with predominantly positive F waves in V1 and inferior leads. Top right and bottom panels show the left atrial activation map, depicting a dual-loop re-entry with one perimitral loop and a second roof-dependent loop around the left pulmonary veins. A narrow common isthmus is present at the anterior mitral isthmus. A narrow secondary isthmus is present at the left atrial roof. White arrows indicate the path of the leading wavefront. Black markers indicate existing lines of conduction block. Ablation was first targeted at the roof isthmus, resulting in slight cycle length prolongation (from 240 to 254 ms). The anterior mitral isthmus was then ablated, resulting in termination to sinus rhythm. Complete conduction block across both lines was then confirmed.

4. Discussion

Dual-loop re-entry was the underlying mechanism in more than half of AFLs. The most common circuit path involved a perimitral loop with a second roof-dependent loop. Compared to single-loop re-entry, dual-loop re-entry was characterized by isthmuses exhibiting greater minimum width, faster local conduction velocity, and higher bipolar electrogram voltage. In case of dual-loop re-entry, ablation more frequently resulted in termination to sinus rhythm when targeting an isthmus on the segment common to both loops, with a termination rate similar to that observed in single-loop AFL ablation. In contrast, ablation of a secondary isthmus more frequently resulted in TCL increase or modification of the atrial activation sequence without arrhythmia termination to sinus rhythm.

4.1. Characteristics of Single- and Dual-Loop Atypical Atrial Flutter

Our results show a higher rate of dual-loop AFL (52% of AFLs in 63% of patients) compared to previous studies. In the largest study to specifically investigate multiple-loop macro-re-entrant atrial tachycardias, Takigawa et al. [1] identified 42 dual-loop and 2 triple-loop re-entries in 41 of 193 (21%) consecutive patients undergoing catheter ablation of post-AF ablation atrial tachycardia. In another study on post-AF ablation atrial tachycardia, Chae et al. [3] reported multiple-loop re-entry in 17 of 78 (22%) patients. Likewise, Derval et al. [2] studied 132 patients undergoing catheter ablation of atrial tachycardia using high-density electroanatomical mapping. They identified 27 dual-loop AFLs in 24 (18%) patients. The lower prevalence of dual-loop re-entry in those previous cohorts might be partly explained by the inclusion, in all three samples, of all patients with atrial tachycardia scheduled for ablation with a high-density mapping system. While patients with clinical presentation as CTI-dependent atrial flutter were excluded, a proportion of patients were eventually diagnosed with CTI-dependent atrial flutter as well as non-re-entrant atrial tachycardias. In contrast, these cases were not included in our series. Small sample sizes may also explain some variability in the prevalence of dual-loop AFL.

While the precise circuit path is highly individual, we found that variants of a perimitral loop with a second roof-dependent loop was the most common dual-loop configuration, representing 46% of dual-loop AFLs. Consistent with our findings, Takigawa et al. [1] found this configuration in 19 of 44 (43%) multiple-loop AFLs. Among the remaining circuits, the PVs/carinas were involved in most cases. Likewise, Derval et al. [2] reported that 22 of 27 (81%) dual-loop re-entries were perimitral with a second roof-dependent loop, 4 (15%) were perimitral with a second localized loop, and 1 (4%) was roof-dependent with a second localized loop. In the study by Chae et al. [3], the precise anatomy was not described for all dual-loop circuits, but the mitral isthmus was reported as the most common isthmus location.

The circuit path of dual-loop AFLs tends to differ based on underlying etiology. The majority of AFLs occur following catheter ablation of AF [2,8], in which case re-entry usually takes place in the LA [1–3], with the most common dual-loop anatomy being a combination of perimitral and roof-dependent re-entry, as discussed above. In the remaining cases, combinations of PV ostia and/or acquired lines of block were most commonly involved. Indeed, the existence of multiple anatomical obstacles and orifices in the LA (mitral annulus, PVs, and left atrial appendage) constitutes a baseline anatomical substrate propitious to the development of re-entry. Acquired conduction blocks from ablation scars, especially when in the vicinity of anatomical obstacles, promote re-entrant tachycardias by forming protected channels/isthmuses delimited on one side by an anatomical obstacle and on the other by the acquired scar. Protected channels enable re-entry by preventing re-entrant wavefronts from colliding laterally with their tail. Such channels commonly involve dual-loop re-entry, with each loop revolving around one of the channel-delimiting obstacles (e.g., mitral annulus and circumferential PV isolation lesions). As a result, the majority of post-AF ablation dual-loop AFLs involve one or two anatomical obstacles, as shown in the present analysis (Table 2) as well as previous series [1,2]. Dual-loop atrial re-entry in patients with a history of cardiac surgery have been predominantly reported as RA re-entry with one CTI-dependent loop and a second peri-atriotomy loop [4,5]. As in post-AF ablation AFL, the predominant substrate of dual-loop re-entry therefore consisted of a iatrogenic block in the vicinity of an anatomical obstacle (the tricuspid annulus). AFL in the absence of iatrogenic atrial scars is rarer and has been infrequently studied. In one study on 223 patients undergoing catheter ablation of left atrial tachycardia, Schaeffer et al. identified 15 (6.7%) patients with LA re-entry and no prior LA-modifying cardiac interventions [6]. The authors report a typical phenotype involving a scar on the anterior LA wall which facilitated re-entry, most commonly in the form of perimitral AFL. In that study, 7 of 15 (47%) patients with "idiopathic" AFL exhibited dual-loop re-entry, all of which consisted of a perimitral loop with a second loop around a scar on the anterior LA. Again, the common underlying substrate was a protected channel formed by an anatomical obstacle and a nearby acquired conduction block. In the study by Derval et al. [2] mentioned above, 16 of 132 (12%) patients had no prior history of cardiac intervention. These patients accounted for 3 of 24 (13%) patients with dual-loop re-entrant atrial tachycardias; detailed anatomy was not reported for this subgroup.

In the present study, isthmuses of dual-loop AFLs exhibited greater minimum width, faster conduction velocity, and higher bipolar electrogram voltage compared to single-loop AFLs. While our sample size is too small for outcome comparisons, ablation targets exhibiting such electrophysiological characteristics have been associated with poorer long-term rhythm outcomes [1,2]. These characteristics may be markers of less vulnerable conduction and therefore less readily ablated targets, as opposed to narrow slow-conducting low-voltage isthmuses [7]. The present findings therefore suggest that, in addition to the anatomical complexity, dual-loop AFLs may be more challenging to ablate due to unfavorable characteristics of potential target isthmuses.

4.2. Implications for Mapping and Catheter Ablation

The present data shows dual-loop re-entry as the most common underlying mechanism of AFL after analysis of complete high-density electroanatomical maps. The prevalence of dual-loop re-entry could be underestimated in clinical practice, since failure to identify dual-loop re-entry may occur despite an apparently complete activation map: documentation of the entire TCL can be achieved by mapping only one of the two re-entry loops. In addition, adequate entrainment mapping criteria with PPI-TCL ≈ 0 ms can be obtained along both loops: average PPI-TCL on secondary isthmuses was -2.6 ± 10.9 ms in the present study. Dual-loop re-entry should therefore be kept in mind as a potential pitfall in AFL mapping. The best strategy to avoid this pitfall may be the systematic acquisition and careful analysis of anatomically complete high-density activation maps.

Given the higher acute efficacy of ablation when targeting the common segment of dual-loop AFLs, as opposed to targeting a secondary isthmus along a side loop, our results suggest that systematic identification of dual-loop re-entry and adequate choice of ablation targets should lead to more selective and efficient ablation strategies. In contrast, incorrect classification of one of two loops as a single-loop re-entry may result in ineffective lesion creation and/or tachycardia modification without termination. Indeed, ablation of a secondary isthmus more frequently resulted in TCL increase or activation sequence modification without tachycardia termination, most commonly due to continuation of the arrhythmia along the second unablated re-entry loop (as illustrated in Figure 4). Most importantly, failure to identify dual-loop re-entry may lead to incomplete elimination of the arrhythmia substrate. Indeed, ablation strategies should take into account the risk of arrhythmia recurrence based on arrhythmia mechanism and individual anatomy. In case of dual-loop re-entry, it appears reasonable to consider anatomically complete elimination of all re-entry loops to optimize long-term rhythm outcomes, e.g., ablation of both the common isthmus and a secondary isthmus or ablation of two secondary isthmuses [5]. In addition, to achieve durable results, lesion sets should consist of complete lines of block made of anatomically contiguous lesions and anchored to anatomical (or electrically silent) obstacles. It should also be noted that perimitral re-entry, which was present in most dual-loop AFLs, has been reported to exhibit a high rate of recurrence after ablation [9]. Complete block along mitral lines can be challenging to obtain and often require epicardial ablations within the CS. Likewise, reconnection has been reported to involve epicardial connections in the majority of recurrences [9].

Recently, Santucci et al. [10] proposed a framework to conceptually unify dual- and single-loop re-entry based on the observation that two distinct critical boundaries (obstacles that border $\geq 90\%$ of TCL) could be identified in all cases of macro-re-entrant atrial tachycardias. From that perspective, when the two boundaries are close to each other, the re-entry mechanism is traditionally classified as dual-loop re-entry, and when the two boundaries are on opposite sides of the chamber, the circuit is traditionally classified as single-loop re-entry. The authors tested an ablation strategy based on creating lesions that connect the two critical boundaries (directly or indirectly via non-critical boundaries) and reported arrhythmia termination in 123 (96%) of 128 cases (including single-loop reentry). While the framework is essentially conceptual in nature, these results highlight the benefit of obtaining complete high-density activation maps of the entire chamber of interest, and of pursing an ablation strategy based on detailed assessment of the complete re-entry circuit.

While the prevention of iatrogenic AFL is beyond the scope of the present study, some insight can be gained from our findings. Given that dual-loop AFL frequently arises in the setting of ablation scars close to anatomical obstacles, one may hypothesize that anchoring ablation lesions to nearby anatomical obstacles could decrease pro-arrhythmia. Likewise, optimizing for durable lines of block through the achievement of irreversible, transmural, anatomically contiguous lesions, may help prevent iatrogenic AFL. However, the effects of such strategies on long-term rhythm outcomes have yet to be determined prospectively.

Given the high prevalence of perimitral re-entry in post-AF ablation AFL (often with a second PV-dependent or roof-dependent loop), mitral isthmus ablation lines, among other lesion sets, have been proposed as an adjunct to PV isolation in AF ablation. Of note, systematic ablation lines (including at the mitral isthmus) at de novo AF ablation have failed to improve overall rhythm outcomes in past randomized trials [11]. Other strategies are currently being evaluated prospectively [12]. Pending further data, our current practical approach to de novo AF ablation involves the individualized assessment of arrhythmia inducibility by atrial burst pacing after PV isolation (primarily to assess AF inducibility and to guide anti-AF substrate modification), and thereafter in a stepwise fashion following AF substrate modification. In the presence of induced sustained AFL, AFL is mapped and targeted for ablation, taking into account AFL anatomy and individual factors such as age and AF type (paroxysmal or persistent).

4.3. Limitations

The main limitation of the present study is its small sample size. In addition, given the observational design, any inference regarding ablation endpoints and implications for ablation strategies should be interpreted with the usual caution. Long-term outcome data is reported for descriptive purposes but cannot be used for meaningful statistical analysis. It should also be noted that the respective value of ablation strategies targeting two isthmuses versus one common isthmus have not been established and remain to be evaluated prospectively.

General technical limitations of electroanatomical mapping systems apply to our study. For example, epicardial activation cannot be mapped endocardially, which may result in incomplete or misleading activation maps. Moreover, automated local activation time annotation, cardiac and respiratory movement filters, and catheter stability filters, are all subject to errors that may lead to inaccuracies.

5. Conclusions

Dual-loop re-entry was the underlying mechanism in more than half of macro-re-entrant atrial tachycardias in patients undergoing catheter ablation of AFL. The most common circuit path involved a perimitral loop with a second roof-dependent loop. Compared to single-loop re-entry, dual-loop re-entry was characterized by isthmuses of greater minimum width, faster conduction velocity, and higher bipolar electrogram voltage. Ablation more frequently resulted in tachycardia termination when targeting an isthmus common to both loops, with a termination rate similar to single-loop AFL ablation. In contrast, ablation of a secondary isthmus on a side loop more frequently resulted in TCL increase or activation sequence modification without arrhythmia termination. Given the high prevalence of dual-loop re-entry and the associated pitfalls, careful assessment of complete activation maps should be included in a systematic approach to AFL mapping. Ablation strategies should consider complete elimination of all re-entrant loops.

Author Contributions: Conceptualization, D.C.S.; Methodology, D.C.S., M.N. and N.J.; Formal Analysis, D.C.S., M.N. and N.J.; Investigation, D.C.S., M.N. and N.J.; Writing—Original Draft Preparation, D.C.S., M.N. and N.J.; Writing—Review & Editing, D.C.S., M.N. and N.J.; Supervision, D.C.S.; Funding Acquisition, D.C.S. All authors have read and agreed to the published version of the manuscript.

Funding: This research received no external funding.

Institutional Review Board Statement: The study was approved by the institutional review board: Commission Cantonale d'Ethique de la Recherche (CCER), Geneva, Switzerland (2018-01802) on 18 October 2018.

Informed Consent Statement: Patient consent was waived due to the retrospective nature of the study.

Data Availability Statement: The original data is not readily available due to privacy concerns.

Conflicts of Interest: N.J.: received educational grants from Biosense Webster. M.N.: none. D.S.: speaker and consultancy honoraria from Biosense Webster, Biotronik, Abbott, and Medtronic.

References

1. Takigawa, M.; Derval, N.; Maury, P.; Martin, R.; Denis, A.; Miyazaki, S.; Yamashita, S.; Frontera, A.; Vlachos, K.; Kitamura, T.; et al. Comprehensive Multicenter Study of the Common Isthmus in Post-Atrial Fibrillation Ablation Multiple-Loop Atrial Tachycardia. *Circ. Arrhythmia Electrophysiol.* **2018**, *11*, e006019. [CrossRef]
2. Derval, N.; Takigawa, M.; Frontera, A.; Mahida, S.; Vlachos, K.; Denis, A.; Duchateau, J.; Pillois, X.; Yamashita, S.; Berte, B.; et al. Characterization of Complex Atrial Tachycardia in Patients With Previous Atrial Interventions Using High-Resolution Mapping. *JACC Clin. Electrophysiol.* **2020**, *6*, 815–826. [CrossRef] [PubMed]
3. Chae, S.; Oral, H.; Good, E.; Dey, S.; Wimmer, A.; Crawford, T.; Wells, D.; Sarrazin, J.-F.; Chalfoun, N.; Kuhne, M.; et al. Atrial Tachycardia After Circumferential Pulmonary Vein Ablation of Atrial Fibrillation: Mechanistic Insights, Results of Catheter Ablation, and Risk Factors for Recurrence. *J. Am. Coll. Cardiol.* **2007**, *50*, 1781–1787. [CrossRef] [PubMed]
4. Seiler, J.; Schmid, D.K.; Irtel, T.A.; Tanner, H.; Rotter, M.; Schwick, N.; Delacrétaz, E. Dual-loop circuits in postoperative atrial macro re-entrant tachycardias. *Heart* **2007**, *93*, 325–330. [CrossRef] [PubMed]
5. Shah, D.; Jaïs, P.; Takahashi, A.; Hocini, M.; Peng, J.T.; Clementy, J.; Haïssaguerre, M. Dual-Loop Intra-Atrial Reentry in Humans. *Circulation* **2000**, *101*, 631–639. [CrossRef] [PubMed]
6. Schaeffer, B.; Akbulak, R.Ö.; Jularic, M.; Moser, J.; Eickholt, C.; Schwarzl, J.M.; Klatt, N.; Kuklik, P.; Meyer, C.; Willems, S. High-Density Mapping and Ablation of Primary Nonfocal Left Atrial Tachycardia: Characterizing a Distinct Arrhythmogenic Substrate. *JACC Clin. Electrophysiol.* **2019**, *5*, 417–426. [CrossRef] [PubMed]
7. Johner, N.; Shah, D.C.; Jousset, F.; Dall'Aglio, P.B.; Namdar, M. Electrophysiological and Anatomical Correlates of Sites With Postpacing Intervals Shorter Than Tachycardia Cycle Length in Atypical Atrial Flutter. *Circ. Arrhythmia Electrophysiol.* **2019**, *12*, e006955. [CrossRef]
8. Laţcu, D.G.; Bun, S.-S.; Viera, F.; Delassi, T.; El Jamili, M.; Al Amoura, A.; Saoudi, N. Selection of Critical Isthmus in Scar-Related Atrial Tachycardia Using a New Automated Ultrahigh Resolution Mapping System. *Circ. Arrhythmia Electrophysiol.* **2017**, *10*, e004510. [CrossRef]
9. Takigawa, M.; Derval, N.; Martin, C.A.; Vlachos, K.; Denis, A.; Nakatani, Y.; Kitamura, T.; Cheniti, G.; Bourier, F.; Lam, A.; et al. Mechanism of Recurrence of Atrial Tachycardia: Comparison Between First Versus Redo Procedures in a High-Resolution Mapping System. *Circ. Arrhythmia Electrophysiol.* **2020**, *13*, e007273. [CrossRef]
10. Santucci, P.A.; Bhirud, A.; Vasaiwala, S.C.; Wilber, D.J.; Green, A. Identification of 2 Distinct Boundaries Distinguishes Critical From Noncritical Isthmuses in Ablating Atypical Atrial Flutter. *JACC Clin. Electrophysiol.* **2024**, *10*, 251–261. [CrossRef] [PubMed]
11. Verma, A.; Jiang, C.; Betts, T.R.; Chen, J.; Deisenhofer, I.; Mantovan, R.; Macle, L.; Morillo, C.A.; Haverkamp, W.; Weerasooriya, R.; et al. Approaches to catheter ablation for persistent atrial fibrillation. *N. Engl. J. Med.* **2015**, *372*, 1812–1822. [CrossRef] [PubMed]
12. Pambrun, T.; Denis, A.; Duchateau, J.; Sacher, F.; Hocini, M.; Jaïs, P.; Haïssaguerre, M.; Derval, N. MARSHALL bundles elimination, Pulmonary veins isolation and Lines completion for ANatomical ablation of persistent atrial fibrillation: MARSHALL-PLAN case series. *J. Cardiovasc. Electrophysiol.* **2019**, *30*, 7–15. [CrossRef] [PubMed]

Journal of
Clinical Medicine

MDPI

Article

Early versus Late Radiofrequency Catheter Ablation in Atrial Fibrillation: Timing Matters

Ahmad A. A. Farghaly [1,2], Hussam Ali [1,*], Pierpaolo Lupo [1], Sara Foresti [1], Guido De Ambroggi [1], Salah Atta [2], Ahmed Abdel-Galeel [2], Aly Tohamy [2] and Riccardo Cappato [1]

1 Arrhythmia & Electrophysiology Center, IRCCS MultiMedica, Sesto San Giovanni, 20099 Milan, Italy; ahmadfarghaly@med.aun.edu.eg (A.A.A.F.); pierpaolo.lupo@multimedica.it (P.L.); sara.foresti@multimedica.it (S.F.); guido.deambroggi@multimedica.it (G.D.A.); riccardo.cappato@multimedica.it (R.C.)

2 Department of Cardiovascular Medicine, Assiut University Heart Hospital, Faculty of Medicine, Assiut University, Assiut 71526, Egypt; salah_s_atta@hotmail.com (S.A.); ahmed.galeel@aun.edu.eg (A.A.-G.); ali.tohamy@gmail.com (A.T.)

* Correspondence: hussamali.ep@gmail.com; Tel.: +39-02-24209400

Abstract: Background: Despite the progressive course of atrial fibrillation (AF), the optimal timing of radiofrequency catheter ablation (RFCA) during disease course is still unknown. We aimed to investigate the impact of early RFCA within a year after AF diagnosis on procedural outcomes. **Methods:** A single-center retrospective study was conducted on symptomatic AF patients (n = 130) referred for RFCA with a 16-month median follow-up. Patients were stratified based on the diagnosis-to-ablation time (DAT) into early (≤1 year) and late (>1 year) RFCA groups. Atrial arrhythmia recurrence after single RFCA was the primary outcome. Secondary outcomes included cardiovascular hospitalizations, AF progression, and antiarrhythmic drug (AAD) use. **Results:** Within a year of AF diagnosis, 33 patients (25.4%) underwent RFCA. In the early-RFCA group, 84.4% of patients did not have recurrent atrial arrhythmia, in contrast to 60.8% in the late-RFCA group ($p = 0.039$). Late RFCA (HR = 2.74, 95% CI = 1.062–7.052, $p = 0.037$) and AF recurrence during the blanking period (HR = 4.57, 95% CI = 2.38–8.57, $p < 0.0001$) were independent predictors of atrial arrhythmia recurrence on multivariate analysis. Compared to the late-RFCA group, the early-RFCA group had significantly lower rates of cardiovascular hospitalizations (18% vs. 42%, $p = 0.023$), AF progression (0.0% vs. 11.3%, $p = 0.044$), and AAD use (45.4% vs. 81.4%, $p < 0.001$). **Conclusions:** Early RFCA within a year of AF diagnosis is associated with less atrial arrhythmia recurrence, fewer cardiovascular hospitalizations, less AF progression, and less AAD use. DAT of more than one year and AF recurrence during the blanking period are independent predictors of atrial arrhythmia recurrence after single RFCA.

Keywords: atrial fibrillation; radiofrequency catheter ablation; diagnosis-to-ablation time; atrial arrhythmia recurrence; cardiovascular hospitalizations; AF progression

1. Introduction

Catheter ablation (CA) is an effective strategy for symptomatic atrial fibrillation (AF) patients, reducing recurrent atrial arrhythmias and cardiovascular hospitalizations [1,2]. However, reported ablation outcomes are still unsatisfactory, with rates of atrial arrhythmia recurrence varying between 20% to 50% at one year post-ablation [3,4].

During the natural course of the disease, structural and electrical remodeling evolve over time and trigger atrial fibrosis, which initiates a vicious cycle of remodeling and promotes AF progression and adversely affects the ablation outcomes [5–7].

According to the recent AF guidelines of the European Society of Cardiology (ESC 2020), CA is recommended (Class I indication) for symptomatic paroxysmal/persistent AF refractory to or intolerant of at least one class I or III antiarrhythmic drug (AAD) [8].

Moreover, CA should be considered (Class IIa indication) as first-line rhythm control therapy (without prior AAD use) in selected patients with symptomatic paroxysmal AF [8]. However, the optimal timing for CA during the disease course is not yet elucidated.

Prior studies have investigated the impact of CA timing on clinical outcomes [2,9–11]. However, the data were contradictory. In our study, we aimed to assess the impact of early radiofrequency CA (RFCA) within one year after AF diagnosis on procedural outcomes, hypothesizing that early RFCA would obviate the vicious cycle of disease progression and improve procedural outcomes.

2. Materials and Methods

2.1. Study Populations

This was a single-center retrospective study. The study enrolled symptomatic AF patients who were intolerant to or had failed AAD referred to our center for RFCA between September 2020 and September 2022 at IRCCS Multimedica hospital, Sesto San Giovanni, Milan, Italy. The follow-up was finished in March 2023. AF diagnosis was established by electrocardiographic documentation of AF, captured on a standard 12-lead ECG, or lasting at least 30 s on Holter ECG recordings [8]. Diagnosis-to-ablation time (DAT) was defined as the time interval between the first documented AF episode and the ablation procedure. Though arbitrary, a 12-month period was considered a reasonable cutoff for the early-ablation group, allowing for a comprehensive clinical assessment of AF patients, their comorbidities, AAD efficacy, and the arrhythmic burden. Patients were stratified based on the DAT into two groups: early-RFCA group (DAT $\leq$ one year) and late-RFCA group (DAT > one year). Eligible patients had paroxysmal or persistent symptomatic AF with $\geq$2 AF episodes over the 6 months before ablation (AF episode defined as $\geq$30 s). Exclusion criteria were (i) previous AF ablation, (ii) long-lasting persistent or permanent AF, (iii) inability to consent, and (iv) age < 18 years old.

2.2. RFCA Protocol

All clinical characteristics (age, sex, and body mass index (BMI)) were addressed. AF type, EHRA class, previous use of rate-control drugs (beta-blockers, calcium channel blockers, and digoxin), and/or rhythm-control drugs (class I, III AAD), and history of electrical cardioversion were reported. History of comorbidities was mentioned. CHA2DS2VASc, CHADS2, and HAS-BLEED scores were calculated for all patients. Trans-thoracic echocardiography was carried out within a week before the procedures to report the left atrial (LA) diameter and left ventricular ejection fraction (LV EF). Transesophageal echocardiography was performed within 24 h before the procedure to exclude the presence of LA thrombi. AADs were stopped 4 to 5 half-lives before ablation. In patients on vitamin K antagonists, ablation was performed under therapeutic INR values of 2 to 3. Direct oral anticoagulants were stopped on the morning of the procedure.

The procedure was performed under general anesthesia. A quadripolar and a decapolar catheter were placed at the His bundle and into the coronary sinus, respectively. Following transseptal puncture, two long sheaths (8.5 F) were advanced into the LA, and then unfractionated heparin was administered to maintain an activated clotting time of 250–300 s during the procedure. Pulmonary venography was performed by injecting contrast during rapid RV pacing. A circular mapping catheter (Lasso 25–15 catheter) was used to record the pulmonary vein potentials. Ablation was performed by elimination of all potentials at the ostium of the pulmonary veins using a 3.5 mm irrigated catheter (ThermoCool SF Bi-Directional Catheter, Biosense Webster, Inc., Irvine, CA, USA).

Successful pulmonary vein isolation (PVI) was defined as complete elimination or dissociation of potentials inside the pulmonary veins guided by the mapping catheter [8]. In patients who were still in AF post-PVI, electrical cardioversion to sinus rhythm was carried out and followed by PVI confirmation. For patients who had documented or induced typical atrial flutter (AFL), a cavo-tricuspid isthmus (CTI) line was placed and followed by confirmation of bidirectional block as an endpoint. Total procedure time (minutes), fluoroscopy time (minutes) and RF duration (minutes) were recorded in the two groups.

During hospitalization post-ablation, a complete clinical examination of all patients was carried out to detect procedural complications. Telemetry and ECG were performed to detect any arrhythmia. Transthoracic echocardiograms were routinely taken to exclude pericardial effusion. Anticoagulation was continued for at least 3 months and stopped thereafter based on the individual CHA2DS2-VASc score. AADs were continued for 3 months and stopped thereafter at the discretion of the referring physician. Patients were discharged one day after the procedure.

2.3. Follow-Up Management

All patients had scheduled outpatient visits at 3, 6, and 12 months post-ablation and then 6 months thereafter with 12-lead ECG and Holter (24–72 h). Between scheduled visits and in cases of symptoms, patients were encouraged to seek the nearest medical facility to document any arrhythmia. Interrogation of implanted devices (pacemakers or implantable loop recorders (ILRs)) was undertaken to assess recurrences.

2.4. Study Endpoints

The primary effectiveness endpoint was freedom from any atrial arrhythmia (atrial arrhythmia, defined as AF, AFL, or atrial tachycardia (AT) that lasted ≥30 s on/off AAD detected by the monitoring tools during the follow-up period excluding the first three months of the blanking period).

The secondary effectiveness endpoints were cardiovascular hospitalization, AF progression and AAD use during the follow-up period.

Cardiovascular hospitalizations were defined as any hospitalizations due to cardiovascular cause, such as AF-related hospitalizations (such as emergency department (ED) visits, repeat ablation, electrical cardioversion and AV nodal ablation), device implantations, and decompensated HF hospitalization, stroke, myocardial infarction, vascular complications and major bleedings.

AF progression was defined as progression from paroxysmal to persistent/permanent AF or persistent to permanent AF [5]. AAD use was defined as AAD use after the blanking period.

The safety endpoint was the absence of procedural complications, including vascular access-related complications (hematomas, femoral artery pseudoaneurysm, arteriovenous fistula), pericardial effusion, cardiac tamponade, pericarditis, transient ischemic attack, embolic stroke, PV stenosis, atrioesophageal fistula, myocardial infarction, and death.

2.5. Statistical Methods

Categorical variables are summarized as frequencies and percentages. Continuous variables are expressed in terms of means ± standard deviation (SD) if normally distributed or median (interquartile range) if abnormally distributed. Differences in variables between groups were analyzed using chi-squared/Fisher's exact test for categorical variables and Z-test or McNemar test for continuous variables. Kaplan–Meier survival analysis was performed using multiple-direction log-rank tests [12]. In the multivariate regression analysis, we included predefined variables, which were age, DAT > 1 year, persistent AF type, LA diameter > 50 mm, and AF recurrence during the blanking period. Selection of the variables based on clinical and published data [13–16]. The adjusted hazard function was estimated using nonparametric smoothing [17]. The confidence interval was 95%, and a p-value ≤ 0.05 was considered statistically significant. All statistical analysis was performed using R-Cran software version 4.3.0. (R Foundation for Statistical Computing, Vienna, Austria).

3. Results

3.1. Baseline Characteristics (Table 1)

We identified 130 symptomatic AF patients who underwent the first RFCA. The mean patient age was 59.2 ± 10.7 years, and 24.6% of patients were female. Thirty-four (26.2%) patients had persistent AF. Structural heart diseases (SHD) were present in 26 (20%) patients. Thirty-three (25.4%) patients had the ablation procedure performed within one year of documented AF diagnosis. For the entire study group, the mean DAT of the whole cohort was 42.99 ± 4.3 months. Mean DAT was 7.6 ± 1.3 months in the early-RFCA group and 55.02 ± 5.2 months in the late-RFCA group. Baseline characteristics were similar in both groups, apart from previous attempts at rhythm control, either by class I, III AADs or by electrical cardioversion (ECV), which more frequently performed in late-RFCA group (82.5% vs. 66.4%, p 0.033 and 52.1% vs. 36.4%, p 0.049, respectively). Median follow-up duration was 16 months (IQR: 10–21).

Table 1. Baseline characteristics.

	Total (n = 130)	Early RFCA (n = 33)	Late RFCA (n = 97)	p-Value
Age (years)	59.15 ± 10.7	57.30 ± 12.7	59.77 ± 9.9	0.256
Diagnosis-to-ablation time (months)	42.99 ± 4.3	7.64 ± 1.3	55.02 ± 5.2	<0.001
Sex				
• Female	32 (24.6%)	10 (30.3%)	22 (22.7%)	0.380
BMI	26.72 ± 3.6	25.87 ± 4.1	27.03 ± 3.4	0.164
Blood Pressure				
• SBP	126.98 ± 11.7	125.76 ± 10.8	128.83 ± 13.6	0.201
• DBP	76.04 ± 12.2	74.48 ± 13.6	77.63 ± 11.4	0.242
GFR	86.75 ± 15.9	89.42 ± 16.7	84.44 ± 15.2	0.116
Comorbidity				
• DM	5 (3.8%)	3 (9.1%)	2 (2.1%)	0.103
• HTN	71 (54.6%)	16 (48.5%)	55 (56.7%)	0.413
• IHD	10 (7.7%)	1 (3%)	9 (9.3%)	0.224
• History of CHF	7 (5.4%)	3 (9.1%)	4 (4.2%)	0.273
• SHD	27 (20%)	5 (18.2%)	21 (20.6%)	0.762
• OSAS	4 (3.1%)	1 (3%)	3 (3.1%)	0.733
• History of stroke	9 (7%)	2 (6.1%)	7 (7.3%)	0.584
AF type				
• PAF	96 (73.8%)	26 (78.8%)	70 (72.2%)	0.455
CHA2DS2-VASc score				
• 0	36 (27.7%)	11 (33.3%)	25 (25.8%)	
• 1	36 (27.7%)	7 (21.2%)	29 (29.9%)	
• 2	34 (26.2%)	9 (27.3%)	25 (25.8%)	0.472
• 3	20 (15.4%)	4 (12.1%)	16 (16.5%)	
• 4	4 (3.1%)	2 (6.1%)	2 (2.1%)	
✓ Mean ± SD	1.38 ± 1.1	1.36 ± 1.2	1.39 ± 1.1	0.909
CHADS2 score				
• 0	50 (38.5%)	15 (45.5%)	35 (36.1%%	
• 1	64 (49.2%)	11 (33.3%)	53 (54.6%)	0.112
• 2	9 (6.9%)	4 (12.1%)	5 (5.2%)	
• 3	7 (5.4%)	3 (9.1%)	4 (4.1%)	
✓ Mean ± SD	0.79 ± 0.79	0.85 ± 0.97	0.77 ± 0.97	0.932

Table 1. *Cont.*

	Total (n = 130)	Early RFCA (n = 33)	Late RFCA (n = 97)	p-Value
HAS-BLED score				
• 0	68 (52.3%)	20 (60.6%)	48 (49.5%)	
• 1	51 (39.2%)	10 (30.3%)	41 (42.3%)	0.245
• 2	11 (8.5%)	3 (9.1%)	8 (8.2%)	
✓ Mean ± SD	0.56 ± 0.6	0.48 ± 0.7	0.59 ± 0.6	0.444
LA Diameter	39.66 ± 3.9	39.33 ± 3.8	40.44 ± 4.1	0.198
LVEF%	60.75 ± 15.9	59.05 ± 5.8	60.52 ± 4.2	0.127
Beta-blocker use	46 (35.4%)	11 (33.3%)	35 (36.1%)	0.775
CCB use	16 (12.3%)	3 (9.1%)	13 (13.4%)	0.518
Class I, III AAD use	105 (80.7%)	23 (69.7%)	82 (84.5%)	0.033
ACEI use	69 (53.1%)	15 (45.5%)	54 (55.7%)	0.312
Statin use	30 (23.1%)	6 (18.2%)	24 (24.7%)	0.479
MRA	3 (2.31%)	1 (3.03%)	2 (2.02%)	0.738
Previous electrical CV	62 (48.1%)	12 (36.4%)	50 (52.1%)	0.049
Follow-up duration	16.32 ± 6.632	16.39 ± 6.324	16.21 ± 6.622	0.975

AAD, antiarrhythmic drug; ACEI, angiotensin-converting enzyme inhibitor; BMI, body mass index; CCB, calcium channel blocker; CHF, congestive heart failure; CV, cardioversion; DBP, diastolic blood pressure; DM, diabetes mellitus; GFR, glomerular filtration rate; HTN, hypertension; LA, left atrium; LVEF, left ventricular ejection fraction; IHD, ischemic heart disease; MRA, mineralocorticoid receptor agonist; OSAS, obstructive sleep apnea; PAF, paroxysmal atrial fibrillation; SBP, systolic blood pressure; SHD, structural heart disease.

3.2. Procedural Characteristics

Successful PVI was achieved in all patients. CTI ablation was performed in nine (6.9%) patients with documented atrial flutter. Total RF and fluoroscopy times were significantly lower in the early-RFCA group than in the late-RFCA group (25.38 ± 6.4 vs. 30.56 ± 5.1, p 0.012, 35.88 ± 3.5 vs. 44.48 ± 2.2, p 0.031, respectively).

3.3. Follow-Up Rhythm Monitoring (Table 2)

Post-ablation rhythm monitoring was performed with intermittent monitoring (Holter 24–72 h) in the majority of patients (90.8%) and with continuous cardiac monitoring (including ILR or permanent pacemaker) in the rest of the patients (9.2%). The proportion of ICM and Holter monitoring did not show significant differences between the groups.

Table 2. Follow-up rhythm monitoring.

	Total (n = 130)	Early RFCA (n = 33)	Late RFCA (n = 97)	p-Value
• Holter	118 (90.8%)	30 (90.9%)	88 (90.7)	=0.822
• ICM	12 (9.2%)	3 (9.1%)	9 (9.3%)	

ICM, implantable cardiac monitoring.

3.4. Outcomes

3.4.1. Primary Outcome

Documented atrial arrhythmia occurred in 43 patients (33.11%) of the whole cohort. The atrial arrhythmia-free rate was significantly higher in the early-RFCA group than in the late-RFCA group (84.8% vs. 60.8%, p 0.039) (Figure 1).

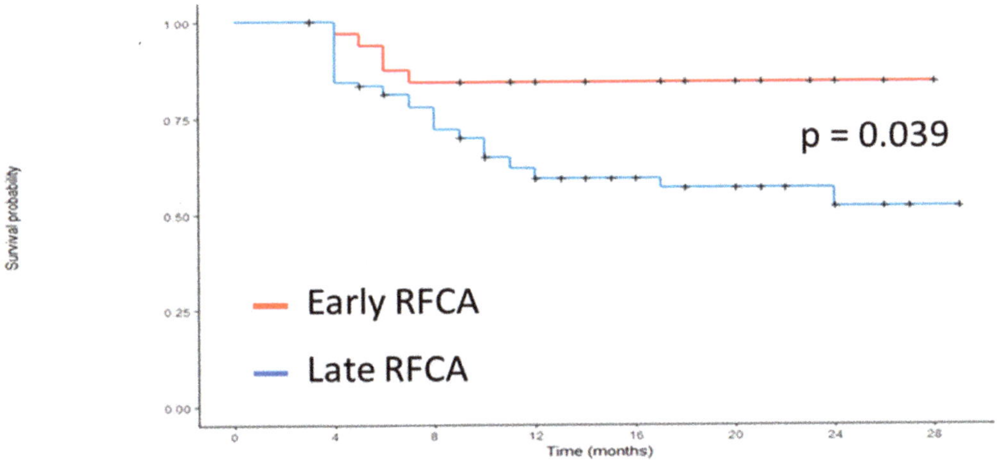

Figure 1. Arrhythmia-free survival after RFAC between early- and late-RFCA groups. RFCA, radiofrequency catheter ablation.

Predictors of Atrial Arrhythmia Recurrence (Table 3)

Using univariate Cox regression analysis, atrial arrhythmia recurrence was significantly associated with age $\geq$ 65 years, DAT > 1 year, persistent AF, CHADS2VASC score $\geq$ 2 and AF recurrence during the blanking period. On multivariate analysis, late RFCA (DAT > 1 year) (HR 2.74, 95% CI 1.062–7.052, *p* 0.037) and AF recurrence during the blanking period (HR 4.57, 95% CI 2.38–8.57, *p* 0.0001) were independent predictors of atrial arrhythmia recurrence after a single AF ablation procedure.

Table 3. Cox regression analysis for prediction of atrial arrhythmia recurrence.

	Univariate Analysis			Multivariate Analysis		
Predictors	**HR**	**95% CI**	***p* Value**	**HR**	**95% CI**	***p* Value**
Age $\geq$ 65	2.238	1.23–4.071	0.008	1.582	0.696–3.616	0.296
DAT (>1 year)	3.001	1.182–7.632	0.021	2.737	1.062–7.052	0.037
Sex (Female)	1.359	0.694–2.659	0.372			
BMI	0.994	0.854–1.104	0.998			
Persistent AF	2.181	1.182–4.022	0.012	1.373	0.649–2.902	0.407
Hypertension	1.139	0.623–2.08	0.672			
DM	1.142	0.764–1.042	0.445			
Ischemic heart disease	0.493	0.119–2.045	0.332			
Heart failure	0.981	0.237–4.061	0.984			
Left ventricular hypertrophy	0.796	0.245–2.579	0.704			
CHADS score $\geq$ 2	1.663	0.73–3.74	0.219			
CHA2DS2VASC score $\geq$ 2	2.251	1.223–4.153	0.001	1.399	0.628–7.133	0.411
Left atrial diameter $\geq$ 50 mm	2.875	0.887–9.318	0.08	1.268	0.359–4.607	0.699
LVEF < 50%	0.988	0.135–7.202	0.991			
AF recurrence during blanking	4.592	2.491–8.466	<0.01	4.517	2.380–8.571	<0.0001

CI, confidence interval; HR, hazard ratio.

3.4.2. Secondary Outcomes (Table 4)

Compared to the late-RFCA group, the early-RFCA group had significantly fewer all cardiovascular hospitalizations (18.2% vs. 42.3%, p 0.023) and lower AAD use (39.4% vs. 77.3%, $p < 0.001$) after a median 16 months of follow-up. AF progression occurred in 11 patients (8.4%) and was observed only in the late-RFCA group. AF progressed from paroxysmal to persistent AF in ten patients, and one patient had progression from persistent to permanent AF. Late RFCA showed a significantly higher rate of AF progression compared to early RFCA (11.3% vs. 0%, p 0.044). No differences were observed in electrical cardioversion (4% vs. 9.3%, p 0.89), emergency department AF-related visits (0.0% vs. 8.2%, p 0.19), or repeat ablation (6.1% vs. 19.6%, p 0.12) between the groups.

Table 4. Secondary outcomes.

	Total (n = 130)	Early RFCA (n = 33)	Late RFCA (n = 97)	p-Value
All cardiovascular hospitalizations	47 (36.2%)	6 (18.2%)	41 (42.3%)	=0.023
Repeat ablation	21 (16.2%)	2 (6.1%)	19 (19.6%)	=0.123
Redo electrical cardioversion	13 (10%)	4 (12.1%)	9 (9.3%)	=0.891
Emergency department AF hospitalizations	8 (6.2%)	0 (0%)	8 (8.2%)	=0.199
AF-related hospitalizations	42 (32.3%)	6 (18.2%)	36 (37.1%)	=0.071
Non-AF-related hospitalizations Pacemaker for bradycardia, 2 cases of HF, PVC ablation and major bleeding	5 (3.1%)	0 (0%)	5 (4.1%)	=0.582
AAD use	94 (72.3%)	15 (45.4)	79 (81.4)	<0.001
AF progression	11 (8.5%)	0 (0%)	11 (11.3%)	=0.044

PVC, premature ventricular contraction.

3.4.3. Safety Outcomes

Two arteriovenous fistulae were reported in 2 patients (1.5%, one complication in each group). Both complications were managed conservatively and did not require surgical intervention, but the hospital stay had been prolonged. There were no serious complications, as there were no cardiac tamponades or atrioesophageal fistulae detected.

4. Discussion

The present study complements the current body of evidence by assessing the influence of DAT on atrial arrhythmia recurrence, AF progression, and hard clinical outcomes such as cardiovascular hospitalizations. A real-world cohort of patients was enrolled and included both paroxysmal and persistent AF types in the presence or absence of structural heart diseases. Furthermore, to mitigate the influence of selection bias on the ablation timing reported in the previous retrospective studies [18–21], which was left to the discretion of the referring physician, the current study included only symptomatic AF patients with two or more AF episodes during the last six months before ablation.

The main findings are as follows. (I) Early RFCA within one year after the first documented AF is associated with less atrial arrhythmia recurrence, cardiovascular hospitalizations, AF progression, and AAD use. (II) Longer DAT (>one year) and AF recurrence during the blanking period are the only independent predictors of atrial tachyarrhythmia recurrence after single RFCA.

4.1. Early RFCA and Atrial Arrhythmia Recurrence

Early RFCA was associated with significantly lower incidence of arrhythmia recurrence, consistent with prior retrospective studies [18–21]. Assessment of RFCA timing has been studied previously by Kawaji et al. [18], where patients were divided into two groups based on DAT: short (≤3 years) DAT (n = 675) and long (≥3 years) DAT (n = 531) with a 5-year mean follow-up. Radiofrequency PVI and CTI ablation were routinely performed for all patients. Notably, the long-DAT-group patients had more history of CHF and stroke. In our study, one year was used as a cutoff to define the early-RFCA group. Patients had comparable baseline characteristics (age), risk factors (CHF and stroke), and AF types in both groups. Additionally, CTI ablation was performed only in patients who had clinically documented or induced atrial flutter.

The impact of DAT on AF recurrence has been recently investigated to demonstrate the upper and lower DAT thresholds [19]. De Greef et al. recommended performing CA within 3 years after first AF diagnosis, where the shorter the DAT (≤3 years), the better the outcome. However, when DAT exceeds three years, it becomes clinically irrelevant. According to De Greef's study, all patients had scheduled visits every six months (only physical examination and ECG were performed). Also, unscheduled visits were conducted if symptoms occurred. In cases of symptoms, ECG, Holter monitoring (1 to 7 days), or event recording was used to report any related arrhythmia. Therefore, the follow-up assessment of asymptomatic recurrences was undetected. In our study, Holter monitoring (1–3 days) was performed in 90% of patients at 3, 6, 12 months, and then every 6 months during follow-up. Continuous cardiac monitoring (cardiac pacemakers and ILR) was used in approximately 10% of our patients. Thus, more precise detection of both asymptomatic and symptomatic recurrent atrial arrhythmia was possible by the use of different monitoring strategies in our study.

In a newly published prospective, randomized, multicenter study of symptomatic paroxysmal and persistent AF patients, an early-ablation strategy (within 1 month post-recruitment) was compared to a delayed ablation strategy (after 12 months post-recruitment, during which AADs were optimized) [22]. Both strategies had similar arrhythmia-free survival, median AF burden, and AAD use at 12 months. The PVI timing was based on the time of referral, not the time of the first AF diagnosis (DAT), as in our study. The study did not report the DAT in the groups. DAT is an evolving indicator of the status of atrial substrate and electrical and structural remodeling that progress during the AF course [5,23]. Missing such a parameter limits the ability to evaluate the procedural outcomes. Moreover, the early-ablation group included patients who had a history of stroke and a higher CHA2DS2VASc score. This could partially explain the lack of difference in ablation outcomes between the groups. In addition, the study did not report the impact of DAT on cardiovascular hospitalizations or AF progression.

4.2. Early RFCA and Secondary Effectiveness Outcomes

The early-RFCA group had significantly fewer cardiovascular hospitalizations compared to the late-RFCA group at a median follow-up of 16 months. Kawaji et al. found the same finding at a longer 5-year follow-up [18]. These findings are in line with the EAST—AFNET 4 trial [24], which supports the initiation of a rhythm-control strategy over a rate-control strategy in reducing hard cardiovascular endpoints (composite risk of cardiovascular death, stroke, or hospitalization for worsening HF or acute coronary syndrome) when applied early (<1 year) during the AF course after a median of 5.1 years of follow-up. However, patients in our cohort were younger and with lower stroke risk (59.15 ± 10.7 years and mean CHA2DS2VASc score 1.38 ± 1.1 in our study vs. 70.2 ± 8.4 years and mean CHA2DS2VASc score 3.4 ± 1.3 in the EAST—AFNET 4 trial). Furthermore, patients who receive RFCA within one year after AF diagnosis are less likely to experience worsening of their medical condition or complications (heart failure, arrhythmia) that may require hospitalizations. In addition, the higher rate of AAD use after ablation might be attributable to longer DAT and higher symptom burden post-ablation (as evident by higher ED visits) in the late-RFCA group.

Repeat RFCA was performed in 21 patients (16.2% of all patients). Reconnected pulmonary veins were found in all patients who underwent repeat RFCA. Three patients in the late-RFCA group also experienced left atrial flutter, which could be attributed to the advanced stage of atrial electrical and structural remodeling among these patients.

Despite being underreported in the literature, the rate of AF progression following CA is an important parameter in the management of AF disease. AF progression is altered by CA, either as an initial rhythm control strategy [25] or after attempts of failed AAD [26]. Interestingly, our study reveals that AF progression was not reported when RFCA was conducted early, but did occur when RFCA was performed more than a year after AF diagnosis. To the best of our knowledge, our study is the first to evaluate the impact of PVI timing on the rate of AF progression in a group of young AF patients with relatively low stroke risk. The 2023 American Heart Association (AHA)–American College of Cardiology (ACC)–Heart Rhythm Society (HRS) AF guidelines recommend performing CA in this group of patients (younger patients with few comorbidities) not only to improve symptoms but also to reduce progression [27]. Wijffels et al. described the "AF begets AF" concept, illustrating potential mechanisms that promote AF initiation, maintenance, and progression [28]. Shortening, spatial dispersion of atrial refractoriness, ion channel dysfunction and slowing of intra-atrial conduction induced by AF itself are major modulators linked to the atrial substrate that promote AF remodeling and fibrosis [28]. Therefore, early restoration and maintenance of sinus rhythm may represent a plausible explanation of the substantially low rate of AF progression in the early-RFCA group in our study. Consequently, initiating and intensifying an effective rhythm-control strategy via early RFCA is crucial to break the vicious cycle of AF progression, especially in younger AF patients with few comorbidities.

4.3. Early RCFA and Safety Outcomes

Despite the growing evidence in favor of adopting an early-ablation strategy during the course of AF disease [2,5], translation into clinical practice may encounter a major concern regarding patient safety. Procedure-related complications should always be considered [8]. We found two small arteriovenous fistulae (1.5%, one fistula in each group), which were managed conservatively. The rate of such complications is comparable to the reported rate (~1%) in a worldwide survey on the safety of CA of AF [29]. In our study, neither mortality nor serious adverse events such as esophageal fistulae or cardiac tamponade were reported.

4.4. DAT as a Predictor of Atrial Arrhythmia Recurrence after Single RFCA

Our study emphasizes the significance of performing PVI early during the AF course, as DAT of more than one year is the only pre-procedural predictor of atrial arrhythmia recurrence. The more frequent and longer the AF episodes, the more cumulative atrial remodeling. These atrial structural and electrical abnormalities render the CA ineffective [5]. In addition, our findings are consistent with an umbrella review of meta-analyses on the predictors of AF recurrence after CA [30]. Of the 28 associations studied between CA and the risk of arrhythmia recurrence, only a DAT of over a year provided highly suggestive evidence [30]. This lends credence to AF being a key driver of atrial remodeling; thus, early RFCA could improve procedural outcomes and halt AF progression.

4.5. Clinical Implications

Our findings may provide valuable insights to optimize patient care by improving clinical practice. Attempts to use more than one AAD should not delay the decision of referral for RFCA. Among the known predictors of worse AF ablation outcomes, such as persistent AF, time to RFCA is a prompt, convenient, and easily adjustable predictor to improve ablation outcomes. Moreover, data-driven approaches have the potential to improve health-care delivery by making it more efficient and effective.

5. Limitations

Different limitations should be addressed. Firstly, our study enrolled a group of relatively young AF patients with few comorbidities. Therefore, our findings should be interpreted with caution when considering older AF patients with multiple comorbidities. Secondly, it is important to acknowledge that administration of mineralocorticoid receptor agonists (MRAs) and sodium–glucose cotransporter 2 (SGLT2) inhibitors lowers the risk of atrial arrhythmia recurrence following AF ablation [31,32]. These beneficial effects received less attention in our analysis. Thirdly, less than 10% of patients had ICMs that are known to provide more accurate detection of AF recurrences, particularly asymptomatic episodes. Nonetheless, the proportion of ICM monitoring did not differ between the groups and was unlikely to affect the findings of our study. Additionally, unmeasured variables (such as patient preference, COVID infection, the need for COVID vaccination, and regional access to ablation-capable centers) could not be excluded and might influence DAT. Despite this, our study suggests that DAT is a reliable predictor of ablation outcomes. Lastly, this study did not incorporate LA parameters using cardiac magnetic resonance or speckle tracking echocardiography. Such advanced imaging modalities can provide valuable data regarding LA function and fibrosis [7] that may influence AF recurrence and progression.

6. Conclusions

Early RFCA within one year of AF diagnosis is associated with less atrial arrhythmia recurrence, cardiovascular hospitalizations, AF progression, and AAD use. Longer DAT (>1 year) and AF recurrence during the blanking period are independent predictors of atrial tachyarrhythmia recurrence after single RFCA.

Author Contributions: Conceptualization, A.A.A.F., S.A. and R.C.; methodology, A.A.-G. and A.T.; software, A.A.-G.; validation, G.D.A.; formal analysis, G.D.A.; investigation, S.F.; resources, S.F.; data curation, H.A. and P.L.; writing—original draft, A.A.A.F.; writing—review and editing, H.A.; supervision, S.A. and R.C. All authors have read and agreed to the published version of the manuscript.

Funding: This research did not receive any specific grant from funding agencies in the public, commercial, or not-for-profit sectors.

Institutional Review Board Statement: The study was approved by the institutional review board of the Faculty of Medicine at Assiut University, Assiut, Egypt (IRB 17200460 on 19 July 2020), and followed the World Medical Association's Declaration of Helsinki.

Informed Consent Statement: All patients enrolled in the study provided written informed consent for participation.

Data Availability Statement: Data are available upon reasonable request.

Conflicts of Interest: The authors declare no conflict of interest.

References

1. Asad, Z.U.A.; Yousif, A.; Khan, M.S.; Al-Khatib, S.M.; Stavrakis, S. Catheter Ablation Versus Medical Therapy for Atrial Fibrillation. *Circ. Arrhythmia Electrophysiol.* **2019**, *12*, e007414. [CrossRef] [PubMed]
2. Kheiri, B.; Simpson, T.F.; Przybylowicz, R.; Merrill, M.; Alhamoud, H.; Osman, M.; Dalouk, K.; Stecker, E.; Henrikson, C.A.; Nazer, B. Ablation versus Antiarrhythmic Drugs as First-Line Treatment of Paroxysmal Atrial Fibrillation: A Meta-Analysis of Randomized Trials. *Circ. Arrhythmia Electrophysiol.* **2021**, *14*, e009692. [CrossRef] [PubMed]
3. Pallisgaard, J.L.; Gislason, G.H.; Hansen, J.; Johannessen, A.; Torp-Pedersen, C.; Rasmussen, P.V.; Hansen, M.L. Temporal trends in atrial fibrillation recurrence rates after ablation between 2005 and 2014: A nationwide Danish cohort study. *Eur. Heart J.* **2017**, *39*, 442–449. [CrossRef] [PubMed]

4. Lévy, S.; Steinbeck, G.; Santini, L.; Nabauer, M.; Maceda, D.P.; Kantharia, B.K.; Saksena, S.; Cappato, R. Management of atrial fibrillation: Two decades of progress—A scientific statement from the European Cardiac Arrhythmia Society. *J. Interv. Card. Electrophysiol.* **2022**, *65*, 287–326. [CrossRef]
5. Gunawardene, M.A.; Willems, S. Atrial fibrillation progression and the importance of early treatment for improving clinical outcomes. *Europace* **2022**, *24* (Suppl. S2), ii22–ii28. [CrossRef] [PubMed]
6. Heijman, J.; Voigt, N.; Nattel, S.; Dobrev, D. Cellular and Molecular Electrophysiology of Atrial Fibrillation Initiation, Maintenance, and Progression. *Circ. Res.* **2014**, *114*, 1483–1499. [CrossRef] [PubMed]
7. Rivner, H.; Mitrani, R.D.; Goldberger, J.J. Atrial Myopathy Underlying Atrial Fibrillation. *Arrhythmia Electrophysiol. Rev.* **2020**, *9*, 61–70. [CrossRef] [PubMed]
8. Hindricks, G.; Potpara, T.; Dagres, N.; Arbelo, E.; Bax, J.J.; Blomström-Lundqvist, C.; Boriani, G.; Castella, M.; Dan, J.-A.; Dilaveris, P.E.; et al. 2020 ESC Guidelines for the diagnosis and management of atrial fibrillation developed in collaboration with the European Association for Cardio-Thoracic Surgery (EACTS): The Task Force for the diagnosis and management of atrial fibrillation of the European Society of Cardiology (ESC) Developed with the special contribution of the European Heart Rhythm Association (EHRA) of the ESC. *Eur. Heart J.* **2021**, *42*, 373–498. [CrossRef] [PubMed]
9. Bunch, T.J.; May, H.T.; Bair, T.L.; Johnson, D.L.; Weiss, J.P.; Crandall, B.G.; Osborn, J.S.; Anderson, J.L.; Muhlestein, J.B.; Lappe, D.L.; et al. Increasing time between first diagnosis of atrial fibrillation and catheter ablation adversely affects long-term outcomes. *Heart Rhythm* **2013**, *10*, 1257–1262. [CrossRef]
10. Lunati, M.; Arena, G.; Iacopino, S.; Verlato, R.; Tondo, C.; Curnis, A.; Porcellini, S.; Sciarra, L.; Molon, G.; Senatore, G.; et al. Is the time between first diagnosis of paroxysmal atrial fibrillation and cryoballoon ablation a predictor of efficacy? *J. Cardiovasc. Med.* **2018**, *19*, 446–452. [CrossRef]
11. Stout, K.; Almerstani, M.; Adomako, R.; Shin, D.; Aroudaky, A.; Tandon, H.; Alziadin, N.; Schleifer, J.W.; Payne, J.; Easley, A.; et al. Prevalence and Impact of Poorly Controlled Modifiable Risk Factors Among Patients Who Underwent Atrial Fibrillation Ablation. *Am. J. Cardiol.* **2023**, *198*, 38–46. [CrossRef] [PubMed]
12. Ditzhaus, M.; Friedrich, S. More powerful logrank permutation tests for two-sample survival data. *J. Stat. Comput. Simul.* **2020**, *90*, 2209–2227. [CrossRef]
13. Kornej, J.; Hindricks, G.; Shoemaker, M.B.; Husser, D.; Arya, A.; Sommer, P.; Rolf, S.; Saavedra, P.; Kanagasundram, A.; Whalen, S.P.; et al. The APPLE score: A novel and simple score for the prediction of rhythm outcomes after catheter ablation of atrial fibrillation. *Clin. Res. Cardiol.* **2015**, *104*, 871–876. [CrossRef] [PubMed]
14. Lycke, M.; Kyriakopoulou, M.; El Haddad, M.; Wielandts, J.-Y.; Hilfiker, G.; Almorad, A.; Strisciuglio, T.; De Pooter, J.; Wolf, M.; Unger, P.; et al. Predictors of recurrence after durable pulmonary vein isolation for paroxysmal atrial fibrillation. *Europace* **2021**, *23*, 861–867. [CrossRef] [PubMed]
15. D'Ascenzo, F.; Corleto, A.; Biondi-Zoccai, G.; Anselmino, M.; Ferraris, F.; di Biase, L.; Natale, A.; Hunter, R.; Schilling, R.; Miyazaki, S.; et al. Which are the most reliable predictors of recurrence of atrial fibrillation after transcatheter ablation?: A meta-analysis. *Int. J. Cardiol.* **2013**, *167*, 1984–1989. [CrossRef] [PubMed]
16. Li, Z.; Wang, S.; Hidru, T.H.; Sun, Y.; Gao, L.; Yang, X.; Xia, Y. Long Atrial Fibrillation Duration and Early Recurrence Are Reliable Predictors of Late Recurrence After Radiofrequency Catheter Ablation. *Front. Cardiovasc. Med.* **2022**, *9*, 864417. [CrossRef]
17. Rebora, P.; Salim, A.; Reilly, M. Bshazard: A flexible tool for nonparametric smoothing of the hazard function. *R J.* **2014**, *6*, 114–122. [CrossRef]
18. Kawaji, T.; Shizuta, S.; Yamagami, S.; Aizawa, T.; Komasa, A.; Yoshizawa, T.; Kato, M.; Yokomatsu, T.; Miki, S.; Ono, K.; et al. Early choice for catheter ablation reduced readmission in management of atrial fibrillation: Impact of diagnosis-to-ablation time. *Int. J. Cardiol.* **2019**, *291*, 69–76. [CrossRef]
19. De Greef, Y.; Bogaerts, K.; Sofianos, D.; Buysschaert, I. Impact of Diagnosis-to-Ablation Time on AF Recurrence: Pronounced the First 3 Years, Irrelevant Thereafter. *JACC Clin. Electrophysiol.* **2023**, *9*, 2263–2272. [CrossRef]
20. De Greef, Y.; Schwagten, B.; Chierchia, G.B.; de Asmundis, C.; Stockman, D.; Buysschaert, I. Diagnosis-to-ablation time as a predictor of success: Early choice for pulmonary vein isolation and long-term outcome in atrial fibrillation: Results from the Middelheim-PVI Registry. *Europace* **2018**, *20*, 589–595. [CrossRef]
21. Hussein, A.A.; Saliba, W.I.; Barakat, A.; Bassiouny, M.; Chamsi-Pasha, M.; Al-Bawardy, R.; Hakim, A.; Tarakji, K.; Baranowski, B.; Cantillon, D.; et al. Radiofrequency ablation of persistent atrial fibrillation: Diagnosis-to-ablation time, markers of pathways of atrial remodeling, and outcomes. *Circ. Arrhythmia Electrophysiol.* **2016**, *9*, e003669. [CrossRef] [PubMed]
22. Kalman, J.M.; Al-Kaisey, A.M.; Parameswaran, R.; Hawson, J.; Anderson, R.D.; Lim, M.; Chieng, D.; A Joseph, S.; McLellan, A.; Morton, J.B.; et al. Impact of early vs. delayed atrial fibrillation catheter ablation on atrial arrhythmia recurrences. *Eur. Heart J.* **2023**, *44*, 2447–2454. [CrossRef] [PubMed]
23. Chew, D.S.; Jones, K.A.; Loring, Z.; Black-Maier, E.; Noseworthy, P.A.; Exner, D.V.; Packer, D.L.; Grant, J.; Mark, D.B.; Piccini, J.P. Diagnosis-to-ablation time predicts recurrent atrial fibrillation and rehospitalization following catheter ablation. *Heart Rhythm. O^2* **2021**, *3*, 23–31. [CrossRef] [PubMed]
24. Kirchhof, P.; Camm, A.J.; Goette, A.; Brandes, A.; Eckardt, L.; Elvan, A.; Fetsch, T.; van Gelder, I.C.; Haase, D.; Haegeli, L.M.; et al. Early Rhythm-Control Therapy in Patients with Atrial Fibrillation. *N. Engl. J. Med.* **2020**, *383*, 1305–1316. [CrossRef] [PubMed]
25. Andrade, J.G.; Deyell, M.W.; Macle, L.; Wells, G.A.; Bennett, M.; Essebag, V.; Champagne, J.; Roux, J.-F.; Yung, D.; Skanes, A.; et al. Progression of Atrial Fibrillation after Cryoablation or Drug Therapy. *N. Engl. J. Med.* **2023**, *388*, 105–116. [CrossRef] [PubMed]

26. Kuck, K.-H.; Lebedev, D.S.; Mikhaylov, E.N.; Romanov, A.; Gellér, L.; Kalējs, O.; Neumann, T.; Davtyan, K.; On, Y.K.; Popov, S.; et al. Catheter ablation or medical therapy to delay progression of atrial fibrillation: The randomized controlled atrial fibrillation progression trial (ATTEST). *Europace* **2021**, *23*, 362–369. [CrossRef] [PubMed]
27. Joglar, J.A.; Chung, M.K.; Armbruster, A.L.; Benjamin, E.J.; Chyou, J.Y.; Cronin, E.M.; Deswal, A.; Eckhardt, L.L.; Goldberger, Z.D.; Gopinathannair, R.; et al. 2023 ACC/AHA/ACCP/HRS Guideline for the Diagnosis and Management of Atrial Fibrillation: A Report of the American College of Cardiology/American Heart Association Joint Committee on Clinical Practice Guidelines. *Circulation* **2024**, *149*, e1–e156. [CrossRef] [PubMed]
28. Wijffels, M.C.; Kirchhof, C.J.; Dorland, R.; Allessie, M.A. Atrial fibrillation begets atrial fibrillation. A study in awake chronically instrumented goats. *Circulation* **1995**, *92*, 1954–1968. [CrossRef] [PubMed]
29. Cappato, R.; Calkins, H.; Chen, S.-A.; Davies, W.; Iesaka, Y.; Kalman, J.; Kim, Y.-H.; Klein, G.; Packer, D.; Skanes, A. Worldwide survey on the methods, efficacy, and safety of catheter ablation for human atrial fibrillation. *Circulation* **2005**, *111*, 1100–1105. [CrossRef]
30. Charitakis, E.; Dragioti, E.; Stratinaki, M.; Korela, D.; Tzeis, S.; Almroth, H.; Liuba, I.; Jönsson, A.H.; Charalambous, G.; O Karlsson, L.; et al. Predictors of recurrence after catheter ablation and electrical cardioversion of atrial fibrillation: An umbrella review of meta-analyses. *Europace* **2023**, *25*, 40–48. [CrossRef]
31. Karakasis, P.; Patoulias, D.; Popovic, D.S.; Pamporis, K.; Theofilis, P.; Nasoufidou, A.; Stachteas, P.; Samaras, A.; Tzikas, A.; Giannakoulas, G.; et al. Effects of mineralocorticoid receptor antagonists on new-onset or recurrent atrial fibrillation: A Bayesian and frequentist network meta-analysis of randomized trials. *Curr. Probl. Cardiol.* **2024**, *49*, 102742. [CrossRef] [PubMed]
32. Stachteas, P.; Karakasis, P.; Karagiannidis, E.; Patoulias, D.; Athanasiadou, P.; Nasoufidou, A.; Papadopoulos, C.; Kassimis, G.; Fragakis, N. Efficacy of sodium-glucose cotransporter 2 inhibitors in preventing atrial fibrillation recurrence after catheter ablation. *Hell. J. Cardiol.* **2024**, *in press*. [CrossRef] [PubMed]

Journal of
Clinical Medicine

MDPI

Article

LA PULSE: Evaluating Left Atrial Function Pre- and Post-Atrial Fibrillation Ablation Using PULSEd Field Ablation

Noha Mahrous [1,*], Florian Blaschke [2,3], Doreen Schöppenthau [2], Gerhard Hindricks [2,3], Leif-Hendrik Boldt [2,3] and Abdul Shokor Parwani [2,3]

1 Department of Cardiothoracic and Vascular Surgery, Deutsches Herzzentrum Der Charité, 13353 Berlin, Germany
2 Department of Cardiology, Angiology and Intensive Care Medicine, Deutsches Herzzentrum Der Charité, 13353 Berlin, Germany
3 DZHK—German Center for Cardiovascular Research, 10785 Berlin, Germany
* Correspondence: noha.mahrous@charite.de

Abstract: Background: Atrial fibrillation (AF) is a common cardiac arrhythmia associated with left atrial dysfunction. The impact of pulmonary vein isolation (PVI) using pulsed field ablation (PFA) on left atrial function has not been previously quantified. This study aims to evaluate the effects of PVI using PFA on left atrial function in patients with AF. **Methods**: Thirty-four patients undergoing PVI with PFA between July 2022 and November 2023 were included. The left atrial function was assessed using echocardiography pre-procedure and at 6 months post-procedure. **Results**: The mean age of the patients was 66.5 ± 9.76 years, with 70.6% being male. The cohort included 44% of patients with paroxysmal AF. PVI was successfully achieved in all patients, with a significant improvement in all aspects of left atrial strain at an average of six-month follow-up. The left atrial strain reservoir (LASr) increased from 12.5 ± 5.8% to 21.7 ± 8.1% ($p < 0.001$). Notably, patients with paroxysmal AF exhibited a greater increase in LASr compared to those with persistent AF. Additionally, pre-procedural sinus rhythm was a significant predictor of better LASr outcomes. **Conclusions**: PFA is associated with significant improvement in left atrial reservoir strain, suggesting a positive impact on atrial function. These findings have important implications for the therapeutic management of AF and warrant further research.

Keywords: atrial fibrillation; pulsed field ablation; left atrial strain; echocardiography; cardiac electrophysiology

1. Introduction

Atrial fibrillation (AF) is the most common cardiac arrhythmia, posing a significant global public health challenge. The incidence and prevalence of AF are rising, with an estimated three million new cases worldwide in 2017 alone. Its occurrence increases with age and additional cardiovascular risk factors, highlighting the need for effective and safe management strategies [1,2].

Beyond its direct health impacts, atrial fibrillation (AF) imposes a considerable economic burden on healthcare systems due to the chronic and recurrent nature of the condition. Frequent hospitalizations, often triggered by AF-related complications such as heart failure exacerbations, strokes, or poorly controlled symptoms, represent a significant proportion of these costs [3].

Rhythm control, particularly through atrial fibrillation (AF) ablation, significantly improves patients' quality of life (QoL) by reducing symptoms. Unlike rate control, rhythm control directly targets the pulmonary triggers of AF, alleviating the physical and mental burden of AF and enhancing overall well-being.

Wokhlu et al. showed that AF ablation provides sustained QoL improvements compared to medications, even in patients with recurrent AF. By reducing AF burden and severity, AF ablation enables patients to regain functional capacity and return to daily activities with fewer limitations [4].

Pulmonary vein isolation (PVI) is the cornerstone of catheter ablation therapy for AF. Traditional PVI techniques, such as radiofrequency and cryoenergy, are not entirely tissue-specific, risking complications by affecting nearby cardiac structures. Pulsed field ablation (PFA) uses biphasic bipolar pulses lasting 2.2 milliseconds at two thousand volts to precisely target heart tissue, potentially reducing risks, shortening procedure times, and lowering pulmonary vein reconnection rates [5,6].

PFA creates lesions with significantly less chronic fibrosis compared to traditional thermal methods. Unlike thermal ablation, which triggers excessive fibrosis through inflammatory responses and microvascular damage, PFA preserves the extracellular matrix and avoids these complications. This unique reparative process is thought to minimize collagen synthesis, possibly leading to improved tissue compliance and better recovery of left atrial mechanical function over time [7].

PFA's tissue-selective nature is also expected to redefine post-ablation protocols, including a shortened blanking period [8].

Pulsed field ablation (PFA), despite being a relatively new technology, has demonstrated a manageable and relatively short learning curve. Ruwald et al. reported significant reductions in procedural and fluoroscopy times during the implementation phase. Furthermore, the integration of high-density voltage mapping enhanced lesion placement accuracy, supporting efficient workflows and demonstrating the feasibility of PFA in real-world clinical settings [9].

The left atrium's role in cardiac function is multifaceted: it serves as a reservoir for blood during ventricular systole, acts passively as a conduit for blood transfer, and functions as a booster pump for ventricular filling during diastole, contributing 15–30% of the LV stroke volume [10,11]. These roles are crucial for maintaining efficient cardiac output, particularly in AF patients, where left atrial function is often compromised [12].

Despite its potential, the impact of PFA on left atrial function remains an area of active research. Left atrial strain, especially the left atrial reservoir strain (LASr), is recognized as a key parameter for assessing atrial function, crucial for evaluating cardiac performance in AF patients [10,12]. This study examines the effect of PFA on LASr as well as on the conduit strain LAScd and the contractile strain LASct.

2. Materials and Methods

2.1. Participant Recruitment

We conducted a retrospective analysis of patients who underwent AF ablation using the FARAPULSE ablation system (Boston Scientific, Marlborough, MA, USA) at our institution in July 2022 and November 2023. Those who consented to a follow-up were subsequently scheduled for an appointment. The follow-up visits included comprehensive echocardiographic evaluations and consultations with a physician. The study's inclusion criteria included all patients aged between 18 and 99 years who underwent PFA for AF.

Consent for post-interventional follow-up and echocardiographic assessment was mandatory.

2.2. Echocardiographic Assessment

Pre- and post-interventional echocardiographic assessments were performed using a standard protocol. Left atrial (LA) strain measurements were conducted using Tomtec software Version (LOT): 41.00 and quantified by two-dimensional speckle-tracking echocardiography with TOMTEC-ARENA post-processing software (Tomtec Imaging Systems GmbH, Unterschleißheim, Germany) (Figure 1). LASr, LAScd, and LASct were assessed using 2D speckle-tracking echocardiography (STE). This technique tracks the motion of myocardial speckles in a frame-by-frame manner, allowing for the assessment of myocardial deformation (strain).

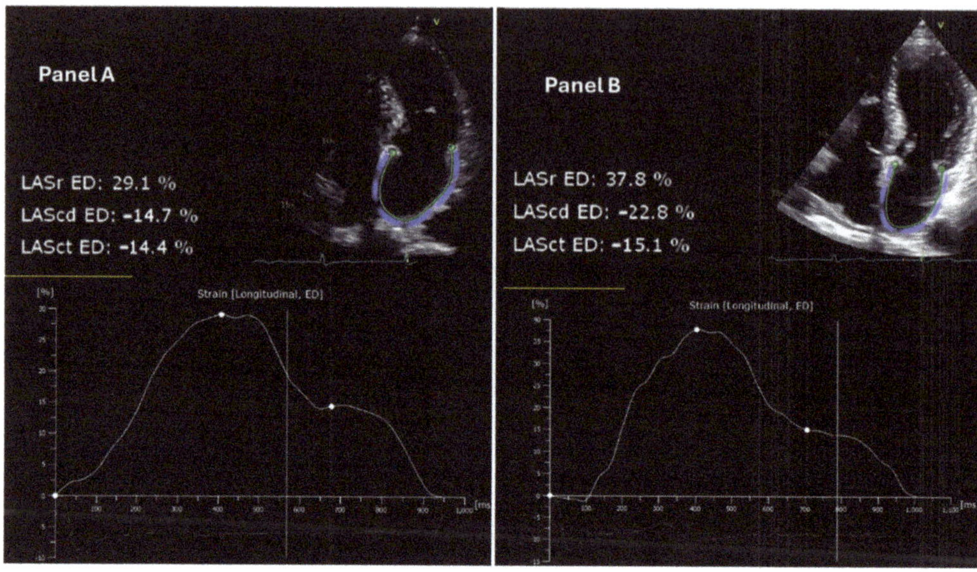

Figure 1. Echocardiographic assessment of left atrial strain reserve in patient 14 before and after pulsed field ablation. The left atrial reservoir strain (LASr), conduit strain (LAScd), and contractile strain (LASct) at the end diastole (ED) are illustrated. (**Panel A**) (left): Pre-ablation two-dimensional speckle-tracking echocardiogram demonstrating a LASr of 29.1%. (**Panel B**) (right): Post-ablation two-dimensional speckle-tracking echocardiogram depicting an increased LASr of 37.8% in the same patient, indicating an improvement in LASr function following the intervention. The strain curves below each echocardiogram reflect the changes in deformation of the left atrial wall over the cardiac cycle, with significant augmentation observed post-ablation.

The LASr was specifically evaluated during the reservoir phase of the cardiac cycle, which corresponds to the period when the left atrium is filling and expanding during ventricular systole.

In addition to LASr, LAScd and LASct were also evaluated. LAScd was measured during the conduit phase of the cardiac cycle, which corresponds to the passive transfer of blood from the left atrium to the left ventricle during early diastole. LASct was assessed during the booster pump phase, reflecting the active contraction of the left atrium in late diastole.

Rhythm status was recorded during both pre- and post-procedural echocardiographic assessments. This determination was performed at the time of strain measurement to ensure accurate interpretation of left atrial strain parameters.

Strain measurements were recorded as a percentage, reflecting the deformation of the left atrium relative to its resting state.

Patients with poor 2D image quality were excluded. Baseline characteristics and echocardiographic parameters were compared before and after the ablation procedure (Figure 1).

A key requirement was the availability of good quality pre-interventional echocardiographic studies. A modified four-chamber view, optimal for LA strain measurements, was preferred; however, a standard four-chamber view was used when the modified view did not provide adequate image quality. Patients without adequate ECG recordings during pre-interventional echocardiography were excluded, regardless of echocardiographic image quality. Both patients presenting with sinus rhythm and atrial fibrillation were included in the study.

All strain measurements were analyzed by a single observer to ensure consistency and eliminate inter-observer variability. While this approach minimizes variability between observers, intra-observer variability was not formally assessed in this study, representing a potential limitation.

2.3. Ablation Procedure

The PFA procedure was performed using the FARAWAVE™ catheter (Boston Scientific, Marlborough, MA, USA) in conjunction with the NAVX™ 3D mapping system (Abbott, Chicago, IL, USA). Pulmonary vein isolation (PVI) was the primary procedural target, aiming to electrically isolate all pulmonary veins. This was the first ablation procedure for all patients. Lesion creation was guided by high-density 3D voltage mapping, and the endpoints of the procedure included confirmation of bidirectional block at all pulmonary veins and non-inducibility of atrial fibrillation, verified through burst atrial pacing at a cycle length of 200 ms.

2.4. Statistical Analysis

Due to the exploratory nature of this research, a formal sample size calculation was not performed. Instead, the cohort size was determined by the availability of eligible patients during the study period, balancing practical constraints with the need for comprehensive data collection.

To interpret our findings, 95% confidence intervals were used to indicate the reliability and generalizability of the estimates. Descriptive p-values are presented to suggest potential patterns within the data, aligning with the aim of hypothesis generation rather than confirmation. Therefore, these p-values should be regarded as preliminary indicators for future research.

For statistical analysis, we utilized IBM SPSS Statistics 29.0 (Armonk, NY, USA). We began by assessing the normality of the distribution for all three parameters, LASr, LAScd, and LASct using the one-sample Kolmogorov-Smirnov test, which is unaffected by sample size. LASr and LASct in our data, comprising 34 observations both pre- and post-intervention (Figure 2), did not significantly deviate from a normal distribution (p-values > 0.05), supporting the use of parametric tests for further analysis.

However, LAScd (conduit strain) significantly deviated from a normal distribution post-intervention ($p = 0.022$).

We applied parametric methods to LASr and LASct in our analysis. The paired t-test was used as our primary method to compare related samples, specifically the pre- and post-intervention measurements.

Nonetheless, we applied non-parametric test methods to all three variables to account for the possibility of non-normal data in LASr and LASct, using a related-samples Wilcoxon signed rank test.

Non-parametric tests were applied to LASr and LASct as part of a sensitivity analysis to confirm the robustness of the results.

To compare the difference in LASr between paroxysmal and persistent AF groups, an independent samples t-test was performed. The difference in LASr was calculated for each group, and the AF type was used as the grouping variable. Cohen's d was calculated to quantify the magnitude of the difference.

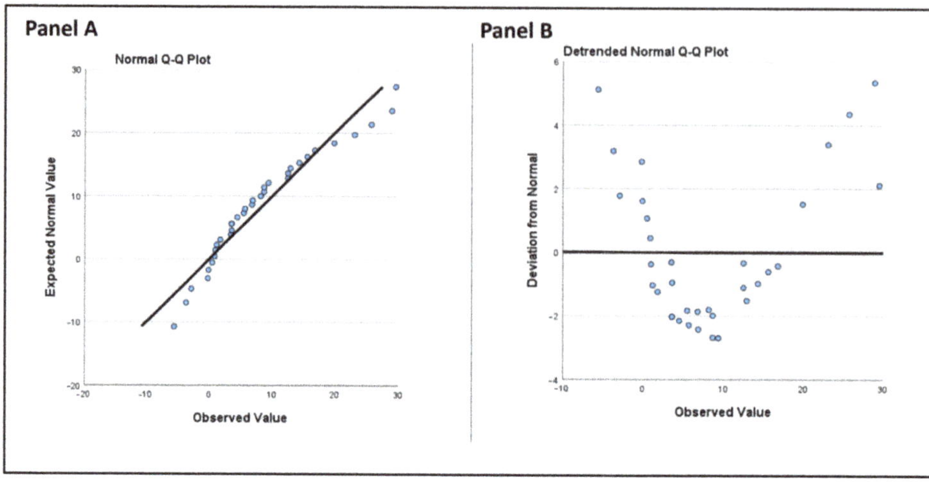

Figure 2. (**Panel A**): Normal QQ plot. The observed values are plotted against expected values from a normal distribution. (**Panel B**): Detrended normal Q-Q plot. This plot displays the deviation of observed values from the expected normal distribution.

An independent *t*-test was used to evaluate the difference in LASr changes between patients with and without AF recurrence. LASr change was calculated as the difference between post-procedural and pre-procedural LASr values. Patients were grouped based on recurrence status. The analysis included the calculation of mean differences, statistical significance (*p*-value), and effect size (Cohen's d) to assess the magnitude of the observed differences.

3. Results

The study cohort comprised 34 patients undergoing PVI using PFA. The mean age of the patients was 66.5 ± 9.76 years, with a predominance of males (70.6%). Among the participants, 44% had paroxysmal AF. The mean Body Mass Index (BMI) was recorded at 26.7 ± 5.0 kg/m^2, and the mean CHA2DS2-VASc score was 2.5 ± 1.5 (Table 1).

Table 1. Baseline characteristics of the study cohort.

Baseline Characteristics (*n* = 34)	
Age (years)	66.5 ± 9.76
Women	10 (29.4%)
Paroxysmal	15 (44%)
TAPSE in mm	18.9 ± 2
BMI (kg/m^2)	26.7 ± 5
Left ventricular ejection fraction (%)	54 ± 10
CHA2 DS2-VASc score	2.5 ± 1.5
LVEDV	117 ± 36
LAVI	45.7 ± 17

This table presents the baseline demographic and clinical characteristics of the 34 patients included in the study. The parameters include age, gender distribution, type of atrial fibrillation (paroxysmal or persistent), tricuspid annular plane systolic excursion (TAPSE), body mass index (B MI), left ventricular ejection fraction (LVEF), CHA2DS2-VASc score, left ventricular end-diastolic volume (LVEDV), and left atrial volume index (LAVI). Values are expressed as mean ± standard deviation (SD) or as absolute numbers with percentages in parentheses.

Echocardiographic evaluations indicated a left ventricular ejection fraction (LVEF) of $54 \pm 10\%$. The mean tricuspid annular plane systolic excursion (TAPSE) was 18.9 ± 2.0 mm. The left ventricular end-diastolic volume (LVEDV) averaged 117 ± 36 mL, and the left atrial volume index (LAVI) was 45.7 ± 17 mL/m^2.

Pre-ablation, the mean LASr was $12.5 \pm 5.8\%$. This increased significantly to $21.7 \pm 8.1\%$ post-ablation ($p < 0.001$), with a mean difference of -8.33 (95% CI: -11.51 to -5.15, $p < 0.001$) and a large effect size (Cohen's d = 0.915) (Figure 3). Subgroup analyses showed that patients with paroxysmal AF experienced an increase in LASr from $24.2 \pm 7.9\%$ to $31.4 \pm 10\%$ ($p < 0.001$) (Table 2). Meanwhile, those with persistent AF showed an increase in LASr from $12.5 \pm 5.8\%$ to $21.7 \pm 8.1\%$ $p < 0.001$.

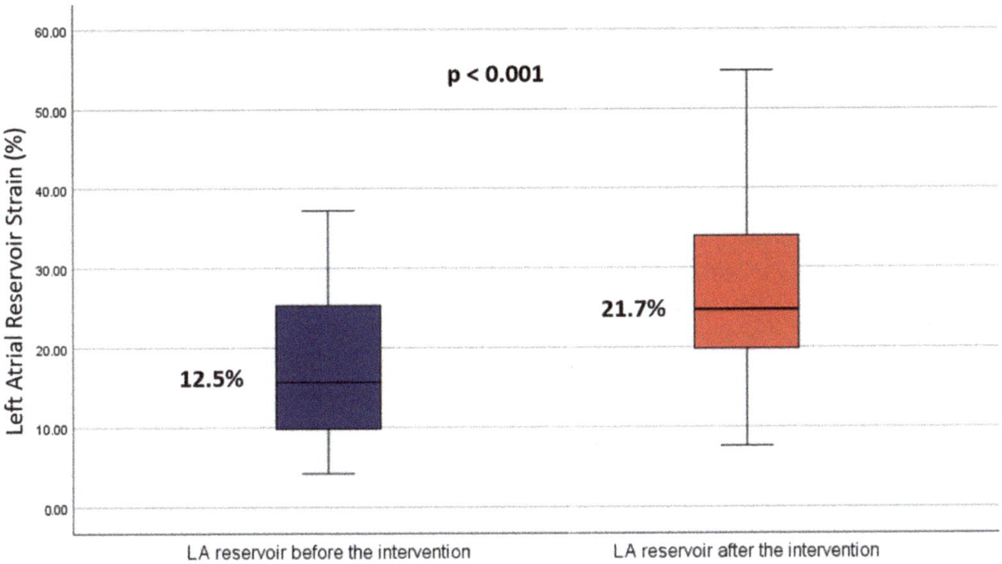

Figure 3. Boxplot comparing left atrial reservoir strain before and after ablation. The blue boxplot represents pre-intervention measurements, while the red boxplot shows post-intervention measurements. This visual comparison highlights the central tendency and variability of the strain measurements before and after the ablation procedure.

Table 2. Left atrial strain reservoir (LASr) in paroxysmal and persistent atrial fibrillation pre- and post-intervention.

	Left Atrial Strain Reservoir Pre-Interventional (Mean ± SD)	Left Atrial Strain Reservoir Post-Interventional (Mean ± SD)	*p*-Value
Paroxysmal AF	24.2 ± 7.9	31.4 ± 10	0.015
Persistent AF	12.5 ± 5.8	21.7 ± 8.1	<0.001

This table compares the left atrial strain reservoir (LASr) measurements before and after pulsed field ablation (PFA) in patients with paroxysmal and persistent atrial fibrillation. The table shows mean ± SD values for pre-interventional and post-interventional LASr, as well as the *p* value.

There was, however, no statistically significant difference in LASr improvement between paroxysmal and persistent AF groups ($p = 0.528$). The effect size was small (Cohen's d = -0.22), indicating a minimal practical difference.

The improvement in LASr was accompanied by corresponding improvements in other echocardiographic parameters, including reductions in left atrial volume. The mean LAVI decreased from 45.7 ± 17 mL/m^2 to 38.2 ± 15 mL/m^2 post-ablation ($p < 0.01$), indicating a reduction in atrial size and potentially less atrial remodeling.

Although gender and type of AF did not predict changes individually (gender, $p = 0.791$; type of AF, $p = 0.530$), a significant interaction ($p = 0.048$) suggested a differential effect of PFA based on these patient characteristics. However, the overall model did not reach statistical significance ($p = 0.920$).

Notably, pre-procedural cardiac rhythm was found to significantly predict improvement in LASr ($p = 0.046$), with better outcomes observed for patients in sinus rhythm before the procedure.

Additionally, a significant increase in contractile strain after the intervention was observed (mean difference = 3.86 ± 6.89, $p = 0.003$) as well as a significant improvement in conduit strain (LAScd) ($p < 0.001$).

The mean LASr change was 9.40 ± 9.51% for patients without recurrence and 4.85 ± 7.08% for those with recurrence. Although patients without recurrence demonstrated a greater improvement in LASr, the difference was not statistically significant ($t(32) = 1.247$, $p = 0.222$). The effect size, as measured by Cohen's d, was 0.50, indicating a moderate but non-significant effect.

4. Discussion

Pulsed field ablation is distinguished by its superior safety profile, tissue selectivity, reduced rates of pulmonary vein reconnection, and shortened procedure times [5,6].

While RF and cryoablation have shown significant improvements in left atrial ejection fraction (LAEF) due to reverse remodeling, they are associated with fibrotic remodeling and a higher risk of impaired atrial compliance [13,14].

In contrast, PFA's tissue-selective mechanism spares surrounding structures and minimizes chronic fibrosis, preserving LA compliance and promoting sustained functional recovery. Furthermore, PFA may reduce the risk of LAEF decline, which has been correlated with arrhythmia recurrence in other modalities. These findings position PFA as a promising alternative to thermal ablation techniques, with the potential to optimize both safety and long-term functional outcomes.

The assessment of left atrial contractile strain serves as a critical surrogate for evaluating left atrial function, reverse remodeling, and cardiac diastolic function. Previous studies have demonstrated improvements in LASr following AF ablation, primarily using traditional energy sources such as radiofrequency and cryoenergy [13,14].

Our study extends these findings by demonstrating that PFA is associated with significant improvements in all left atrial strain aspects in patients with symptomatic AF. The considerable increase in left atrial strain underscores PFA's potential to enhance cardiac function.

4.1. Improvement in Left Atrial Strain

The statistically significant increase in LASr post-PFA highlights the efficacy of this ablation technique in enhancing atrial function. This is particularly noteworthy given the crucial role of the left atrium in overall cardiac performance, especially in AF patients where compromised atrial function is common.

A recently published small study reported similar results, demonstrating improvements in left atrial strain, active emptying fraction, and expansion index at three months post-ablation. These results are in concordance with our findings, reinforcing the potential of PFA to enhance atrial mechanical function [15].

While our findings suggest a significant improvement in LASr following PFA, it is important to note that in the absence of a control group, these results cannot be solely attributed to the specific energy type. The observed effects may also be influenced by the reduction in AF burden or other non-specific benefits of rhythm control achieved through catheter ablation.

In our subgroup analysis, both paroxysmal and persistent AF patients demonstrated significant improvements in LASr following PFA. However, the magnitude of improvement did not differ significantly between the two groups. Given that persistent AF is typically associated with worse clinical outcomes and higher rates of major cardiac events compared to paroxysmal AF [16], the observed improvement in LASr regardless of AF type suggests that PFA remains a viable and effective treatment option even for patients with persistent AF.

The significant improvement in left atrial strain following PFA suggests a dual benefit of this procedure: not only targeting the arrhythmogenic substrate but also promoting better atrial mechanical function. This could translate into improved clinical outcomes for AF patients, potentially reducing the burden of this arrhythmia on the healthcare system.

The interaction between gender and AF type in influencing LASr changes post-PFA is an intriguing aspect of our results. Although our model did not demonstrate strong overall predictive power, this interaction may be attributed to the small sample size or patient-specific factors influencing the efficacy of PFA. These observations warrant further investigation to better tailor PFA to individual patient profiles and optimize outcomes.

Furthermore, the improvement in left atrial strain was not limited to the reservoir function (LASr) but also extended to conduit strain (LAScd) and contractile strain (LASct), indicating enhanced left atrial performance across all functional phases.

The observed non-normal distribution of LAScd post-intervention is likely due to the small sample size, which may have influenced the statistical assessment of normality.

Our analysis indicates a trend toward greater improvement in LASr among patients without AF recurrence compared to those with recurrence; however, this difference was not statistically significant. This lack of statistical significance could be attributed to the limited sample size. Future studies with larger cohorts are needed to confirm these observations.

4.2. Potential Mechanisms

a. Tissue selectivity:

PFA's mechanism of action involves creating pores in the myocyte cell membrane through irreversible electroporation, leading to targeted cell death [5]. This selective tissue ablation spares surrounding non-cardiac tissues, reducing the risk of collateral damage. Studies have shown that PFA induces large acute late gadolinium enhancement (LGE) without microvascular damage or intramural hemorrhage. This selective ablation contributes to improved atrial mechanical function and reduced complications, making PFA a promising alternative to thermal ablation techniques.

b. Anti-remodeling effect:

A study comparing PFA with thermal ablation found that PFA prevented chronic atrial fibrotic changes and restrictive mechanics, with most LGE lesions disappearing in the chronic stage, indicating a specific reparative process [7]. These long-term benefits highlight PFA's potential to improve patient outcomes and reduce the burden of AF on the healthcare system.

Recent evidence also suggests that the traditional 3-month blanking period may not fully apply to PFA due to its lower inflammatory response, with a shortened blanking period of 1 month proposed based on its predictive value for late arrhythmia recurrence. These findings highlight PFA's potential to improve procedural safety, preserve atrial function, and redefine post-ablation management protocols [8].

4.3. Implications of the Findings

Our study has demonstrated that PFA is associated with a statistically significant improvement in all aspects of left atrial strain (LASr, LAScd, and LASct), an indicator of enhanced atrial function. This finding can have significant implications, as improved left atrial strain post-ablation could translate into better overall cardiac function for patients, potentially leading to reduced symptoms, improved exercise capacity, and quality of life. Moreover, the observed improvement in left atrial strain may also have prognostic implications, as previous studies have linked it to lower rates of atrial fibrillation recurrence [10]. Hence, our results suggest that PFA may not only serve as an effective treatment for rhythm control but also confer long-term structural benefits to the atrium, which could influence future AF management strategies.

4.4. Study Limitations

A key limitation of our study is the small sample size and the short follow-up period. While our results are statistically significant, larger studies with longer follow-up are needed to confirm these findings and assess the long-term impact of PFA on atrial function. Additionally, our study was conducted at a single center, which may limit the generalizability of the findings. Future multicenter studies could provide a more comprehensive understanding of the effects of PFA on left atrial function.

Furthermore, the ablations were performed using the FARAPULSE ablation system (Boston Scientific, Marlborough, MA, USA), which is not representative of all systems using pulsed field ablation. Additional studies using other systems for pulsed field ablation are needed to generalize these findings.

Another limitation of our study is the absence of AF burden estimation in the patient cohort. As AF burden increasingly emerges as a critical determinant of procedural success and long-term outcomes, its quantification could have provided valuable insights into the relationship between recurrence, LASr changes, and atrial remodeling. Incorporating AF burden in future studies would allow for a more comprehensive evaluation of the factors influencing left atrial functional recovery and overall efficacy of AF ablation.

Another limitation was the variability in echocardiographic image quality, common in clinical settings. Although we aimed to use a modified four-chamber view optimal for left atrial strain measurements, this was not always feasible, and in such cases, a standard four-chamber view was used.

4.5. Future Research Directions

Future research should focus on exploring the long-term outcomes of PFA on LA function and examining the impact of this procedure on patients' quality of life and long-term rhythm control as well as exploring patient-specific predictors of response to PFA.

5. Conclusions

In conclusion, our explorative study provides evidence that pulsed field ablation is associated with significant improvement in left atrial reservoir strain among patients with atrial fibrillation. Given the study's observational design and considering these promising results, further randomized trials are needed to elucidate the relationships between pulsed field ablation and improved atrial function in patients with atrial fibrillation and to solidify PFA's place in the AF management continuum.

Author Contributions: N.M.: Concept and design of the study, data acquisition, statistical analysis, drafting of the manuscript, journal submission, and corresponding author. F.B. and D.S.: Data analysis and interpretation, statistical analysis, and manuscript revision. L.-H.B. and G.H.: Supervision of the study and critical revision of the manuscript. A.S.P.: Concept and design of the study, data collection, supervision of the study, drafting of the manuscript, and approval of the final version. All authors have read and agreed to the published version of the manuscript.

Funding: This research did not receive any specific grant from funding agencies in the public, commercial, or not-for-profit sectors.

Institutional Review Board Statement: This study was conducted in accordance with the ethical standards of the Charite Research Ethics Committee. The study received ethics approval from Charite Research Ethics Committee, reference number [EA1/284/21] on 29 September 2021.

Informed Consent Statement: Written informed consent was obtained from study participants. All procedures performed in studies involving human participants were in accordance with the ethical standards of the institutional research committee and with the Declaration of Helsinki. Patient confidentiality and privacy were maintained throughout the study.

Data Availability Statement: The datasets generated and/or analyzed during the current study are not publicly available due to privacy or ethical restrictions but are available from the corresponding author on request. De-identified data can be made available while maintaining confidentiality.

Conflicts of Interest: The authors declare that there are no conflicts of interest regarding the publication of this paper. No financial or personal relationships have influenced the work reported in this manuscript.

References

1. Lloyd-Jones, D.; Adams, R.J.; Brown, T.M.; Carnethon, M.; Dai, S.; De Simone, G.; Ferguson, T.B.; Ford, E.; Furie, K.; Gillespie, C. Heart disease and stroke statistics—2010 update: A report from the American heart association. *Circulation* **2010**, *121*, 948–954. [PubMed]
2. Lippi, G.; Sanchis-Gomar, F.; Cervellin, G. Global epidemiology of atrial fibrillation: An increasing epidemic and public health challenge. *Int. J. Stroke* **2021**, *16*, 217–221. [CrossRef] [PubMed]
3. Wolowacz, S.E.; Samuel, M.; Brennan, V.K.; Jasso-Mosqueda, J.G.; Van Gelder, I.C. The cost of illness of atrial fibrillation: A systematic review of the recent literature. *Europace* **2011**, *13*, 1375–1385. [CrossRef] [PubMed]
4. Wokhlu, A.; Monahan, K.H.; Hodge, D.O.; Asirvatham, S.J.; Friedman, P.A.; Munger, T.M.; Bradley, D.J.; Bluhm, C.M.; Haroldson, J.M.; Packer, D.L. Long-Term Quality of Life After Ablation of Atrial Fibrillation. The Impact of Recurrence, Symptom Relief, and Placebo Effect. *J. Am. Coll. Cardiol.* **2010**, *55*, 2308–2316. [CrossRef] [PubMed]
5. Reddy, V.Y.; Dukkipati, S.R.; Neuzil, P.; Anic, A.; Petru, J.; Funasako, M.; Cochet, H.; Minami, K.; Breskovic, T.; Sikiric, I.; et al. Pulsed Field Ablation of Paroxysmal Atrial Fibrillation: 1-Year Outcomes of IMPULSE, PEFCAT, and PEFCAT II. *Clin. Electrophysiol.* **2021**, *7*, 614–627. [CrossRef] [PubMed]
6. Della Rocca, D.G.; Marcon, L.; Magnocavallo, M.; Menè, R.; Pannone, L.; Mohanty, S.; Sousonis, V.; Sorgente, A.; Almorad, A.; Bisignani, A.; et al. Pulsed electric field, cryoballoon, and radiofrequency for paroxysmal atrial fibrillation ablation: A propensity score-matched comparison. *Europace* **2024**, *26*, euae016. [CrossRef] [PubMed]
7. Nakatani, Y.; Sridi-Cheniti, S.; Cheniti, G.; Ramirez, F.D.; Goujeau, C.; André, C.; Nakashima, T.; Eggert, C.; Schneider, C.; Viswanathan, R.; et al. Pulsed field ablation prevents chronic atrial fibrotic changes and restrictive mechanics after catheter ablation for atrial fibrillation. *Europace* **2021**, *23*, 1767–1776. [CrossRef] [PubMed]
8. Mohanty, S.; Torlapati, P.G.; Casella, M.; Della Rocca, D.G.; Schiavone, M.; Doty, B.; La Fazia, V.M.; Pahi, S.; Pierucci, N.; Valeri, Y.; et al. Redefining the blanking period after pulsed-field ablation in patients with atrial fibrillation. *Heart Rhythm* 2024, *in press*. [CrossRef] [PubMed]
9. Ruwald, M.H.; Johannessen, A.; Hansen, M.L.; Haugdal, M.; Worck, R.; Hansen, J. Pulsed field ablation in real-world atrial fibrillation patients: Clinical recurrence, operator learning curve and re-do procedural findings. *J. Interv. Card. Electrophysiol.* **2023**, *66*, 1837–1848. [CrossRef] [PubMed]
10. Hoit, B.D. Assessment of Left Atrial Function by Echocardiography: Novel Insights. *Curr. Cardiol. Rep.* **2018**, *20*, 96. [CrossRef] [PubMed]
11. Blume, G.G.; Mcleod, C.J.; Barnes, M.E.; Seward, J.B.; Pellikka, P.A.; Bastiansen, P.M.; Tsang, T.S. Left atrial function: Physiology, assessment, and clinical implications. *Eur. J. Echocardiogr.* **2011**, *12*, 421–430. [CrossRef] [PubMed]
12. Jarasunas, J.; Aidietis, A.; Aidietiene, S. Left atrial strain—An early marker of left ventricular diastolic dysfunction in patients with hypertension and paroxysmal atrial fibrillation. *Cardiovasc. Ultrasound* **2018**, *16*, 29. [CrossRef] [PubMed]

13. Giannopoulos, G.; Kossyvakis, C.; Vrachatis, D.; Aggeli, C.; Tsitsinakis, G.; Letsas, K.; Tsiachris, D.; Tsoukala, S.; Efremidis, M.; Katritsis, D.; et al. Effect of cryoballoon and radiofrequency ablation for pulmonary vein isolation on left atrial function in patients with nonvalvular paroxysmal atrial fibrillation: A prospective randomized study (Cryo-LAEF study). *J. Cardiovasc. Electrophysiol.* **2019**, *30*, 991–998. [CrossRef] [PubMed]
14. Tops, L.F.; Delgado, V.; Bertini, M.; Marsan, N.A.; Den Uijl, D.W.; Trines, S.A.; Zeppenfeld, K.; Holman, E.; Schalij, M.J.; Bax, J.J. Left atrial strain predicts reverse remodeling after catheter ablation for atrial fibrillation. *J. Am. Coll. Cardiol.* **2011**, *57*, 324–331. [CrossRef] [PubMed]
15. Banai, A.; Sliman, H.; Feder, O.; Chorin, E.; Schwartz, L.A.; Topilsky, Y.; Rosso, R. PO-04-139 Impact of Pulsed Field Ablation on Left Atrial Function in Patients with Persistent Atrial Fibrillation. *Heart Rhythm* **2024**, *21*, S440–S441. [CrossRef]
16. De Vos, C.B.; Pisters, R.; Nieuwlaat, R.; Prins, M.H.; Tieleman, R.G.; Coelen, R.J.S.; van den Heijkant, A.C.; Allessie, M.A.; Crijns, H.J. Progression from Paroxysmal to Persistent Atrial Fibrillation. Clinical Correlates and Prognosis. *J. Am. Coll. Cardiol.* **2010**, *55*, 725–731. [CrossRef] [PubMed]

Journal of
Clinical Medicine

MDPI

Article

Electrographic Flow Mapping Provides Prognosis for AF Ablation Outcomes Across Two Independent Prospective Patient Cohorts

Kent R. Nilsson [1,2,†], Amitesh Anerao [2,†], Melissa H. Kong [3], Pawel Derejko [4], Tamás Szili-Török [5], Sandeep Goyal [1], Mohit Turagam [6], Atul Verma [7] and Steven Castellano [3,*]

1 Department of Cardiac Electrophysiology, Piedmont Heart Institute, Athens, GA 30309, USA; nilsson@uga.edu (K.R.N.); sandeep.goyal@piedmont.org (S.G.)
2 Medical College of Georgia, Augusta University/University of Georgia Partnership, Athens, GA 30602, USA; amitesh.anerao@uga.edu
3 Cortex, Inc., Menlo Park, CA 94025, USA; mhkong1@gmail.com
4 Department of Cardiology, Medicover Hospital Warsaw, 02-972 Warsaw, Poland; pawel.derejko@medicover.pl
5 Cardiology Center, Department of Internal Medicine, University of Szeged, 6720 Szeged, Hungary; szilitorok@hotmail.com
6 Icahn School of Medicine at Mount Sinai, New York, NY 10029, USA; mohit.turagam@mountsinai.org
7 McGill University Health Centre, Montreal, QC H4A 3J1, Canada; atul.verma@mcgill.ca
* Correspondence: steven.castellano@gmail.com; Tel.: +1-732-500-0303
† These authors contributed equally to the work.

Abstract: Background/Objectives: Electrographic flow (EGF) mapping allows for the visualization and quantification of atrial fibrillation (AF) wavefront propagation patterns. EGF-identified sources were shown in the randomized controlled *FLOW-AF* trial to significantly increase the likelihood of AF recurrence within 1 year if left unablated. Electrographic flow consistency (EGFC) additionally measures the stability of observed wavefront patterns, such that patients with more organization have a healthier substrate and lower recurrence. Source presence and EGFC can be used collectively to assign mechanistic phenotypes to AF patients. **Methods:** The patient phenotypes, treatment modalities, and outcomes in *FLOW-AF* were compared with those of patients in the ensuing *AF-FLOW Global Registry*, which was conducted by separate physicians at discrete clinical centers. **Results:** Patients with low EGFC (≤0.62) had a 12-month freedom from AF (FFAF) of 46%, while those with a high mean EGFC (>0.62) had a FFAF of 81%. Right atrial EGFC was correlated with left atrial EGFC, and the highest recurrence occurred in those with biatrial low EGFC. Source presence also affected the recurrence rates in both trials, such that the presence of EGF-identified sources in PVI-only patients lowered the FFAF from 65% to 36%, but the elimination of sources produced a 30% absolute increase in FFAF from 36% to 66%. **Conclusions:** Patient outcomes by EGF-based AF phenotype were consistent across two cohorts of patients from separate clinical trials at distinct centers. Patients with a high EGFC and no sources post-procedure had the best outcomes. EGF mapping provides insights into underlying disease pathophysiology and may be employed prospectively to predict recurrence.

Keywords: ablation; arrythmias; atrial fibrillation; basket catheter; cardiac; electrographic flow mapping; panoramic mapping

1. Introduction

Atrial fibrillation (AF) is the most common arrhythmia and is associated with significant morbidity and mortality and a rising prevalence worldwide [1–4]. AF patients have a high risk for thromboembolism, stroke, myocardial infarction, hospitalization, and death, which is not significantly reduced even among asymptomatic patients [5]. This is because asymptomatic patients—who account for up to 40% of the diagnosed population of AF patients [6]—more often progress to permanent AF in the absence of appropriate anti-arrhythmic drugs or ablation therapy, which often curtail complications [5].

While the need for more widespread AF screening and treatment is growing, there remains a ceiling of efficacy observed in the effectiveness of AF therapies. Pulmonary vein isolation (PVI) has, thus far, emerged as the cornerstone of management for both paroxysmal AF (PAF) and persistent AF (PeAF). Though recurrence rates following PVI are significantly higher for PeAF than for PAF, empiric standardized endocardial ablation lesion sets for PeAF have failed to improve clinical outcomes beyond PVI alone [7,8]. As a result, PVI without adjunctive ablation has remained the gold standard for the treatment of PeAF.

Given the challenges of managing patients with PeAF, multiple mapping and ablation strategies have been proposed to improve patient outcomes. Some have focused on improving the effectiveness of PVI ablations. For example, the recent CHARISMA trial showed that successful PVI could be predicted when local impedance dropped by at least 21 Ω at anterior sites and 18 Ω at posterior sites, and that higher contact forces were non-linearly correlated with increased impedance drops [9]. Such findings add to the prior understanding of the importance of good contact in preventing recurrence from the TOCCATA study [10]. Additionally, pulsed field ablation (PFA) has been vetted as a novel, tissue-selective alternative to radiofrequency (RF) ablation with a selectivity for cardiac tissue that reduces the risk for esophageal injuries, pulmonary vein (PV) stenosis, and phrenic nerve palsy [11–17]. Moreover, PFA trials have, thus far, shown a high 76% durability of PVIs among recurring patients, as well as similar efficacy, with 60% ± 10% freedom from arrythmias after one year for PeAF patients [11,18,19].

Other strategies for improving AF ablation outcomes have, instead, emphasized additional lesion sets that could improve outcomes beyond PVI. These include complex fractionated atrial electrogram ablation [20], rotor ablation [21], charge density mapping [22], dispersion mapping [23], image-guided fibrosis [24], and artificial-intelligence-driven lesions [22]. However, each method has substantial limitations and variable clinical results.

To this end, electrographic flow (EGF) mapping has been shown to be a promising modality that rapidly (1) localizes extra-PV drivers of persistent AF and (2) quantifies the health of the underlying substrate as electrographic flow consistency (EGFC). Most mapping technologies suffer from a poor spatial resolution, difficulty in identifying the true source of the arrhythmia due to complex electrical patterns, susceptibility to noise and artifacts, a lack of real-time mapping capabilities, operator dependence in interpreting data, and inconsistent results across different mapping techniques or a lack of reproducibility on repeat mappings [25–27]. However, EGF mapping creates a full, near-real-time spatiotemporal reconstruction of organized atrial electrical wavefront propagation in order to reveal reproducible patterns pertaining to a patient's rhythm-dependent map properties [28–31].

While avoiding many of the weaknesses of conventional mapping systems, EGF mapping has also led to improved procedural efficacy. The recent multicenter, randomized, controlled *FLOW-AF* clinical trial of 85 PeAF and long-standing PeAF (LS-PeAF) patients showed that EGF mapping identified sources in 60% of patients. The ablation of these sources in addition to PVI improved freedom from AF (FFAF) (68% vs. 17%, $p = 0.042$) and freedom from AF/Atrial Tachycardia (AT)/Atrial Flutter (AFL) (51% vs. 14%, $p = 0.103$) at

12 months [32]. Furthermore, source presence and EGFC could be used to phenotypically classify patients into four categories that had treatment-dependent outcomes post-ablation. The phenotypes were as follows: Type I—no extra-PV sources and a high EGFC; Type II—sources and a high EGFC; Type III—sources and a low EGFC; and Type IV—no sources and a low EGFC [32–34].

Subsequently, the *AF-FLOW Global Registry* study was performed to gather information on how physicians would employ EGF mapping in their clinical procedures and again assess post-procedure outcomes. The study consisted of 25 patients from five clinical centers with PAF, PeAF, and LS-PeAF. It again demonstrated that patients with a high EGFC (Types I and II) had higher rates of FFAF than those with a low EGFC (Types III and IV), and that patients with sources remaining post-procedure had a lower FFAF than those with no sources [35].

Here, we seek to compare outcomes across both *FLOW-AF* and the *AF-FLOW Global Registry*. We aim to use both studies to collectively analyze the predictive power of EGF mapping properties for post-procedure FFAF with a focus on (1) the impact of EGFC—both overall and by atrium—on 12-month outcomes, (2) the association between phenotype and outcome among patients receiving PVI-only procedures, and (3) the effect of source ablation on modulating these PVI-only outcomes.

2. Materials and Methods

2.1. Trial Overview

The details of the trials have been previously outlined for *FLOW-AF* (ClinicalTrials.gov identifier number NCT04473963) and the *AF-FLOW Global Registry* (NCT05481359). *FLOW-AF* enrolled 85 patients and was powered to test safety and map reproducibility for EGF-mapped patients [32]. The *AF-FLOW Global Registry* enrolled 25 patients and was powered to test source detection and ablation rate in an open clinical setting [35].

2.2. PVI Ablation Procedure

All procedures were performed under sedation after obtaining informed consent. The patients underwent 3-dimensional electroanatomic mapping with either Ensite NavX (Abbott, Abbott Park, IL, USA) or CARTO (Biosense Webster, Diamond Bar, CA, USA), followed by PVI using an irrigated-tip RF ablation catheter. The ablation catheter power and temperature settings were at the operator's discretion. Intravenous heparin was administered for systemic anticoagulation to maintain an activated clotting time of >300 s prior to the insertion of the 64-pole basket mapping catheter. For any ablation of PVs, confirmation of PVI (entrance or exit block) was performed after a mandatory minimum 20-min wait following the last RF application.

2.3. EGF Mapping

EGF mapping was performed both pre- and post-PVI using the Ablamap® v9.0.4-v11.1.0.56 software (Ablacon, Wheat Ridge, CO, USA). Unipolar electrograms (EGMs) were recorded using a commercially available 64-electrode basket mapping catheter connected to a proprietary, CE-marked recording system (EP Map, Herdecke, Germany). Each recording was 1 min long, and the unipolar signals were processed using a proprietary algorithm to remove the QRS complex, noise, baseline fluctuations, and far-field signals. Using a biharmonic spline interpolation based on Green's function, the electrical field was estimated, and a Horn–Schunck flow estimation of the Green's interpolation frames was performed to visualize atrial wavefront propagation over time. Haines et al. published an in-depth explanation of the theoretical basis for EGF mapping and details of the EGF mapping algorithm [36], which were more recently summarized by Castellano and Kong [34]. The dominant patterns of wavefront propagation over time were displayed as flow vectors in EGF Segment Maps, enabling the visualization of the origins of excitation, representing extra-PV AF triggers, called sources. Active sources exhibited divergent flow fields.

EGF mapping was typically performed by obtaining 1-min recordings from the 64-pole basket catheter placed in multiple standardized positions within each atrium, as well as additional recordings after any source ablations to confirm elimination. In the left atrium (LA), there were the following two standardized basket positions: (1) posterosuperior LA with the dome of the basket aiming toward the left PVs and LA appendage (LAA) and (2) lateral LA with the basket dome pointing toward the LAA and mitral valve. In the right atrium (RA), there were the following three standardized basket positions: (1) superior vena cava (SVC)/RA junction with the basket position halfway into the SVC; (2) central RA with the basket dome pointing to the SVC with a vertical catheter shaft orientation and the basket expanded to fill the RA; and (3) anterolateral RA with the basket dome pointing to the RA appendage and tricuspid valve and the catheter deflected anteriorly and laterally from the SVC. Mapping in additional basket positions in either atrium was performed if necessary to obtain complete endocardial atrial coverage.

2.4. EGF-Guided Ablation

If EGF mapping identified an extra-PV source with a source activity (SAC) of $\geq$ 26.5% based on the prespecified threshold for clinical significance, EGF-guided ablation at the target location of the focal source was required for patients in the treatment groups, though not for those in the control groups. Repeat EGF mapping was recommended to confirm the elimination of the source via reduction in the SAC below the SAC threshold. If additional sources were unmasked during repeat mapping, additional ablation was advised until all sources were eliminated.

2.5. EGFC Calculations from EGF Maps

EGFC was computed for each recording from the Euclidean length of vector field estimates across all basket electrodes over time, thereby providing a measure of the overall magnitude of the flow across the mapping catheter, averaged in arbitrary units. Importantly, electrodes with low contact were removed from the calculation because of artificially low local EGFC values that were observed at non-contacting electrode positions.

After calculating the EGFC for each recording, an overall EGFC was then computed for each patient in AF and/or SR. To perform this, the EGFCs from each of a patient's recordings in a given basket position during the chosen rhythm were first averaged to compute positional EGFC means per rhythm per patient. These positional EGFCs were then averaged within each atrium to generate a mean EGFC per atrium per patient. Such a method allowed for all recording positions to be given equal weight. Lastly, each patient's two atrial EGFCs were then averaged again to generate an overall mean EGFC per patient. A threshold of 0.62 for the overall mean EGFC was used for phenotyping high vs. low EGFC, as derived from prior studies [32,33].

2.6. Statistical Analysis

Summary data are expressed as mean value $\pm$ one standard deviation. p-values for group comparisons were computed using two-tailed, independent t-tests for continuous variables and two-tailed z-tests for proportions, as appropriate. For all statistical tests, the null hypothesis was rejected at the level of $p < 0.05$ (bolded).

3. Results

3.1. Trial Design and Demographics

The two trials that were analyzed were *FLOW-AF* and the *AF-FLOW Global Registry*. *FLOW-AF* was a multi-centered, randomized trial evaluating EGF mapping prospectively for the first time. Redo and PeAF or LS-PeAF patients were analyzed from Homolka Hospital (Prague, Czech Republic), Praxisklinik Herz und Gefaesse (Dresden, Germany), the Erasmus MC Department of Cardiology (Rotterdam, The Netherlands), and the University Medical Center Hamburg-Eppendorf (Hamburg, Germany). Patients with sources with an SAC of $\geq$ 26.5% were randomized to either treatment, where the sources were ablated, or control where the sources were left unablated.

Subsequently, the *AF-FLOW Global Registry* was conducted as a follow-up study to explore the implications of EGF mapping in a broader patient population. The *AF-FLOW Global Registry* consisted of 25 prospective all-comers, including de novo and PAF patients. Patients were enrolled from University Health Center, the University of Georgia (Athens, Georgia), Piedmont Athens Regional Hospital (Athens, Georgia), Mount Sinai Hospital (New York, NY, USA), the Erasmus MC Department of Cardiology (Rotterdam, The Netherlands), and Medicover Hospital (Warsaw, Poland). The *AF-FLOW Global Registry* also gave physicians the liberty to treat EGF-identified sources in a way they saw fit, and patients were not randomized to have all sources with an SAC of $\geq$ 26.5% ablated or left unablated as they were in the *FLOW-AF* study arms.

Patient demographics by trial are shown in Table 1. There were no significant differences among any of the demographic variables between the two trials.

Table 1. Patient demographics in *FLOW-AF* and the *AF-FLOW Global Registry*. There were no significant differences observed between the patient populations of the two trials.

Patient Demographics	*FLOW-AF*	*AF-FLOW Global Registry*	*p*-Value
Age (years)	65.6 ± 9.3	63.9 ± 11.2	0.445
Female sex, n (%)	31/85 (36%)	9/25 (36%)	0.968
LA diameter (cm)	4.4 ± 0.6	4.4 ± 0.5	1.000
Left ventricular ejection fraction (%)	57.2 ± 6.4	55.0 ± 2.5	0.096
Body mass index (kg/m^2)	29.1 ± 4.6	27.9 ± 3.9	0.239
CHA_2DS_2VASc score, mean ± SD	2.4 ± 1.3	2.7 ± 1.9	0.367
Diabetes, n (%)	15/85 (18%)	4/25 (16%)	0.849
Hypertension, n (%)	63/85 (74%)	16/25 (64%)	0.322
History of AFL, n (%)	15/85 (18%)	6/23 (26%)	0.363

3.2. EGFC Was Related to AF Recurrence Rates Across All Patient Cohorts

Substrate health was first studied across the FFAF vs. recurrence patients in the two studies. When analyzing the EGFCs across all patients, those who experienced FFAF had mean EGFC values of 0.52 ± 0.11 and 0.59 ± 0.15 in *FLOW-AF* and the *AF-FLOW Global Registry*, respectively. By contrast, patients who experienced AF recurrence had mean EGFC values of 0.49 ± 0.09 and 0.47 ± 0.12. The pooled total EGFCs across the two studies demonstrated that patients who experienced FFAF had a mean EGFC of 0.54 ± 0.12, while recurring patients had a mean EGFC of 0.49 ± 0.09 (***p* = 0.022**). EGFC differences by outcome are shown in Table 2.

Moreover, the recurrence rates were similar across the two trials based on the EGFC classification of all-comers. Patients with a low overall EGFC ($\leq$0.62) demonstrated FFAF rates of 42% (n = 48) and 59% (n = 17) in *FLOW-AF* and the *AF-FLOW Global Registry*, respectively, while those with a high mean EGFC (>0.62) had FFAF rates of 79% (n = 28) and 100% (n = 4). Pooled data across both trials showed that those with a low overall EGFC had a total FFAF rate of 46% (n = 65) vs. 81% (n = 32) for those with a high overall EGFC (**p = 0.005**), as shown in Figure 1.

Table 2. EGFC for patients experiencing 12-month FFAF vs. AF recurrence in *FLOW-AF* and the *AF-FLOW Global Registry*. The FFAF EGFC was significantly higher than the recurrence EGFC (p = 0.022).

Trial	FFAF Patient EGFC	Recurrence Patient EGFC
FLOW-AF	0.52 ± 0.11 (n = 42)	0.49 ± 0.09 (n = 34)
AF-FLOW Global Registry	0.59 ± 0.15 (n = 14)	0.47 ± 0.12 (n = 7)
Pooled total	0.54 ± 0.12 (n = 56)	0.49 ± 0.09 (n = 41)

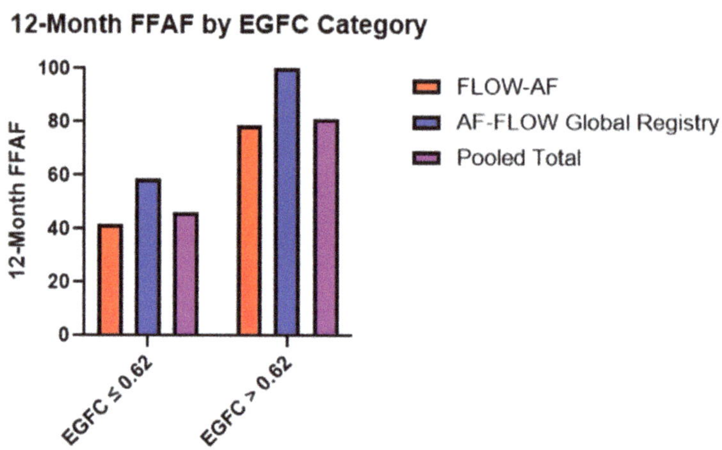

Figure 1. Twelve-month FFAF rates based on EGFC categorization. Patients with healthier substrate (EGFC > 0.62) demonstrated better outcomes (p = 0.005) in a consistent pattern across both *FLOW-AF* and the *AF-FLOW Global Registry*.

Further analysis was conducted on EGFC by atrium among patients with sources ablated by the end of the procedure. Patients with a high atrial EGFC were defined as having a mean RA EGFC ≥ the population mean RA EGFC or a mean LA EGFC ≥ the population mean LA EGFC for each atrium, respectively. Those with a high EGFC in both the right and left atria showed the highest FFAF of 87% (n = 15). For patients who presented with a high mean EGFC in just the right or left atrium, their FFAF rates were 67% (n = 9) and 63% (n = 8), respectively. Lastly, patients who had a low EGFC in both right and left atria had an FFAF rate of 55% (n = 31). Therefore, patients with a high mean EGFC in both atria showed a 32% increase in FFAF compared with those with a low mean EGFC in both atria (**p = 0.034**). Recurrence by mean EGFC in each atrium is shown in Figure 2 alongside dashed lines indicating the population mean EGFC for each atrium.

Across all patients, the mean EGFC was lower in the LA than the RA (0.53 ± 0.19 vs. 0.60 ± 0.23, **p = 0.026**). A linear relationship was also established between the mean RA EGFC and mean LA EGFC of patients (m = 0.51, r = 0.42, **p < 0.001**), which was unaffected by trial or recurrence status.

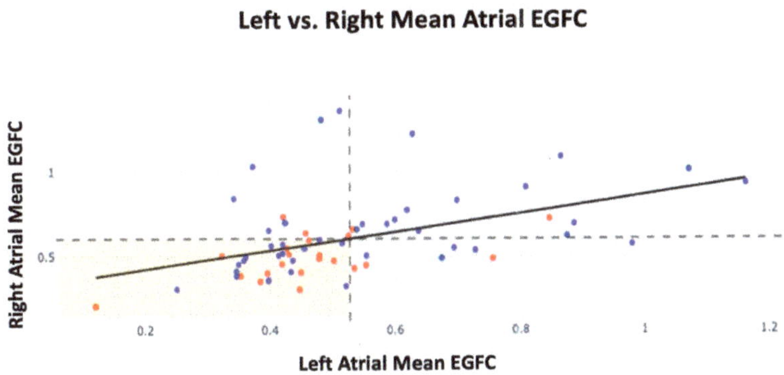

Figure 2. Mean EGFC and outcomes by atrium across all patients in *FLOW-AF* and the *AF-FLOW Global Registry*. FFAF patients are depicted in blue; recurrence patients are depicted in red. The horizontal dashed line indicates the population mean RA EGFC; the vertical dashed line indicates the population mean LA mean EGFC. A linear relationship was established between RA and LA EGFC means (m = 0.51, r = 0.42, $p < 0.001$). Slope and r were unaffected by recurrence status of patients.

3.3. Phenotyping by EGFC and Source Presence Can Aid in Predicting Procedure Outcomes

The four phenotypes and the characteristic appearances of their EGF Summary Maps and EGF Segment Maps are shown in Figure 3, and overall outcomes by phenotype are shown in Figure 4. Table 3 follows with outcomes by phenotype and treatment modality.

Table 3. FFAF by phenotype and treatment modality for patients enrolled in *FLOW-AF* and the *AF-FLOW Global Registry*. Among PVI-only patients, FFAF decreased significantly between Type I patients with neither sources nor low EGFC to Type II and Type IV patients with either sources or low EGFC ($p = 0.003$) and decreased further between Type I patients and Type III patients with both sources and low EGFC ($p < 0.001$).

Patient Phenotype and Treatment	*FLOW-AF* FFAF	*AF-FLOW Global Registry* FFAF
Type I—PVI-only	10/10 (100%)	1/1 (100%)
Type II—PVI-only	5/10 (50%)	n/a
Type III—PVI-only	3/13 (23%)	1/2 (50%)
Type IV—PVI-only	11/22 (50%)	4/7 (57%)
Type II—PVI + EGF-guided ablation	7/8 (88%)	3/3 (100%)
Type III—PVI + EGF-guided ablation	6/13 (46%)	5/8 (63%)

Trends in the 12-month FFAF rates among the four phenotypes remained consistent across both trials. Among PVI-only patients noted in Table 3, Type I patients with no EGF-identified sources and a healthy substrate had 100% FFAF rates in both *FLOW-AF* and the *AF-FLOW Global Registry*. Type II patients with sources but a healthy substrate had a worse FFAF rate of 50% in *FLOW-AF*, though no Type II patients received PVI-only in the *AF-FLOW Global Registry*. This outcome was similar to that of Type IV patients with no sources but an unhealthy substrate, who had FFAF rates of 50% and 57%, respectively. Lastly, Type III patients with EGF-identified sources and an abnormal substrate had the worst outcomes in both trials, with FFAF rates of 23% and 50%. The pooled data of the two trials showed Type I patients to have 100% FFAF, Type IV having 52% FFAF, Type II having 50% FFAF, and Type III having 27% FFAF. Therefore, as PVI-only patients demonstrated either sources or a low EGFC in moving from Type I with neither to Types II or IV with one such factor, the FFAF significantly decreased (***p* = 0.003**). It decreased further in Type III patients with both factors compared to Types II or IV with just one, such that the overall differences in FFAF were most pronounced in Type I vs. Type III (***p* < 0.001**).

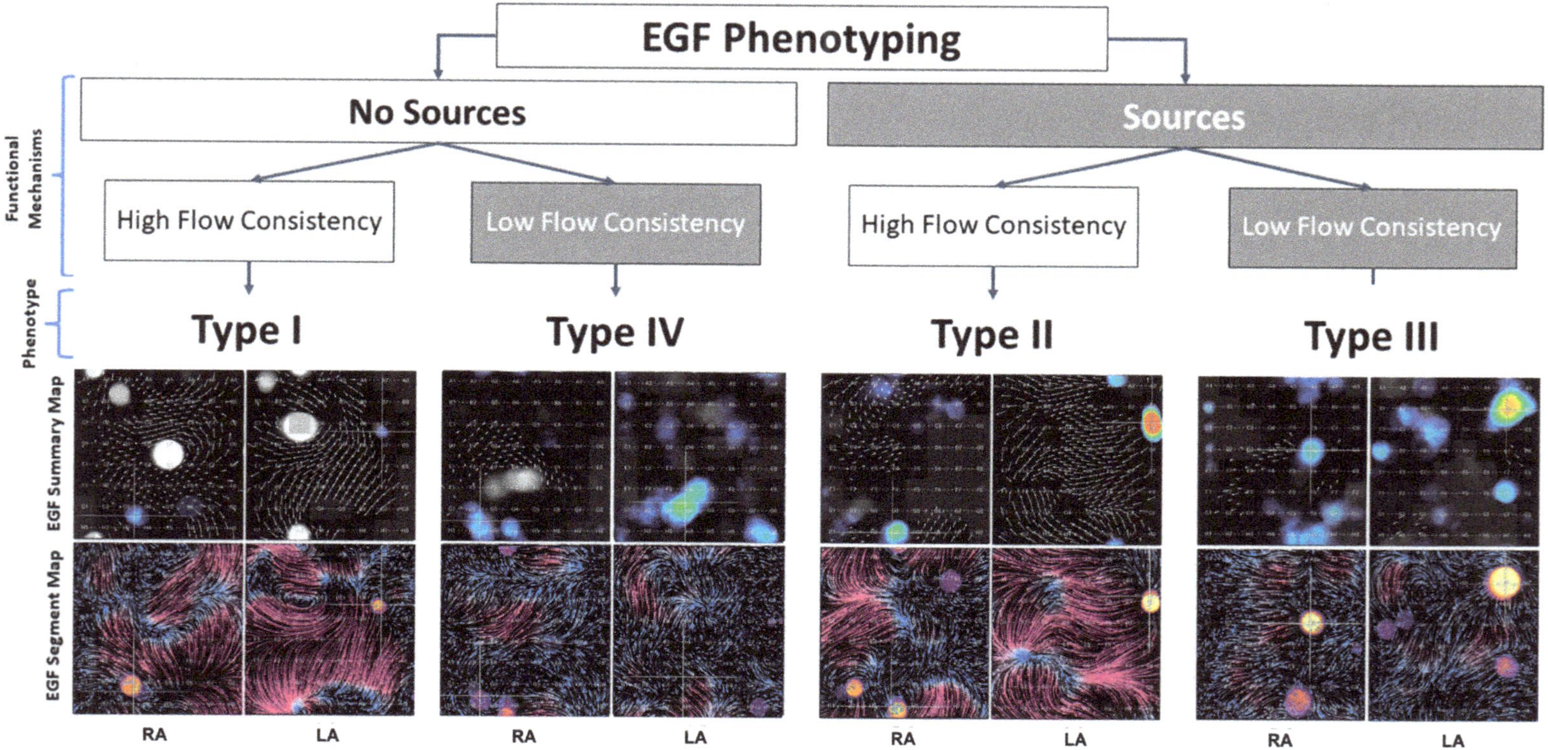

Figure 3. Four phenotypes were characterized based on the presence or absence of EGF-identified sources coupled with the presence of high or low EGFC. Active sources appear as yellow-red spots on summary maps and often localize to focal regions of divergent flow (yellow) on segment maps. EGFC is visualized as high-magnitude flow in a consistent direction over time, so regions with high EGFC are seen as vectors of longer length on summary maps and as purple regions on segment maps. Shorter vectors and more blue regions are areas of disorganized flow with low EGFC.

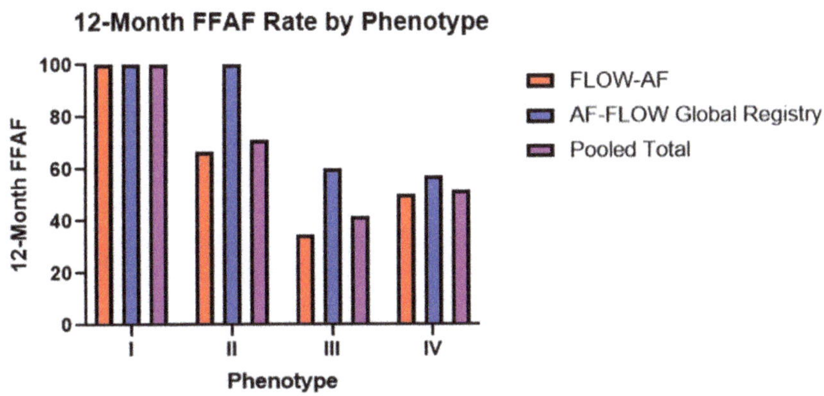

Figure 4. Twelve-month FFAF rates by phenotype across both trials. Trends from the *AF-FLOW Global Registry* help to validate those initially reported in *FLOW-AF* with improved Type II and Type III outcomes in the *AF-FLOW Global Registry* buoyed by the higher rate of EGF-guided source ablation among *AF-FLOW Global Registry* patients.

3.4. Source Ablation Improves FFAF in Both Independent Studies

When the outcomes by phenotype across the two studies shown in Figure 4 were analyzed, the *AF-FLOW Global Registry* FFAF rates were similar to the *FLOW-AF* FFAF rates among Type I and Type IV patients without sources, but the FFAF was noticeably higher among *AF-FLOW Global Registry* Type II and Type III patients with sources. Moreover, within the *AF-FLOW Global Registry*, Type I outcomes were identical to Type II outcomes at 100% FFAF, while Type III and Type IV outcomes were also highly similar at 60% and 57% FFAF, respectively. These diverging results between the trials were believed to predominantly result from procedural differences. In contrast with the *FLOW-AF* protocol requiring the randomization of source patients to PVI-only or PVI + EGF-guided ablation of sources, the *AF-FLOW Global Registry* patients predominantly received PVI plus targeted adjunctive source ablation when sources were observed.

Data were consequently also broken down by the combination of source presence and treatment modality. Among patients receiving PVI-only, source presence lowered the FFAF from 65% in pooled Type I and Type IV patients to 36% in pooled Type II and Type III patients (***p* = 0.023**). Moreover, among the source-containing Type II and Type III patients, those who received EGF-guided source ablation in addition to PVI demonstrated significantly improved outcomes, with 91% (10/11) Type II patients and 52% (11/21) Type III patients having FFAF, up from 50% (5/10) and 27% (4/15) after PVI alone. Combined data across both studies accordingly showed a 30% absolute increase in the FFAF from 36% to 66% (***p* = 0.026**) among source patients receiving PVI + EGF-guided ablation vs. PVI-only. Furthermore, since Type II and Type III patients with sources ablated had 66% FFAF, their outcomes mirrored and non-significantly differed from the Type I and Type IV patients who had 65% FFAF after PVI-only (p = 0.953). These data are shown in Table 3 and Figure 5.

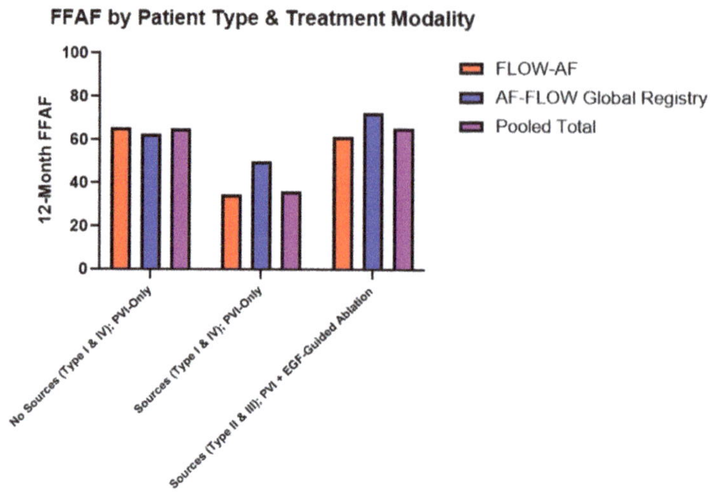

Figure 5. Twelve-month FFAF by patient type and treatment modality. Patients who received extra-PV ablation of EGF-identified sources showed higher rates of FFAF across both trials (p = 0.026), bringing FFAF to similar levels observed in patients without sources. Trends in improved outcomes due to source ablation in the *AF-FLOW Global Registry* align with those of *FLOW-AF*.

4. Discussion

The randomized, controlled *FLOW-AF* clinical trial represented the first attempt to determine if EGF mapping could be employed in a clinical setting to provide prognostic information and guide the targeted ablation of AF sources in difficult-to-treat redo and PeAF patients. After accomplishing these goals, the *AF-FLOW Global Registry* was subsequently designed to observe utilization of EGF mapping across a wider cohort of physicians treating AF all-comers and to validate the findings from *FLOW-AF*. Over these two studies of different AF populations from different clinical centers, EGF mapping successfully categorized patients into distinct phenotypes based on the presence of extra-PV sources and the quantification of substrate health.

Patients who recurred had a lower mean EGFC in both *FLOW-AF* and the *AF-FLOW Global Registry*. The presence of an abnormal substrate alone (overall EGFC of $\leq$0.62) also resulted in a 37% and 41% reduction in FFAF in the two trials, respectively. The relationship established between EGFC and patient outcomes in *FLOW-AF*, therefore, remained consistent among the *AF-FLOW Global Registry* patients.

These differences in FFAF rates based on EGFC can likely be attributed to the importance of tissue homogeneity in propagating a stable electrical wavefront. Substrate complexion can be altered by a variety of different mechanisms, such as abnormal myocyte hypertrophy, fibroblast proliferation, or even rapid inflammation. When such factors are not present, maps have higher EGFC whereby both the overall magnitude of flow vectors are higher and their directionality is more consistent over time, so that when segments are summed over the timescale of a 60 s recording, the net magnitude of flow in each location is minimally cancelled out by changes in direction in subsequent frames. Such patterns of rapid, consistent flow through the substrate suggest that a patient's AF is more organized and less chaotic, which we find to be a good prognostic sign. To support these findings, correlations have already been found between EGFC and bipolar voltage [31,35], which is also generally linked to improved outcomes; however, it remains a future goal to determine if associations exist between EGFC and localized regions of fibrosis or cardiomyopathy via cardiac MRI. It is also of interest whether SGLT2 inhibitors improve EGFC, as they have been shown to potentially reduce atrial fibrosis and remodeling, as well as decrease AF recurrence [37,38]. Nevertheless, through EGF mapping, physicians can already quantify the structural homogeneity of each patient via their overall EGFC, giving a prognostic assessment of the patient's level of AF organization or atrial health.

When further analyzing EGFC by atrium across both trials, it followed intuitively that patients had the best prognosis when they had EGFC values above the population mean in both their left and right atria. Accordingly, patients suffered a decreased FFAF when their EGFC was lower in either atrium, and the FFAF rates were the lowest when both the right and left atria concurrently had an EGFC below the population mean. The data also showed that categorizing patients based on the location of low EGFC zones was not as useful as collectively classifying them as either low or high EGFC based on an overall threshold, as previously described in *FLOW-AF* [32]. When overall EGFC is employed as a prognostic metric in this manner, the percentage of healthy substrate over the entire endocardial surface is quantified irrespective of anatomical location. As such, all tissue appears equally important in contributing to the conduction pathways propagating AF and the consequent likelihood of recurrence.

The pooled data comparing LA and RA EGFCs also demonstrated that the LA EGFC was significantly lower than the RA EGFC across all patients; however, there was a correlation between the LA EGFC and RA EGFC, which suggests that the substrate health of one atrium is not independent from the other. The slope of 0.51 further indicates that the already higher EGFC in the RA decreased from patient-to-patient at half the rate as it did in the LA. As such, these observations may collectively reflect that, pathophysiologically, disease originates in the LA near the PVs and spreads to the RA [39]. It thus follows that biatrial disease with maximal substrate remodeling is associated with the worst outcomes.

The ability to prognosticate patient outcomes increased when EGFC quantification was paired with noting the presence or absence of extra-PV sources. These sources were shown to decrease the rates of FFAF in both *FLOW-AF* and the *AF-FLOW Global Registry* after PVI-only therapy. Accordingly, through combining source presence and overall EGFC, four phenotypes were outlined in *FLOW-AF*, and they were again employed in the *AF-FLOW Global Registry* for validation.

Though small adjustments to the software, phenotype cutoffs, and mapping and ablation strategies have emerged over time, careful efforts were made to align the patients between the two trials when comparing them for the analysis presented here. When first using EGF mapping as a strictly diagnostic tool, we studied patients who did not receive ablation of EGF-identified sources to predict PVI-only outcomes. In both trials, Type I patients had a 100% FFAF at 12 months. Since Type I patients have a healthy substrate and no extra-PV sources, they are predominantly patients who can be treated solely with PVI with reliably good outcomes. When then looking at Type II and Type IV patients, the presence of either extra-PV sources or a low EGFC independently dropped the FFAF rate by a similar magnitude. This trend was maintained across the two trials. Lastly, when comparing the FFAF in Type II and Type IV patients with Type III patients who have both prognostic factors, a multiplicative drop in FFAF was noted due to the presence of both factors. Type III patients were shown to have the lowest rates of FFAF across both studies, likely due to the compounding effects of having a low EGFC and extra-PV sources after PVI-only.

Beyond using EGF as a predictive tool for the prognosis of PVI-only patients, both trials also had a separate treatment population defined as patients who received EGF-guided ablation of extra-PV sources. In *FLOW-AF*, there was a strict cutoff requiring multiple maps to show an SAC of $\geq 26.5\%$ for ablation in the treatment-arm patients, while the mapping and SAC thresholds for extra-PV source ablation varied from patient to patient in the *AF-FLOW Global Registry* based on physician discretion. Still, patients could be aligned to define treated Type II and Type III patients as those with at least one source with SAC $\geq$ 26.5% ablated, and this EGF-guided ablation of sources increased the FFAF rates in both trials to produce an absolute increase of 30% FFAF. Type II and Type III patients receiving source ablation also had similar and non-significantly different outcomes than those of Types I and Type IV patients who never had sources identified in the first place. Therefore, the ability for targeted ablation to negate the deleterious effects of extra-PV sources indicates that EGF-detected sources may play a significant role in propagating the AF circuits beyond the PVs and suggests that their ablation is necessary for optimal treatment. When combined with improved ablation strategies [9,11], the targeting of all such AF triggers in this manner should continue to improve the effectiveness of therapeutic strategies while providing greater insights into each patient's mechanism of disease.

A weakness in these comparisons between *FLOW-AF* and the *AF-FLOW Global Registry* is that the patients in the *AF-FLOW Global Registry* were healthier because they included de novo and PAF patients. The sample sizes for PVI-only patients in the Registry were also very small, and even included zero PVI-only Type II patients; however, similar trends in FFAF by phenotype were still present between the two studies, despite the high propensity for population differences or noise. EGF mapping itself also brought limitations, including the need for good wall contact to best assess the health of the substrate and the acute locations of sources. Physicians using the technology additionally needed to be able to steer the basket into a series of positions that covered the full endocardial surface. Still, a diverse group of physicians distinct from those in *FLOW-AF* used EGF mapping in the *AF-FLOW Global Registry* and were able to quickly learn these techniques. Consequently, it seems likely that, with training and skilled use, EGF mapping can provide physicians with an assessment of a patient's overall substrate health and their presence or absence of extra-PV sources. This information can in turn inform users on a patient's AF mechanism and how effective a PVI-only or PVI + source ablation approach may be for that patient.

By contrast, current guidelines for classifying AF are based on temporal persistence, where PAF indicates that the longest AF episode lasted fewer than 7 days and PeAF signifies that the longest episode lasted more than 7 days. This framework has been used for outlining inclusion and exclusion criteria for clinical trials and for selecting therapies, but it does not adequately reflect either the actual temporal persistence of AF nor any inherent pathophysiological characteristics, and it is not tied to AF burden or mechanism [40–43]. We consequently believe that EGF phenotyping provides a superseding means of binning patients based on their pathophysiology that will be more useful in directing treatments. We also expect future efforts to work on refining phenotype cutoffs and the therapeutic strategies employed within each category, particularly in regard to developing an ablation strategy for patients with a low EGFC (Type III and Type IV) that targets the substrate to improve outcomes beyond PVI + source ablation [38,44]. At the same time, tuning an ablation strategy to a patient's individual phenotype will likely allow for fewer unnecessary ablations and for targeting the minimally necessary treatment to an individual's specific mechanism of AF.

5. Conclusions

The *AF-FLOW Global Registry* was a multicenter trial that validated the results of the randomized, controlled *FLOW-AF* trial. In analyzing both trials, trends were established that demonstrated the efficacy of EGF mapping in providing prognostic information and guiding treatment for AF. Evidence for the following was found: (1) EGFC can be an effective marker of substrate health, and high EGFC values are tied to a higher 12-month FFAF; (2) LA EGFC is lower than but correlated with RA EGFC, suggestive of general substrate remodeling progressive from the LA to the RA; (3) EGF-identified extra-PV sources may be potent drivers of AF, whose presence decreases FFAF rates if left unablated; and (4) phenotyping patients based on EGFC and source presence may be useful in predicting patient recurrence and designing optimal mechanism-specific ablation strategies.

Author Contributions: Conceptualization, K.R.N., M.H.K., A.V. and S.C.; methodology, K.R.N., M.H.K., A.V. and S.C.; software, S.C.; validation, M.H.K. and S.C.; formal analysis, S.C.; investigation, K.R.N., P.D., T.S.-T., S.G. and M.T.; resources, K.R.N., M.H.K., P.D., T.S.-T., S.G. and M.T.; data curation, A.A. and S.C.; writing—original draft preparation, A.A. and S.C.; writing—review and editing, K.R.N., M.H.K. and S.C.; visualization, A.A. and S.C.; supervision, M.H.K., A.V. and S.C.; project administration, K.R.N., M.H.K., A.V. and S.C.; funding acquisition, M.H.K. All authors have read and agreed to the published version of the manuscript.

Funding: This research was funded by Cortex, Inc., formerly Ablacon, Inc. Three physicians at the Czech Republic who participated in *FLOW-AF* were supported by a Scientific Grant by the Ministry of Health Czech Republic, DRO (NNH, IG 180504).

Institutional Review Board Statement: *FLOW-AF* (NCT04473963) was conducted according to the guidelines of the Declaration of Helsinki and approved by the Institutional Review Board of Nemocnice Na Homolce Hospital, Prague (protocol code CP-001/002 and date of approval 27 September 2019) and subsequently by other participating centers. The *AF-FLOW Global Registry* (NCT05481359) was conducted according to the guidelines of the Declaration of Helsinki and approved by the Institutional Review Board of Medicover Hospital, Warsaw (protocol code CP-005 and date of approval 5 August 2022) and subsequently by other participating centers.

Informed Consent Statement: Informed consent was obtained from all subjects involved in the study.

Data Availability Statement: Data from both *FLOW-AF* (NCT04473963) and the *AF-FLOW Global Registry* (NCT05481359) are available on clinicaltrials.gov.

Conflicts of Interest: K.R.N. and A.V. are members of the scientific advisory board for Cortex, Inc. M.H.K. is a former employee of Cortex, Inc. T.S.-T. consulted for product development with Cortex, Inc. S.C. is a current employee of Cortex, Inc.

Abbreviations

The following abbreviations are used in this manuscript:

AF	Atrial fibrillation
AFL	Atrial flutter
AT	Atrial tachycardia
EGF	Electrographic Flow
EGFC	Electrographic Flow Consistency
EGM	Electrogram
FFAF	Freedom from atrial fibrillation
LA	Left atrium
LAA	Left atrial appendage
LS-PeAF	Long-standing persistent atrial fibrillation
PAF	Paroxysmal atrial fibrillation
PeAF	Persistent atrial fibrillation
PFA	Pulsed field ablation
PV	Pulmonary vein
PVI	Pulmonary vein isolation
RA	Right atrium
RF	Radiofrequency
SAC	Source activity
SVC	Superior vena cava

References

1. Kornej, J.; Börschel, C.S.; Benjamin, E.J.; Schnabel, R.B. Epidemiology of atrial fibrillation in the 21st century: Novel methods and new insights. *Circ. Res.* **2020**, *127*, 4–20. [CrossRef] [PubMed]
2. Roth, G.A.; Mensah, G.A.; Johnson, C.O.; Addolorato, G.; Ammirati, E.; Baddour, L.M.; Barengo, N.C.; Beaton, A.Z.; Benjamin, E.J.; Benziger, C.P. Global burden of cardiovascular diseases and risk factors, 1990–2019: Update from the GBD 2019 study. *J. Am. Coll. Cardiol.* **2020**, *76*, 2982–3021. [CrossRef] [PubMed]
3. Krijthe, B.P.; Kunst, A.; Benjamin, E.J.; Lip, G.Y.; Franco, O.H.; Hofman, A.; Witteman, J.C.; Stricker, B.H.; Heeringa, J. Projections on the number of individuals with atrial fibrillation in the European Union, from 2000 to 2060. *Eur. Heart J.* **2013**, *34*, 2746–2751. [CrossRef] [PubMed]
4. Linz, D.; Gawalko, M.; Betz, K.; Hendriks, J.M.; Lip, G.Y.; Vinter, N.; Guo, Y.; Johnsen, S. Atrial fibrillation: Epidemiology, screening and digital health. *Lancet Reg. Health–Eur.* **2024**, *37*, 100786. [CrossRef]
5. Karakasis, P.; Pamporis, K.; Siontis, K.C.; Theofilis, P.; Samaras, A.; Patoulias, D.; Stachteas, P.; Karagiannidis, E.; Stavropoulos, G.; Tzikas, A. Major clinical outcomes in symptomatic vs. asymptomatic atrial fibrillation: A meta-analysis. *Eur. Heart J.* **2024**, ehae694. [CrossRef] [PubMed]
6. Boriani, G.; Laroche, C.; Diemberger, I.; Fantecchi, E.; Popescu, M.I.; Rasmussen, L.H.; Sinagra, G.; Petrescu, L.; Tavazzi, L.; Maggioni, A.P. Asymptomatic atrial fibrillation: Clinical correlates, management, and outcomes in the EORP-AF Pilot General Registry. *Am. J. Med.* **2015**, *128*, 509–518.e502. [CrossRef]
7. Schmidt, B.; Brugada, J.; Arbelo, E.; Laroche, C.; Bayramova, S.; Bertini, M.; Letsas, K.P.; Pison, L.; Romanov, A.; Scherr, D. Ablation strategies for different types of atrial fibrillation in Europe: Results of the ESC-EORP EHRA Atrial Fibrillation Ablation Long-Term registry. *EP Eur.* **2020**, *22*, 558–566. [CrossRef]
8. Verma, A.; Jiang, C.-y.; Betts, T.R.; Chen, J.; Deisenhofer, I.; Mantovan, R.; Macle, L.; Morillo, C.A.; Haverkamp, W.; Weerasooriya, R. Approaches to catheter ablation for persistent atrial fibrillation. *N. Engl. J. Med.* **2015**, *372*, 1812–1822. [CrossRef] [PubMed]
9. Lepillier, A.; Maggio, R.; De Sanctis, V.; Malacrida, M.; Stabile, G.; Zakine, C.; Champ-Rigot, L.; Anselmino, M.; Segreti, L.; Dell'Era, G. Insight into contact force local impedance technology for predicting effective pulmonary vein isolation. *Front. Cardiovasc. Med.* **2023**, *10*, 1169037. [CrossRef]
10. Reddy, V.Y.; Shah, D.; Kautzner, J.; Schmidt, B.; Saoudi, N.; Herrera, C.; Jaïs, P.; Hindricks, G.; Peichl, P.; Yulzari, A. The relationship between contact force and clinical outcome during radiofrequency catheter ablation of atrial fibrillation in the TOCCATA study. *Heart Rhythm* **2012**, *9*, 1789–1795. [CrossRef] [PubMed]
11. Schaack, D.; Schmidt, B.; Tohoku, S.; Bordignon, S.; Urbanek, L.; Ebrahimi, R.; Hirokami, J.; Efe, T.H.; Chen, S.; Chun, K.J. Pulsed field ablation for atrial fibrillation. *Arrhythmia Electrophysiol. Rev.* **2023**, *12*, e11. [CrossRef] [PubMed]
12. Reddy, V.Y.; Dukkipati, S.R.; Neuzil, P.; Anic, A.; Petru, J.; Funasako, M.; Cochet, H.; Minami, K.; Breskovic, T.; Sikiric, I. Pulsed field ablation of paroxysmal atrial fibrillation: 1-year outcomes of IMPULSE, PEFCAT, and PEFCAT II. *Clin. Electrophysiol.* **2021**, *7*, 614–627. [CrossRef] [PubMed]
13. Reddy, V.Y.; Anic, A.; Koruth, J.; Petru, J.; Funasako, M.; Minami, K.; Breskovic, T.; Sikiric, I.; Dukkipati, S.R.; Kawamura, I. Pulsed field ablation in patients with persistent atrial fibrillation. *J. Am. Coll. Cardiol.* **2020**, *76*, 1068–1080. [CrossRef] [PubMed]
14. Schmidt, B.; Bordignon, S.; Chen, S.; Bologna, F.; Urbanek, L.; Pansera, F.; Ernst, M.; Chun, K.J. 5S study: Safe and simple single shot pulmonary vein isolation with pulsed field ablation using sedation. *Circ. Arrhythmia Electrophysiol.* **2022**, *15*, e010817. [CrossRef] [PubMed]
15. Pansera, F.; Bordignon, S.; Bologna, F.; Chen, S.; Urbanek, L.; Schmidt, B.; Chun, K.-R.J. Catheter ablation induced phrenic nerve palsy by pulsed field ablation—Completely impossible? A case series. *Eur. Heart J.-Case Rep.* **2022**, *6*, ytac361. [CrossRef] [PubMed]
16. van Driel, V.J.; Neven, K.G.; van Wessel, H.; du Pré, B.C.; Vink, A.; Doevendans, P.A.; Wittkampf, F.H. Pulmonary vein stenosis after catheter ablation: Electroporation versus radiofrequency. *Circ. Arrhythmia Electrophysiol.* **2014**, *7*, 734–738. [CrossRef]
17. Howard, B.; Haines, D.E.; Verma, A.; Packer, D.; Kirchhof, N.; Barka, N.; Onal, B.; Fraasch, S.; Miklavčič, D.; Stewart, M.T. Reduction in pulmonary vein stenosis and collateral damage with pulsed field ablation compared with radiofrequency ablation in a canine model. *Circ. Arrhythmia Electrophysiol.* **2020**, *13*, e008337. [CrossRef] [PubMed]
18. Chun, K.J.; Bordignon, S.; Chen, S.; Schaack, D.; Urbanek, L.; Ebrahimi, R.; Hirokami, J.; Bologna, F.; Schmidt, B. Findings from repeat ablation using high-density mapping after pulmonary vein isolation with pulsed field ablation. *Europace* **2023**, *25*, 433–440.
19. Lemoine, M.D.; Fink, T.; Mencke, C.; Schleberger, R.; My, I.; Obergassel, J.; Bergau, L.; Sciacca, V.; Rottner, L.; Moser, J. Pulsed-field ablation-based pulmonary vein isolation: Acute safety, efficacy and short-term follow-up in a multi-center real world scenario. *Clin. Res. Cardiol.* **2023**, *112*, 795–806. [CrossRef]
20. Scott, P.A.; Silberbauer, J.; Murgatroyd, F.D. The impact of adjunctive complex fractionated atrial electrogram ablation and linear lesions on outcomes in persistent atrial fibrillation: A meta-analysis. *Europace* **2016**, *18*, 359–367. [CrossRef]

21. Narayan, S.M.; Krummen, D.E.; Shivkumar, K.; Clopton, P.; Rappel, W.-J.; Miller, J.M. Treatment of atrial fibrillation by the ablation of localized sources: CONFIRM (Conventional Ablation for Atrial Fibrillation with or Without Focal Impulse and Rotor Modulation) trial. *J. Am. Coll. Cardiol.* **2012**, *60*, 628–636. [CrossRef]
22. Seitz, J.; Durdez, T.M.; Albenque, J.P.; Pisapia, A.; Gitenay, E.; Durand, C.; Monteau, J.; Moubarak, G.; Théodore, G.; Lepillier, A. Artificial intelligence software standardizes electrogram-based ablation outcome for persistent atrial fibrillation. *J. Cardiovasc. Electrophysiol.* **2022**, *33*, 2250–2260. [CrossRef]
23. Marrouche, N.F.; Greene, T.; Dean, J.M.; Kholmovski, E.G.; Boer, L.M.d.; Mansour, M.; Calkins, H.; Marchlinski, F.; Wilber, D.; Hindricks, G. Efficacy of LGE-MRI-guided fibrosis ablation versus conventional catheter ablation of atrial fibrillation: The DECAAF II trial: Study design. *J. Cardiovasc. Electrophysiol.* **2021**, *32*, 916–924. [CrossRef] [PubMed]
24. Willems, S.; Verma, A.; Betts, T.R.; Murray, S.; Neuzil, P.; Ince, H.; Steven, D.; Sultan, A.; Heck, P.M.; Hall, M.C. Targeting nonpulmonary vein sources in persistent atrial fibrillation identified by noncontact charge density mapping: UNCOVER AF trial. *Circ. Arrhythmia Electrophysiol.* **2019**, *12*, e007233. [CrossRef]
25. Duchateau, J.; Sacher, F.; Pambrun, T.; Derval, N.; Chamorro-Servent, J.; Denis, A.; Ploux, S.; Hocini, M.; Jaïs, P.; Bernus, O. Performance and limitations of noninvasive cardiac activation mapping. *Heart Rhythm* **2019**, *16*, 435–442. [CrossRef]
26. Gianni, C.; Mohanty, S.; Di Biase, L.; Metz, T.; Trivedi, C.; Gökoğlan, Y.; Güneş, M.F.; Bai, R.; Al-Ahmad, A.; Burkhardt, J.D. Acute and early outcomes of focal impulse and rotor modulation (FIRM)-guided rotors-only ablation in patients with nonparoxysmal atrial fibrillation. *Heart Rhythm* **2016**, *13*, 830–835. [CrossRef]
27. Hemam, M.E.; Dave, A.S.; Rodríguez-Mañero, M.; Valderrábano, M. Epiphenomenal re-entry and spurious focal activation detection by atrial fibrillation mapping algorithms. *Clin. Electrophysiol.* **2021**, *7*, 923–932. [CrossRef] [PubMed]
28. Kong, M.H.; Castellano, S.; Ruppersberg, P.; Lizama, K.S.; Avitall, B. Visualization of electrographic flow fields of increasing complexity and detection of simulated sources during spontaneously persistent AF in an animal model. *Front. Cardiovasc. Med.* **2023**, *10*, 1223481. [CrossRef]
29. Reddy, V.Y.; Kong, M.H.; Petru, J.; Maan, A.; Funasako, M.; Minami, K.; Ruppersberg, P.; Dukkipati, S.; Neuzil, P. Electrographic flow mapping of persistent atrial fibrillation: Intra-and inter-procedure reproducibility in the absence of 'ground truth'. *Europace* **2023**, *25*, euad308. [CrossRef] [PubMed]
30. Sommer, P.; Castellano, S.; Kong, M.H.; Haines, D.E. PO-04-093 Characterization of Egf-Identified Source Signatures in Sinus Rhythm and Atrial Fibrillation. *Heart Rhythm* **2023**, *20*, S521. [CrossRef]
31. Sommer, P.; Castellano, S.; Ahapov, K.; Jansen, M.M.; Mehta, N.K.; Kong, M.H. A single-center trial of electrographic flow mapping and concomitant voltage mapping in sinus rhythm and atrial fibrillation (FLOW EVAL-AF). *J. Interv. Card. Electrophysiol.* **2024**, 1–11. [CrossRef] [PubMed]
32. Reddy, V.Y.; Langbein, A.; Petru, J.; Szili-Torok, T.; Funasako, M.; Dinshaw, L.; Wijchers, S.; Rillig, A.; Spitzer, S.G.; Bhagwandien, R. A Randomized Trial of Electrographic Flow-Guided Redo Ablation for Nonparoxysmal Atrial Fibrillation (FLOW-AF). *JACC Clin. Electrophysiol.* **2024**, *10*, 1856–1869. [CrossRef] [PubMed]
33. Verma, A.; Castellano, S.; Kong, M.H.; Neuzil, P.; Szili-Torok, T.; Spitzer, S.G.; Rillig, A.; Reddy, V.Y. PVI-Only is Not Enough for All Persistent AF Patients: A FLOW-AF Subgroup Analysis. *Heart Rhythm* **2024**. [CrossRef]
34. Castellano, S.; Kong, M.H. Electrographic flow mapping of atrial fibrillation. *Curr. Opin. Cardiol.* **2025**, *40*, 8–14. [CrossRef] [PubMed]
35. Nilsson, K.R.; Castellano, S.; Kong, M.H.; Derejko, P.; Szili-Torok, T.; Goyal, S.K.; Wijchers, S.; Turagam, M.; Reddy, V.Y.; Verma, A.; et al. AF-FLOW Global Registry Confirms Validity of Electrographic Flow Mapping as a Phenotyping Tool for Atrial Fibrillation. *J. Cardiovasc. Electrophysiol.* 2025, *ahead of print*.
36. Haines, D.E.; Kong, M.H.; Ruppersberg, P.; Haeusser, P.; Avitall, B.; Szili-Torok, T.; Verma, A. Electrographic flow mapping for atrial fibrillation: Theoretical basis and preliminary observations. *J. Interv. Card. Electrophysiol.* **2023**, *66*, 1015–1028. [CrossRef]
37. Shao, Q.; Meng, L.; Lee, S.; Tse, G.; Gong, M.; Zhang, Z.; Zhao, J.; Zhao, Y.; Li, G.; Liu, T. Empagliflozin, a sodium glucose co-transporter-2 inhibitor, alleviates atrial remodeling and improves mitochondrial function in high-fat diet/streptozotocin-induced diabetic rats. *Cardiovasc. Diabetol.* **2019**, *18*, 165. [CrossRef] [PubMed]
38. Pandey, A.K.; Okaj, I.; Kaur, H.; Belley-Cote, E.P.; Wang, J.; Oraii, A.; Benz, A.P.; Johnson, L.S.; Young, J.; Wong, J.A. Sodium-glucose co-transporter inhibitors and atrial fibrillation: A systematic review and meta-analysis of randomized controlled trials. *J. Am. Heart Assoc.* **2021**, *10*, e022222. [CrossRef] [PubMed]
39. Lin, W.-S.; Prakash, V.; Tai, C.-T.; Hsieh, M.-H.; Tsai, C.-F.; Yu, W.-C.; Lin, Y.-K.; Ding, Y.-A.; Chang, M.-S.; Chen, S.-A. Pulmonary vein morphology in patients with paroxysmal atrial fibrillation initiated by ectopic beats originating from the pulmonary veins: Implications for catheter ablation. *Circulation* **2000**, *101*, 1274–1281. [CrossRef] [PubMed]
40. Calkins, H. HRS/EHRA/ECAS/APHRS/SOLAECE expert consensus statement on catheter and surgical ablation of atrial fibrillation. *Europace* **2017**, *2018*, e1.

41. January, C.T.; Wann, L.S.; Alpert, J.S.; Calkins, H.; Cigarroa, J.E.; Cleveland Jr, J.C.; Conti, J.B.; Ellinor, P.T.; Ezekowitz, M.D.; Field, M.E. 2014 AHA/ACC/HRS guideline for the management of patients with atrial fibrillation: Executive summary: A report of the American College of Cardiology/American Heart Association Task Force on practice guidelines and the Heart Rhythm Society. *Circulation* **2014**, *130*, 2071–2104. [CrossRef]
42. Charitos, E.I.; Pürerfellner, H.; Glotzer, T.V.; Ziegler, P.D. Clinical classifications of atrial fibrillation poorly reflect its temporal persistence: Insights from 1,195 patients continuously monitored with implantable devices. *J. Am. Coll. Cardiol.* **2014**, *63*, 2840–2848. [CrossRef] [PubMed]
43. Zaman, J.A.; Baykaner, T.; Clopton, P.; Swarup, V.; Kowal, R.C.; Daubert, J.P.; Day, J.D.; Hummel, J.; Schricker, A.A.; Krummen, D.E. Recurrent post-ablation paroxysmal atrial fibrillation shares substrates with persistent atrial fibrillation: An 11-center study. *Clin. Electrophysiol.* **2017**, *3*, 393–402. [CrossRef]
44. Huo, Y.; Gaspar, T.; Schönbauer, R.; Wójcik, M.; Fiedler, L.; Roithinger, F.X.; Martinek, M.; Pürerfellner, H.; Kirstein, B.; Richter, U. Low-voltage myocardium-guided ablation trial of persistent atrial fibrillation. *NEJM Evid.* **2022**, *1*, EVIDoa2200141. [CrossRef] [PubMed]

Journal of
Clinical Medicine

MDPI

Article

Prediction of Ablation Index and Lesion Size Index for Local Impedance Drop-Guided Ablation

Lukas Sprenger [1,*], Fabian Moser [1], Vera Maslova [1], Adrian Zaman [1], Marc Nonnenmacher [1], Sven Willert [1], Derk Frank [1,2] and Evgeny Lian [1,2]

1 Department of Internal Medicine III (Cardiology and Intensive Care Medicine), University Hospital Schleswig-Holstein (UKSH), Arnold-Heller-Str. 3, 24105 Kiel, Germany
2 German Centre of Cardiovascular Research (DZHK), Partner Site Hamburg/Kiel/Lübeck, Arnold-Heller-Str. 3, 24105 Kiel, Germany
* Correspondence: Lukas.Sprenger@uksh.de

Abstract: (1) **Background**: The effectiveness of RF ablation for PVI depends on the lesion location and size to achieve continuous and durable lesion lines. AI and LSI are widely accepted lesion metrics for guiding the ablation procedure. LI dynamics is another parameter that guides PVI and does not rely on input variables. Limited data are available on a direct comparison between lesion metrics. Our study aims to compare RF application durations and influencing factors during index-guided (AI and LSI) and LI-guided approaches by predicting lesion metrics using machine learning. (2) **Methods**: While the coefficients in AI and LSI formulas are not disclosed, we trained custom machine-learning models based on Random Forest and Gradient Boosting Regressors to predict AI and LSI metrics for LI-guided ablations. (3) **Results**: The median RF application durations differed significantly between the lesion metrics, with 7.32, 19.91, and 11.92 s for AI-, LSI-, and LI-guided procedures, respectively. Mean CF was found to be an important predictor of RF application duration for the AI- and LSI-guided approaches. (4) **Conclusions**: Depending on the metric used, the significant differences in RF application durations suggest that an AI-guide approach may allow for shorter RF application durations, followed by LSI-guided and LI-guided procedures. Further studies are needed to evaluate the safety and efficacy of these results in a clinical setting.

Keywords: atrialfibrillation (AF); pulmonary vein isolation (PVI); radiofrequency ablation (RFA); ablation index (AI); lesion size index (LSI); local impedance (LI)

1. Introduction

Radiofrequency (RF) catheter ablation is an established treatment option for atrial fibrillation (AF) [1]. Ablation success highly depends on the location and size of the lesion created by the ablation catheter, thereby leading to a continuous and durable lesion set forming an ablation line between the pulmonary vein (PV) and the left atrium. The main reason for AF recurrence after ablation is the electrical reconnection of the PV and the left atrium [2], whereas prolonged RF application duration bears the risk of complications, such as steam pops, pericardial effusion, or atrioesophageal fistula [3]. Aiming at creating durable ablation results while mitigating complications emphasizes the importance of precise lesion size prediction.

The Ablation Index (AI) and Lesion Size Index (LSI) are widely accepted, easy-to-use lesion metrics for estimating the RF lesion size and help guiding the ablation procedure. Depending on the physicist's discretion, they are available in their corresponding 3D mapping systems: CARTO© 3 (Biosense Webster, Irvine, CA, USA) and EnSite™ (Abbott, Abbott Park, MA, USA). The feasibility of both AI and LSI has been shown in previous studies [4–6]. Both metrics are dependent on their input parameters, such as contact force (CF), delivered power (P), radiofrequency current (I), and application duration (τ). Local impedance (LI) is another parameter that guides catheter ablation and does not depend on further input parameters. LI dynamics measurement was implemented in the RHYTHMIA HDx™ (Boston Scientific, Marlborough, MA, USA) platform with DIRECTSENSE™ technology. The LOCALIZE trial showed that LI dynamic predicts acute and chronic PV segment conduction block, even without CF monitoring [7]. Next-generation ablation catheters (IntellaNav Stablepoint™ with DIRECTSENSE™ technology) integrate both LI and CF measurement, but the current RHYTHMIA HDx™ platform neither provides AI nor LSI indices to guide the ablation procedure.

Currently, there are a lack of data on the direct comparison of lesion metrics, such as AI-, LSI-, and LI-drop-guided ablations. Most studies have reviewed lesion metrics individually regarding their acute efficacy and long-term success. For example, they show shorter procedure times and fewer PV gaps for an LSI-guided approach than an LI-drop-guided ablation procedure [8]. However, a direct comparison regarding RF application duration and influencing factors for lesion creation is particularly required.

Our study aims to provide insights into RF application durations and influencing factors by comparing index-guided (AI and LSI) and LI-guided approaches, which is achieved by predicting AI and LSI metrics using a machine learning approach and by showing the feasibility of their applicability in a clinical setting.

2. Methods

While CF and LI monitoring (Stablepoint™, RHYTHMIA HDx™ with DIRECTSENSE™ technology, Boston Scientific, Marlborough, MA, USA) are available simultaneously during ablation, AI and LSI formulas contain proprietary coefficients, which are not disclosed (see Equations (1) and (2)).

$$\text{Ablation Index} = \left\{K \cdot \int_0^{\tau} CF^{a}_{(\tau)}\, P^{b}_{\tau}\, d\tau\right\}^{c}, \quad (1)$$

$$\text{Lesion Size Index} = b_0\left(1 - e^{\frac{-F}{b_1}} + b_2\right)\left(1 - e^{\frac{-I^2}{b_3^2}}\right)\left(1 - b_4 + \frac{b_4\left(1 - e^{\frac{-\tau}{b_5}}\right)}{1 - e^{\frac{-60}{b_5}}}\right). \quad (2)$$

Equation (1) shows how the Ablation Index (AI) is calculated, while Equation (2) shows how the Lesion Size Index (LSI) is calculated. Ablation Index (AI, arbitrary units): CF = contact force; P = power; τ = application duration; and K, a, b, c represent constants (proprietary data). Lesion Size Index (LSI, arbitrary units): F = 6 s sliding window of average contact force; I = 6 s sliding window of average radiofrequency current; τ = time; and $b_0, b_1, b_2, b_3, b_4, b_5$ represent constants (proprietary data).

We performed a two-step approach to estimate the AI and LSI for the lesions created by the RHYTHMIA HDx™ system, as these indices are not provided by the system. In the first step, as predicting lesion indices can be comprehended as a regression problem, we trained two machine learning algorithms for AI and LSI predictions using collected ablation data. In the second step, we retrospectively analyzed the atrial ablation data of patients undergoing LI-drop-guided ablation, utilizing our pre-trained models to predict AI and LSI lesion metrics.

Data preparation, model generation, and statistics were conducted in Python using Numpy [9], Pandas [10], scikit-learn [11], Scipy [12], Statsmodel [13], pyGAM [14], and

Miceforest. Matplotlib [15] and Seaborn [16] were used for visualization. For the software library version used, see Table A1.

2.1. Patient Population

Patient data, both for model generation and data analysis, were provided and anonymized at the time of export from its specific ablation system, with baseline patient characteristics attached. For model generation, patients undergoing radiofrequency PVI for the ablation of paroxysmal or persistent AF using either AI-guided (Carto© 3 system, Biosense Webster, Irvine, CA, USA) or LSI-guided (EnSiteX™ system, Abbott, Abbott Park, MA, USA) approaches were selected. Data were exported from the RHYTHMIA HDx™ system with DIRECTSENSE™ technology for data analysis.

All procedures were carried out in accordance with the current guidelines [1]. SmartTouch® and TactiCath™ ablation catheters were used for index-guided ablation while using the CARTO© 3 system (Biosense Webster, Irvine, CA, USA) and EnSite™ system (Abbott, Abbott Park, MA, USA) accordingly. The energy was delivered using an IntellaNav Stablepoint™ ablation catheter (RHYTMIA HDx™ system, Boston Scientific, Marlborough, MA, USA) for the LI drop-guided procedures.

2.2. Model Generation

We gathered two training datasets by exporting the ablation data from ten patients that had been undergoing ablation for paroxysmal or persistent atrial fibrillation from their respective mapping systems. This resulted in a total of 553 (AI) and 22 (LSI) lesions. As we aimed to be able to predict the lesion indices for every time point τ during the ablation process, we further separated the independent and dependent variables during lesion creation, with a total of 529,684 (AI) and 42,538 (LSI) data points for training purposes. Furthermore, using the Simpsons' rule [17] during data preparation, we calculated the force–time integral for every time point τ during lesion creation. For the parameter space of both models, refer to Tables 1 and 2.

Table 1. The training parameters for the Ablation Index Model (the AI training dataset used).

Parameter	Median (IQR)
Contact Force, g·s	12.096 (12.178)
Power, W	50.0 (9.8)
Ablation Index	362.259 (196.058)

Table 2. The training parameters for the Lesion Size Index Model (the LSI training data set used).

Parameter	Median (IQR)
Contact Force, g·s	11.500 (9.800)
Power, W	40.0 (0.0)
RF current, mA	526.134 (33.021)
Lesion Size Index	2.591 (1.097)

We used the Shapiro–Wilkins and Anderson–Darling tests as normality tests. For both training datasets, the Shapiro–Wilkins and Anderson–Darling tests indicated a non-Gaussian distribution. Additionally, the variance inflation factors (VIFs) and correlation coefficients suggested the existence of multicollinearity, potentially affecting the stability of the models. To address these challenges, we compared a Random Forest Regressor [18,19] and a Gradient Boosting Regressor [19] alongside three linear models—Ridge, Lasso, and ElasticNet [19]. During the training of the LSI model, we employed quantile transform to handle the non-Gaussian distribution and skewness of the LSI training data.

Furthermore, we conducted hyperparameter [20] tuning to improve the performance of all models using *GridSearchCV* with a 10-fold cross-validation. We chose the hyperparameters to be optimized based on our own conducted early experiments to account for both simple and more complex models. For the optimized hyperparameters and their value ranges, refer to Table A2.

To evaluate our final models, we used the coefficient of determination (R^2) and the mean absolute error (MAE) while applying a 30% split for cross-validation. Regarding our AI prediction model, the Random Forest model performed best with an R^2 of 0.85 and an MAE of 6.62. For our LSI prediction, we chose the Gradient Boosting model, as it showed the best performance with an R^2 of 0.97 and an MAE of 0.10. The three linear models also performed less successfully, most likely due to their inability to model the non-linear relationship of the underlying data (refer to Table 3 for the complete test results).

Table 3. Performance metrics (R^2 and MAE) for the AI and LSI prediction models during cross-validation when applying a 30% split.

Model	R^2	MAE
AI prediction		
Random Forest	0.972	6.617
Gradient Boosting	0.924	15.422
Ridge	0.807	41.044
Lasso	0.807	41.043
ElasticNet	0.807	41.044
LSI prediction		
Random Forest	0.940	0.132
Gradient Boosting	0.969	0.103
Ridge	0.925	0.163
Lasso	0.925	0.159
ElasticNet	0.925	0.161

2.3. Data Analysis

Subsequently, we analyzed the atrial ablation data of 27 patients who underwent LI-drop-guided ablation. For patient demographics, refer to Table 4. To our knowledge, no patients suffered from procedural complications or had to undergo a redo procedure. The data exported from the RHYTHMIA HDx™ mapping system (Boston Scientific, Marlborough, MA, USA) contained raw LI, CF, and power measurements. We used linear interpolation to transfer to a standard time base and sampling frequency of 997 Hz for every ablation trace. According to the LOCALIZE trial's approach, raw LI measurements were first filtered through a moving mean filter with a window length of 1.5 s (see Figure 1) [7]. We based all further calculations on the filtered LI, which we refer to as LI in the following sections. In analogy to Ohm's law for alternating current, the RF current was calculated from the LI and power measurements.

The data contained three-dimensional coordinates of the ablation catheter's tip location. Using the k-nearest neighbor algorithm [21,22], we calculated the linear interlesion distance (ILD) between two adjacent lesions. Therefore, the tip's mean position was calculated for each lesion.

We then calculated the predicted indices for every time point τ on the ablation trace using our earlier trained AI and LSI prediction models (Figure 2). The local impedance drop plateau was defined as the local minimum. While only lesions that reached the operator's desired LI-drop target were exported, we visually confirmed a correctly set LI drop point/plateau for each lesion. AI targets were set to ≥ 400, and LSI targets were set to ≥ 4.

Table 4. Patient demographics for the exported data used during data analysis, n = 27 (LI-guided), are reported as count and percentage.

Patient Characteristics	
Age (years)	66 ± 14.0 [1]
Male, n (%)	12 (43)
Ejection fraction ≤ 55%, n (%)	9 (32)
Hypertension, n (%)	16 (57)
Diabetes, n (%)	4 (14)
Chronic kidney disease [2], n (%)	15 (54)
Indication	
Atrial fibrillation (AF)	13 (48.2)
Atrial flutter (AFL)	12 (44.4)
Atrial tachycardia	2 (7.4)

[1] M ± SD: Mean ± Standard Deviation. [2] KDIGO 2012 ≥ G2

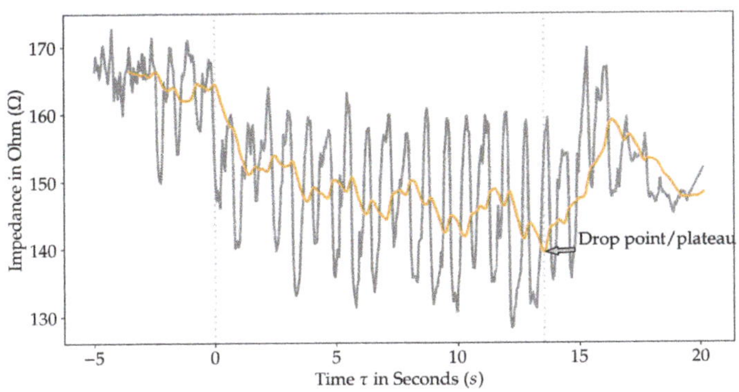

Figure 1. According to the LOCALIZE trial, raw LI measurements were first filtered through a moving mean filter with a window length of 1.5 s [7]. The figure shows both raw (grey) and filtered LI (orange), as well as the LI drop point/plateau. Data integrity was ensured by trimming the left edge of the filtered LI data. This was due to using a moving mean filter extending over the initial data points with a window size of 1.5 s.

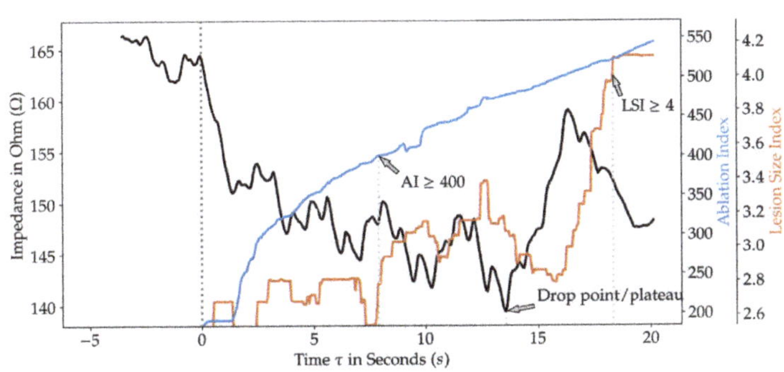

Figure 2. The filtered local impedance (LI), the predicted Ablation Index (AI), and the predicted Lesion Size Index (LSI) during an ablation procedure for every time point τ. The arrows mark the AI- and LSI-targets and the LI drop plateau. Note the AI and LSI prediction start for time points was $\tau \geq 0$ seconds (s). The LI drop plateau was defined as the local minimum. While only lesions that reached the operator's desired LI-drop target were exported, we visually confirmed a correctly set LI drop point/plateau for each lesion.

Lesion metrics were then exported for further statistical analysis.

2.4. Statistics

During data preparation, we excluded lesions with missing values for the AI prediction model. We used Little's MCAR (Missing Completely at Random) test to address missing values for our LSI prediction model. With the test yielding a chi-square statistic of 12.93 and a p-value of 0.166, we employed Multiple Imputation by Chained Equations (MICE) with five iterations to handle the missing values for the LSI ablation duration. Subsequently, to further provide robustness to our results, a sensitivity analysis of the imputation process was performed. We compared MICE against the mean, median, and k-nearest neighbor (KNN) imputations with consistent results of 0.802 for R^2 and 0.974 for MAE. Also, we tested for different iteration counts for MICE (5, 10, and 15), with stable performance metrics ranging from 0.713 to 0.748 for R^2 and 1.078 to 1.130 for MAE. We, therefore, opted to use MICE as our imputation method for the LSI duration data. Additionally, lesions with RF application durations over 30 s and ILD over 6 mm were excluded beforehand according to the CLOSE-Protocol [4] and Kanamori et al. [23]. Overall, a total of 13% of all lesions were excluded.

We reported continuous variables as the median with inter-quartile range (Q1–Q3) or mean $\pm$ standard deviation, and the categorical variables were summarized as count and percentage. We tested against a Gaussian distribution using Shapiro–Wilkins and Anderson–Darling tests. In addition, we utilized Q-Q plots and histograms for visual evaluation.

The Friedman and post-hoc Wilcoxon signed-rank tests were used to compare the ablation durations between groups.

The residuals were not normally distributed, and the Lagrange Multiplier test indicated signs of heteroscedasticity. Since the Gauss–Markov assumptions were violated, we used Generalized Additive Models (GAMs) to capture the potential non-linear relationships and Random Forests as a robust, non-parametric approach to regression analysis.

3. Results

Our main findings are presented in Table 5. The results indicate that the median RF application duration differed significantly depending on the lesion metric used (Friedman-Test: $\chi^2(2) = 1418.95$, $p \leq 0.001$, and n=1090). While the median RF application duration guided by an AI target of ≥400 was 7.32 (IQR = 5.05–9.57) s, the median RF application duration guided by an LSI target of ≥4 was 19.91 (IQR = 17.59–22.95) s. The LI drop plateau was reached after a median RF application duration of 11.92 (IQR = 8.02–16.72) s.

There is a moderate difference when comparing an LI-guided approach and an AI-guided approach in significantly shorter RF application durations for AI-guided procedures, $W = 116,012.00$, $p_{Bonferroni} < 0.001$, r (Cohen, 1992) = -0.53. In contrast, the LI plateau is achieved more quickly than an LSI target of ≥4, $W = 31,720.00$, $p_{Bonferroni} < 0.001$, r (Cohen, 1992) = -0.77. Comparison of the AI-guided and LSI-guided RF application durations also revealed a substantial difference with shorter RF application durations for AI guided procedures, $W = 116.00$, $p_{Bonferroni<0.001}$, r (Cohen, 1992) = -0.87.

In predicting the RF application duration for an AI-guided procedure, GAMs and Random Forests consistently identified the mean CF, starting CF, LI drop, and LI starting impedance as critical predictors. While all parameters were significant (GAMs $ps < 0.001$), the mean CF had the highest importance (0.811) in prediction RF application duration, followed by starting CF (importance 0.110). In contrast, in an AI-guided approach, ILD had no predictive value for RF application duration.

Table 5. The main results with the lesion metrics (n = 1090) for all lesions created. Continuous variables are reported as the median with inter-quartile range (IQR). The LI drop plateau was defined as the local minimum, and only the lesions that reached the operator's desired LI-drop target were exported. AI and LSI targets were set to AI ≥ 400 and LSI ≥ 4.

Lesion Metric	Median (IQR)	*p*
RF application duration LI, s	11.92 (8.02–16.72) [1]	<0.001 [3]
RF application duration AI, s	7.32 (5.05–9.57) [1]	<0.001 [3]
RF application duration LSI, s	19.91 (17.59–22.95) [1]	<0.001 [3]
LI drop, Ω	20.36 (14.32–27.69)	-
LI start impedance, Ω	146.59 (135.96–158.96)	-
CF mean, g·s	18.18 (11.67–25.51)	-
Start CF, g·s	16.87 (10.26–24.23)	-
Ablation Index at LI plateau	476.46 (387.49–533.69) [1]	-
Lesion Size Index at LI plateau	3.17 (2.47–3.55) [1]	-
Interlesion distance, mm	3.66 (2.78–4.52) [2]	-

[1] Our machine learning models calculated the values. [2] Calculated using the k-nearest neighbor algorithm [21,22]. [3] *p*-values for Friedman test: $\chi^2(2) = 1418.95$. Post-hoc Wilcoxon signed-rank test between different metrics, all $ps_{Bonferroni} < 0.001$.

Regarding the predictors for the RF application duration in LSI-guided procedures, the mean CF, LI start, and drop values were significant factors influencing the RF application duration (GAMs $ps < 0.001$). However, their importance differed, with the mean CF values having the highest importance (importance 0.617), as identified by Random Forest. Contrary to an AI-guided approach, the interlesion distance was a significant (GAMs $ps < 0.001$) factor; however, it was a less important factor (importance 0.067) than the mean CF in predicting RF application durations.

In contrast to AI- and LSI-guided procedures, GAMs and Random Forest identified the LI drop and LI start values as significant (GAMs $ps < 0.001$) and important (0.325 and 0.195) predictors, respectively, for RF application duration in LI-guided procedures. While GAMs and Random Forest identified significant and important predictors, they were put into perspective by emphasizing the Random Forest metrics. As the mean squared error was considered high (mean CV MSE = 38.432) and the coefficient of determination ($R^2 = 0.064$) was low, the Random Forest model was less reliable, possibly compromising the identified values of the predictors.

4. Discussion

This study provides new insights into the level of lesion creation during catheter ablation, showing significant differences in the RF application durations between the AI-, LSI-, and LI-guided ablation strategies with AI and LSI targets set to 400 and 4, respectively. The data analysis based on our trained machine learning models predicted the AI and LSI values and, thus, the presented data are based on our models' reliance in the context of machine learning. The AI and LSI metrics remain proprietary to their respective mapping systems. This retrospective cohort study with a comparative analysis is the first to provide a direct comparison to such an extent.

With RF catheter ablation already providing an established treatment option, especially in AF, to an aging population in Europe and the consecutively rising burden of arrhythmias for individuals, as well as the healthcare system, its importance will increase. While recent analysis, such as the study conducted by Wita et al., shows regional differences in ablation rates [24], it is essential to understand and compare the current metrics to optimize outcomes across different healthcare systems.

Published data showed longer RF application durations in LSI-guided procedures compared to LI-guided procedures, which might result in more durable lesions [8]. Regarding RF application duration and energy delivery, HPSD ablation is currently being reviewed [3,25], with recent studies, such as La Fazia et al., showing the impact of the power setting in achieving transmural lesions and their effect on arrhythmia recurrence [26].

This current study had its main focus on the level of lesion creation. We report significant differences in the RF application duration between AI-, LSI-, and LI-guided approaches. The significantly shorter RF application duration observed with an AI-guided ablation approach compared to an LSI-guided approach was one of the most notable outcomes. Similarly, the RF application duration for an LI-guided approach was significantly shorter than an LSI-guided approach. While the exact clinical impact of different RF application durations remains unclear, our findings may suggest that shorter RF application durations with an AI-guided approach lead to shorter, more efficient procedures while mitigating complications such as atrio-esophageal fistula. On the other hand, LSI-guided ablations with longer RF application durations may subsequently result in more durable lesions, as suggested by Lian et al. [8].

Predictors for RF application durations vary between approaches, with the mean CF having the highest relative importance for AI- (0.811) and LSI-guided (0.617) approaches. As the AI formula already incorporates CF as one input variable and the LSI formula contains a 6 s sliding window of mean CF, the finding of the mean CF as the most important predictor does not seem to have much novelty. However, this proves that our machine learning model predictions work as expected, as AI and LSI rely on their input variables. Furthermore, the results underline the necessity of stable tissue–catheter contact for durable lesions. However, the variability in CF between cases may depend on anatomical differences, such as atrial wall thickness, or operator techniques.

LI drop and starting LI values were identified with regression analysis as important predictors (0.325 and 0.195) for RF application duration during LI-guided procedures. These results are in line with the findings of the LOCALIZE trial [7] while also linking them with RF application duration. The results of the LOCALIZE trial [7] may provide a reference for our machine learning models as the findings of influencing factors are assumed to be of close similarity. In contrast to the LOCALIZE trial [7], the relative importance of LI drop and starting LI as a predictor for RF application duration when compared to the mean CF for AI- and LSI-guided procedures, as a predictor, showed a considerably lower predictive performance. This suggests that LI, as a real-time indicator, lacks the ability to fully capture the complexity of lesion creation. The Random Forest model's lower predictive performance ($R^2 = 0.064$) further underlines these findings as it may influence the operator's choice of metric to guide the procedure.

More studies are needed to evaluate the safety and efficacy of these results in a clinical setting. Assessment of different machine learning techniques and the incorporation of more procedural and periprocedural parameters will help to construct a more patient-tailored ablation approach [27–29].

Study Limitations

Our study has several fundamental limitations that primarily arise from using a two-step approach. First, the limitations that apply when using machine learning. Second, the limitations arise from methodological and underlying data challenges.

While the AI and LSI metrics are proprietary, the exact formula coefficients have not been publicly disclosed. Thus, our approach relies on our models correctly predicting their according indices. Although we used Random Forest and Gradient Boosting for our underlying models, the small training data size of 52,968 (AI) and 4253 (LSI) for every time point τ during lesion creation can lead to overfitting. In particular, this is problematic when applying lesion metric prediction to unseen data. However, Random Forest is less susceptible to overfitting due to its nature of reducing variance compared to Gradient Boosting. This especially applies to a limited training data parameter space. On the other hand, Gradient Boosting reduces bias, thus leading to a better fit within the parameter space. Regarding outliers, Random Forest tends to be more resistant as the averaging effect across many trees reduces their impact. For the training data parameter space on which our models were trained, refer to Tables 1 and 2. For example, as shown by La Fazia et al., different power settings affect transmural lesion creation [26]. This is assumed not to be a concern with Random Forest as the effect of a different power setting is averaged in certain trees as long as the specific power setting is included in our training data parameter space. In addition, it has to be acknowledged that our models were trained on data exported from PVI procedures, while the data analysis included all atrial ablation procedures.

Thus, future studies using a similar machine learning approach must primarily address the below challenges. In particular, this means larger and more specific training datasets, for instance, only on PVI data, to enhance robustness and transferability. A refined model training process would also provide benefits, such as evaluating different ensemble learning techniques or neuronal networks.

In the second step of our approach, we analyzed the data from patients who underwent LI-guided ablation alongside our predicted AI and LSI metrics. While this is a retrospective study, data were provided anonymously during export. Thus, the potential for unmeasured confounders affecting the outcomes cannot be excluded. Our dataset represents a heterogeneous patient population, with a relatively small sample size of only 27 patients who underwent LI-guided ablation for different atrial arrhythmias. Likewise, data analysis was not conducted separately for different segments, such as anterior/superior or posterior/inferior. In addition, our dataset lacks periprocedural baseline characteristics, such as echocardiographic parameters, operator variability regarding experience and techniques used, and procedural characteristics such as procedural time. Also, our study did not examine the effect of different RF application durations on the mitigation of complications and long-term clinical outcomes. Thus, the potential for unmeasured confounders affecting the outcomes cannot be excluded, and the likelihood of statistical bias is also increased.

As already stated, the lower performance of our LSI prediction model leads to missing values for our LSI RF application duration. We, therefore, had to rely on MICE to deal with missing data. While we performed Little's MCAR test and sensitivity analysis, we assumed that our data were not Missing Completely at Random (MCAR) and likely Missing at Random (MAR). This also comes with the assumption that our data were not Missing Not at Random (MNAR) as no other confirmation of MNAR, like comparing to different parameters like CF, was applicable. In addition to the already lower performance of our LSI model, this procedure may introduce bias. While the beforehand exclusion of lesions with RF application duration over 30 s and ILD over 6 mm admits established practices, similar aspects of bias are applicable.

As already acknowledged above, future studies would benefit from more specific and larger datasets that allow for subpopulation analysis, such as different types of arrhythmias or adjusting AI and LSI targets for anterior/superior and posterior/inferior segments.

5. Conclusions

This is the first retrospective cohort study with a comparative analysis comparing predicted AI and LSI metrics for LI-guided procedures. Our study reveals significant differences in median RF application durations depending on the lesion metric used. Moreover, the feasibility of using machine learning to predict lesion metrics was shown. Further studies are needed to assess different machine learning approaches and to evaluate the safety and efficacy of these results in a clinical setting.

Author Contributions: Conceptualization, E.L.; methodology, E.L. and L.S.; software, L.S.; validation, D.F. and E.L.; investigation, F.M., V.M., A.Z., M.N. and S.W.; writing—original draft preparation, L.S.; writing—review and editing, F.M. and E.L.; visualization, L.S.; supervision, E.L. and D.F.; project administration, E.L. All authors have read and agreed to the published version of the manuscript.

Funding: This research received no external funding.

Institutional Review Board Statement: This study was conducted in accordance with the guidelines detailed in the Declaration of Helsinki, and it was approved by the Institutional Review Board (or Ethics Committee) of Medizinische Fakultät der Christian-Albrechts-Universität zu Kiel (D 592/24; 7 October 2024).

Informed Consent Statement: Informed consent was obtained from all the subjects involved in this study.

Data Availability Statement: The data presented in this study are available on request from the corresponding authors due to legal reasons.

Conflicts of Interest: The authors declare no conflicts of interest.

Abbreviations

The following abbreviations are used in this manuscript:

AF	Atrial fibrillation
AFL	Atrial flutter
AI	Ablation Index
CF	Contact force
GAMs	Generalized additive models
HPSD	high-power short-duration
ILD	Interlesion distance
LI	Local impedance
LSI	Lesion Size Index
MAE	Mean absolute error
Mean CV MSE	Mean squared error (MSE) from the coefficient of variation (CV)
MICE	Multiple imputation by chained equations
PV	Pulmonary vein
PVI	Pulmonary vein isolation
R^2	Coefficient of determination
RF	Radiofrequency
VIF	Variance inflation factors

Appendix A

Table A1. Software library and versions used.

Python Library	Version
Numpy	1.26.4
Pandas	2.2.2
Scikit-learn	1.2.2
Scipy	1.11.4
Statsmodel	0.14.0
pyGAM	0.9.1
Miceforest	6.0.3
Matplotlib	3.7.1
Seaborn	0.12.2

Table A2. Hyperparameters and the value ranges used during the training process.

Model	Hyperparameters and Value Range
Random Forest	min_samples_split: 2,4,6 min_samples_leaf: 1,2,3
Gradient Boosting	alpha: 0.001, 0.005, 0.01, 0.05, 0.1, 0.5, 0.99
Ridge	alpha: 0.001, 0.005, 0.01, 0.05, 0.1, 0.5, 0.99
Lasso	alpha: 0.001, 0.005, 0.01, 0.05, 0.1, 0.5, 0.99
ElasticNet	alpha: 0.001, 0.005, 0.01, 0.05, 0.1, 0.5, 0.99

References

1. Van Gelder, I.C.; Rienstra, M.; Bunting, K.V.; Casado-Arroyo, R.; Caso, V.; Crijns, H.J.G.M.; Potter, T.J.R.D.; Dwight, J.; Guasti, L.; Hanke, T.; et al. 2024 ESC Guidelines for the Management of Atrial Fibrillation Developed in Collaboration with the European Association for Cardio-Thoracic Surgery (EACTS). *Eur. Heart J.* **2024**, *45*, 3314–3414.
2. Calkins, H.; Hindricks, G.; Cappato, R.; Kim, Y.-H.; Saad, E.B.; Aguinaga, L.; Akar, J.G.; Badhwar, V.; Brugada, J.; Camm, J.; et al. 2017 HRS/EHRA/ECAS/APHRS/SOLAECE Expert Consensus Statement on Catheter and Surgical Ablation of Atrial Fibrillation. *Heart Rhythm.* **2017**, *14*, e275–e444. [CrossRef]
3. Chieng, D.; Segan, L.; Sugumar, H.; Al-Kaisey, A.; Hawson, J.; Moore, B.M.; Nam, M.C.Y.; Voskoboinik, A.; Prabhu, S.; Li, L.; et al. Higher Power Short Duration vs. Lower Power Longer Duration Posterior Wall Ablation for Atrial Fibrillation and Oesophageal Injury Outcomes: A Prospective Multi-Centre Randomized Controlled Study (Hi-Lo HEAT Trial). *EP Eur.* **2023**, *25*, 417–424. [CrossRef]
4. Phlips, T.; Taghji, P.; El Haddad, M.; Wolf, M.; Knecht, S.; Vandekerckhove, Y.; Tavernier, R.; Duytschaever, M. Improving Procedural and One-Year Outcome after Contact Force-Guided Pulmonary Vein Isolation: The Role of Interlesion Distance, Ablation Index, and Contact Force Variability in the 'CLOSE'-Protocol. *EP Eur.* **2018**, *20*, f419–f427. [CrossRef] [PubMed]
5. Venkatesh Prasad, K.; Bonso, A.; Woods, C.E.; Goya, M.; Matsuo, S.; Padanilam, B.J.; Kreis, I.; Yang, F.; Williams, C.G.; Tranter, J.H.; et al. Lesion Index–Guided Workflow for the Treatment of Paroxysmal Atrial Fibrillation Is Safe and Effective—Final Results from the LSI Workflow Study. *Heart Rhythm O2* **2022**, *3*, 526–535. [CrossRef] [PubMed]
6. Hussein, A.; Das, M.; Riva, S.; Morgan, M.; Ronayne, C.; Sahni, A.; Shaw, M.; Todd, D.; Hall, M.; Modi, S.; et al. Use of Ablation Index-Guided Ablation Results in High Rates of Durable Pulmonary Vein Isolation and Freedom from Arrhythmia in Persistent Atrial Fibrillation Patients: The PRAISE Study Results. *Circ. Arrhythm. Electrophysiol.* **2018**, *11*, e006576. [CrossRef] [PubMed]
7. Das, M.; Luik, A.; Shepherd, E.; Sulkin, M.; Laughner, J.; Oesterlein, T.; Duffy, E.; Meyer, C.; Jais, P.; Duchateau, J.; et al. Local Catheter Impedance Drop During Pulmonary Vein Isolation Predicts Acute Conduction Block in Patients with Paroxysmal Atrial Fibrillation: Initial Results of the LOCALIZE Clinical Trial. *EP Eur.* **2021**, *23*, 1042–1051. [CrossRef] [PubMed]
8. Lian, E.; Pantlik, R.; Maslova, V.; Willert, S.; Moser, F.; Remppis, A.; Frank, D.; Demming, T. Local Impedance Drop–Guided versus Lesion Size Index–Guided Pulmonary Vein Isolation. *J. Interv. Card. Electrophysiol.* **2024**, *67*, 2051–2058. [CrossRef] [PubMed]
9. Harris, C.R.; Millman, K.J.; van der Walt, S.J.; Gommers, R.; Virtanen, P.; Cournapeau, D.; Wieser, E.; Taylor, J.; Berg, S.; Smith, N.J.; et al. Array Programming with NumPy. *Nature* **2020**, *585*, 357–362. [CrossRef] [PubMed]
10. McKinney, W. Data structures for statistical computing in python. In Proceedings of the 9th Python in Science Conference, Austin, TX, USA, 28 June–3 July 2010; Volume 445, pp. 56–61.
11. Pedregosa, F.; Varoquaux, G.; Gramfort, A.; Michel, V.; Thirion, B.; Grisel, O.; Blondel, M.; Prettenhofer, P.; Weiss, R.; Dubourg, V.; et al. Scikit-Learn: Machine Learning in Python. *J. Mach. Learn. Res.* **2011**, *12*, 2825–2830.
12. Virtanen, P.; Gommers, R.; Oliphant, T.E.; Haberland, M.; Reddy, T.; Cournapeau, D.; Burovski, E.; Peterson, P.; Weckesser, W.; Bright, J.; et al. SciPy 1.0: Fundamental Algorithms for Scientific Computing in Python. *Nat. Methods* **2020**, *17*, 261–272. [CrossRef]
13. Skipper, S.; Perktold, J. statsmodels: Econometric and statistical modeling with python. In Proceedings of the 9th Python in Science Conference, Austin, TX, USA, 28 June–3 July 2010.
14. Servén, D.; Brummitt, C.; Abedi, H. *dswah/pyGAM*, v0.8.0; Zenodo: Geneva, Switzerland, 2018.
15. Hunter, J.D. Matplotlib: A 2D Graphics Environment. *Comput. Sci. Eng.* **2007**, *9*, 90–95. [CrossRef]
16. Waskom, M. seaborn: Statistical Data Visualization. *J. Open Source Softw.* **2021**, *6*, 3021. [CrossRef]
17. Cartwright, K.V. Simpson's Rule Cumulative Integration with MS Excel and Irregularly-Spaced Data. *J. Math. Sci. Math. Educ.* **2017**, *12*, 1–9.
18. Breiman, L. Random Forests. *Mach. Learn.* **2001**, *45*, 5–32. [CrossRef]
19. Hastie, T.; Tibshirani, R.; Friedman, J. *The Elements of Statistical Learning*; Springer: Berlin/Heidelberg, Germany, 2009.
20. Bergstra, J.; Bengio, Y. Random Search for Hyper-Parameter Optimization. *J. Mach. Learn. Res.* **2012**, *13*, 281–305.
21. Fix, E.; Hodges, J.L. Discriminatory Analysis—Nonparametric Discrimination: Consistency Properties. *Int. Stat. Rev.* **1989**, *57*, 238. [CrossRef]

22. Cover, T.M.; Hart, P.E. Nearest Neighbor Pattern Classification. *IEEE Trans. Inf. Theory* **1967**, *13*, 21–27. [CrossRef]
23. Kanamori, N.; Kato, T.; Sakagami, S.; Saeki, T.; Kato, C.; Kawai, K.; Chikata, A.; Takashima, S.; Murai, H.; Usu, S.; et al. Optimal Lesion Size Index to Prevent Conduction Gap during Pulmonary Vein Isolation. *J. Cardiovasc. Electrophysiol.* **2018**, *29*, 1616–1623. [CrossRef]
24. Wita, K.; Dyrbuś, M.; Kowalski, O.; Wita, M.; Myrda, K.; Hoffmann, A.; Błachut, A.; Jadczyk, T.; Mizia-Stec, K.; Gołba, K.; et al. The regional distribution of catheter ablations of atrial fibrillation and atrial flutter in Poland in 2023. *Pol. Heart J.* 2024, *online ahead of print*. [CrossRef]
25. Winkle, R.A. HPSD ablation for AF high-power short-duration RF ablation for atrial fibrillation: A review. *J Cardiovasc Electrophysiol.* **2021**, *32*, 2813–2823. [CrossRef] [PubMed]
26. la Fazia, V.M.; Pierucci, N.; Schiavone, M.; Compagnucci, P.; Mohanty, S.; Gianni, C.; della Rocca, D.G.; Horton, R.; Al-Ahmad, A.; di Biase, L.; et al. Comparative effects of different power settings for achieving transmural isolation of the left atrial posterior wall with radiofrequency energy. *Europace* **2024**, *26*, euae265. [CrossRef]
27. Muffoletto, M.; Qureshi, A.; Zeidan, A.; Muizniece, L.; Fu, X.; Zhao, J.; Roy, A.; Bates, P.A.; Aslanidi, O. Toward Patient-Specific Prediction of Ablation Strategies for Atrial Fibrillation Using Deep Learning. *Front. Physiol.* **2021**, *12*, 674106. [CrossRef] [PubMed]
28. Ogbomo-Harmitt, S.; Muffoletto, M.; Zeidan, A.; Qureshi, A.; King, A.P.; Aslanidi, O. Exploring interpretability in deep learning prediction of successful ablation therapy for atrial fibrillation. *Front. Physiol.* **2023**, *14*, 1054401. [CrossRef] [PubMed]
29. Razeghi, O.; Kapoor, R.; Alhusseini, M.I.; Fazal, M.; Tang, S.; Roney, C.H.; Rogers, A.J.; Lee, A.; Wang, P.J.; Clopton, P.; et al. Atrial fibrillation ablation outcome prediction with a machine learning fusion framework incorporating cardiac computed tomography. *J. Cardiovasc. Electrophysiol.* **2023**, *34*, 1164–1174. [CrossRef]

Journal of
Clinical Medicine

MDPI

Article

Spontaneous Resolution of Ventricular Pre-Excitation During Childhood: A Retrospective Study

Antonio Sanzo [1], Alessandro Seganti [1,2], Andrea Demarchi [3], Riccardo Simone Fino [4], Irene Raso [5], Alessia Claudia Codazzi [6], Barbara Petracci [1], Andrea Bongiorno [1,2], Roberto Rordorf [1,*,†] and Savina Mannarino [5,†]

1 Arrhythmia and Electrophysiology Unit, Division of Cardiology, Fondazione IRCCS Policlinico S. Matteo, 27100 Pavia, Italy; antonio.sanzo@gmail.com (A.S.)
2 Department of Molecular Medicine, University of Pavia, 27100 Pavia, Italy
3 Cardiocentro Ticino Institute, Ente Ospedaliero Cantonale, 6900 Lugano, 6500 Bellinzona, Switzerland; andrea.demarchi@eoc.ch
4 Independent Researcher, 20100 Milano, Italy; riccardo.s.fino@gmail.com
5 Cardiology Unit, Paediatric Department, Buzzi Children's Hospital Milano, 20154 Milano, Italy; irene.raso@asst-fbf-sacco.it (I.R.)
6 Paediatric Cardiology Department, Fondazione IRCCS Policlinico San Matteo, 27100 Pavia, Italy
* Correspondence: r.rordorf@smatteo.pv.it; Tel.: +39-0382-501276
† Last shared authorship.

Abstract: Background/Objectives: Ventricular pre-excitation (VP) increases the risk of sudden cardiac death among children. While transcatheter ablation could potentially be therapeutic, it is not without risk, especially in smaller children. Accessory pathways (APs) may spontaneously lose anterograde conduction properties over time, making invasive treatment unnecessary. We aim to investigate the probability of spontaneous loss of VP during childhood, as well as the potential factors that may be associated with VP resolution. **Methods:** We conducted a retrospective study of patients with VP diagnosed before 12 years of age and referred to two Northern Italian tertiary care hospitals between 1993 and 2021. Patients with complex congenital heart disease were excluded. Our primary objective was to determine the likelihood of spontaneous resolution of VP. **Results:** Overall, 153 patients were included, with a median age at first diagnosis of 4.9 years (25th–75th percentile: 75 days–8.4 years) and a median follow-up of 4.9 years (25th–75th percentile: 1.8–8 years). Through left truncated Kaplan–Meier analysis, we estimated that anterograde conduction would persist in 53% and 33.8% of patients at the age of 1 and 16 years, respectively. Our findings revealed that the absence of symptoms and intermittent VP were associated with a higher likelihood of VP resolution. It is noteworthy that no major arrhythmic events were reported. **Conclusions:** Our study strongly supports the implementation of a conservative strategy in younger children with VP. Our findings indicate that a significant proportion of pediatric patients may experience spontaneous resolution of VP in the early years of their lives, making any invasive treatment unnecessary.

Keywords: ventricular pre-excitation; pediatric electrophysiology; sudden cardiac death; arrhythmic risk stratification; Wolf–Parkinson–White syndrome; arrhythmias

1. Introduction

Ventricular pre-excitation (VP) is a congenital condition characterized by the conduction of impulses from the atrial to the ventricular myocardium through an accessory pathway (AP) in addition to conduction across the atrioventricular (AV) node. The prevalence of this condition is estimated to be between 0.1% and 0.3% [1,2]. For a long time, it has been studied in the context of Wolf–Parkinson–White (WPW) syndrome, which is characterized by VP and arrhythmia-related symptoms. VP has been associated with a higher risk of sudden cardiac death (SCD) of about 0.15% per year and may approach 3–4% over a lifetime, particularly during childhood and adolescence [3]. Transcatheter ablation of the AP is the cornerstone treatment as it has been shown to be highly effective with low risk in adults [4]. However, transcatheter ablation may carry a higher risk of complications with slightly lower efficacy in the first years of life, particularly in low-weight children (less than 15 kg) [5,6]. As a result, recent European guidelines indicate that transcatheter ablation should only be considered after the age of 8 [4].

The hypothesis that patients younger than 21 years carry a higher risk of major arrhythmic events (MAEs) is supported by previous studies that also included patients with congenital heart disease (CHD—a subgroup with an inherently higher risk profile) [7,8]. Moreover, some of those patients were treated with outdated pharmacological therapies such as blockers of the AV node, which ultimately favors anterograde conduction over the AP, and only a minority of patients under the age of 8 were included. It is known that during growth, a proportion of APs may spontaneously lose anterograde conduction, particularly before the first year of age. However, the natural history of VP in childhood remains poorly understood and, given the conflicting literature, determining the most suitable treatment for these patients remains a challenge [9–11]. Our study aims to describe the likelihood of the persistence of anterograde conduction from birth to the end of the pediatric period in a contemporary pediatric cohort without CHD, analyzing the factors that may influence the spontaneous resolution of VP. The primary endpoint of the study was the spontaneous loss of VP, defined as the disappearance of the manifest delta wave on at least two consecutive electrocardiograms (ECGs) and/or on one 24 h Holter monitoring ECG. We also describe the management strategy we pursued in these patients.

2. Methods

As part of this study, we retrospectively recruited patients diagnosed with VP between ages 0 and 12 years and referred to two high-volume, tertiary care hospitals in Lombardy, Italy (Fondazione Policlinico San Matteo, Pavia, and Ospedale dei Bambini "Vittore Buzzi", Milano), from 1993 to 2021. The review board of both hospitals approved the publication of the anonymized retrospective data of the patients, using information collected for routine clinical practice, and waived the requirement for specific informed consent; however, since these are research hospitals, each parent or guardian signed a generic consent form for their child to participate in clinical research using anonymized data. The study was conducted in accordance with the Declaration of Helsinki Patient age at diagnosis was defined by the earliest available pre-excited electrocardiogram. The patients enrolled were evaluated and the diagnostic ECG was performed as part of screening for long QT syndrome, screening for sports medicine, preoperative screening, symptoms, or as a recommendation by pediatricians. Patients were enrolled through an electrocardiogram performed either for the presence of symptoms or as part of ECG screening.

All ECGs were reviewed by at least two investigators to confirm the diagnosis of VP and estimate the location of the APs following the Arruda algorithm [12]. All patients underwent an echocardiogram to exclude CHD. The duration of follow-up was defined as the time from presentation to the last clinical follow-up. Spontaneous loss of VP was defined as the absence of the delta wave on a 24 h Holter ECG, ensuring a reliable assessment of conduction loss through the accessory pathway (AP). Patients with spontaneous loss of VP underwent annual re-evaluation and if a delta wave reappeared on subsequent assessments, they were reassigned to the persistent VP group.

Follow-up ended when patients reached the age of 16 or were lost to follow-up.

Patients with significant or complex CHD and double APs, either suspected during non-invasive screening (ECG and 24 h Holter ECG) or confirmed during an invasive electrophysiological study, were excluded.

Data collected included demographics, medical history, presence of persistent or intermittent VP, spontaneous resolution of manifest VP, and clinical events during follow-up. Atrial fibrillation (AF) with rapid conduction over an AP, arrhythmic syncope, SCD, and death were considered major arrhythmic events (MAEs).

2.1. Risk Stratification Tools

Risk stratification for arrhythmia was performed using both non-invasive and invasive methods. Non-invasive risk stratification was conducted using resting a 12-lead ECG, 24 h Holter ECG, and exercise stress testing. All patients underwent 24 h Holter ECG both at baseline and during follow-up, while the exercise stress test was only performed on subjects deemed able to cooperate in the performance of the test. Individuals who showed both pre-excited and non-pre-excited beats on the 24 h Holter ECG were considered to have intermittent VP. Patients with baseline intermittent VP on Holter ECG or abrupt beat-to-beat loss of VP during the exercise test were considered to possess non-invasive, low-risk characteristics. In the present paper, these patients are indicated as "low risk" to simplify readability.

Invasive risk stratification was performed using either transesophageal or intracavitary electrophysiological studies. Individuals with accessory pathway refractoriness at baseline greater than 250 ms or a shortest pre-excited RR interval (SPERRI) greater than 250 ms, with refractoriness during beta-adrenergic stimulation greater than 220 ms or a SPERRI greater than 220 ms, were considered not at high risk [13,14], even though it is known that non-invasive stratification tools in pediatric patients do not demonstrate very high negative predictive value [15,16].

2.2. Management

Patients were managed following the most recent Consensus Statements and Clinical practice guidelines [6,13,17]. Chronic drug therapy was initiated in symptomatic patients when needed. Transcatheter ablation was performed when the risk–benefit ratio was considered acceptable as stated by international documents and after acceptance of informed consent provided by the parents or a legal guardian.

2.3. Statistical Analysis

Given the time-to-event dependency of the congenital condition under study and because the observation often started after birth, we considered that the left truncation resulted from the design of the study to delineate the survival curve of VP [18,19]. The results are presented as the mean $\pm$ SD for normally distributed continuous variables (tested with the Shapiro–Wilk normality test), as the median (25th and 75th percentiles) for continuous variables without normal distribution, and as numbers (%) for categorical data. One-way analysis of variance and Student's unpaired *t*-test were used to compare normally distributed continuous variables. For non-normally distributed continuous variables, the Wilcoxon rank-sum test was used. Chi-square and Fisher's exact tests were used to compare categorical variables. By the term "event", we considered the occurrence of the spontaneous loss of VP, and by the term "survival", we meant the persistence of manifest VP. Patients that underwent effective catheter ablation were right-truncated. Freedom from events was reported using the Kaplan–Meier method and comparisons were performed using the logrank test. A two-tailed p-value < 0.05 was considered statistically significant. Univariate analysis of predictors of the primary endpoint was performed with Cox proportional hazards regression. All variables with a p-value < 0.10 and those considered clinically relevant were inserted into a multivariate Cox regression model to assess the hazard ratio (HR) and 95% confidence intervals (CIs) of the relationship between predictors and the primary endpoint. The rule of limiting the number of independent variables to 1 for every 10 events was followed. All statistical analyses, including Kaplan–Meier curves and the graphs, were performed with the use of R Project software (version 4.2.2) and its package "ggsurvfit" and "gtsummary".

3. Results

3.1. Patient Characteristics

In this study, 153 patients were enrolled with a median age of 4.9 years (range: 75 days–8.4 years) at the first diagnosis; of these patients, 64 (41.9%) were female. The median follow-up time was 4.9 years (range: 1.6–8 years). Table 1 summarizes the main population characteristics. According to electrocardiographic criteria [12], the most common location of the AP insertion was the right free wall and the right posteroseptal area (26.6% each), as detailed in Table 1.

Table 1. Characteristics of the patients ("d" stands for "days", whereas the rest of the variables are expressed in years).

	Total (n = 153)	VP Persistence (n = 111)	VP Loss (n = 42)	p-Value
Female sex (n,%)	64 (41.8)	44 (39.6)	20 (47.6)	0.372
Age at diagnosis (years)	4.9 (75 d–8.4)	6 (1.3–9.2)	61 d (24 d–4.3)	<0.001
Follow-up time (days)	4.9 (1.7–8)	4.9 (1.6–7.2)	1954.5 (5.4–8.6)	0.550
CHD	8 (5.2)	6 (5.4)	2 (4.8)	0.121
Atrial septal defects (n,%)	3 (1.8)	1 (0.9)	2 (4.8)	0.122
Ventricular septal defects (n,%)	5 (3.3)	5 (4.5)	0 (0)	0.163
LV dyssynchrony (n,%)	8 (5.2)	6 (5.3)	2 (4.8)	0.897
Symptoms (n,%)	47 (30.7)	39 (35.1)	8 (19)	0.054
Palpitations	32 (68.1)	30 (76.8)	2 (25)	
Chest pain	1 (2.1)	1 (2.6)	0 (0)	
Dizziness	1 (2.1)	1 (2.6)	0 (0)	
Vomiting	3 (6.3)	1 (2.6)	2 (25)	
Poor oral intake	1 (2.1)	1 (2.6)	0 (0)	
Slow growth	1 (2.1)	0 (0)	1 (12.5)	
Heart failure	7 (14.9)	5 (12.8)	2 (25)	
SVT (n,%)	31 (20.3)	23 (20.7)	8 (19)	0.818

Arrhythmia-related symptoms were reported in 30.7% of children or by their caregivers. The most common symptom was palpitations, occurring in 32 cases (68%), followed by acute heart failure during SVT in 7 cases (14.9%). Notably, patients who experienced acute heart failure during SVT were predominantly younger children, particularly infants. Other reported symptoms included vomiting in three cases (6.3%), and chest pain, dizziness, poor oral intake, or slow growth in one case each (2.1%). None of the patients experienced syncope, chronic heart failure, or symptoms related to AF. Tachyarrhythmias were documented in 31 patients (20.3%), all of which were orthodromic atrioventricular re-entrant tachycardia (AVRT). Neither antidromic AVRT nor atrial fibrillation (AF) was observed in our study. No cases of antidromic tachycardia were detected.

None of the included patients had significant CHD. There were 10 (6.5%) patients with non-complex CHD, specifically small self-resolving ventricular septal defects, and hemodynamically insignificant atrial septal defects. In eight patients (5.2%), echocardiographic evaluation revealed interventricular dyssynchrony, which was attributed to accessory pathway conduction. These children were monitored with serial echocardiograms, and none developed chronic ventricular dysfunction. At the time of the electrophysiological study, the ejection fraction values were within the normal range (>55%), despite the presence of echocardiographic evidence of ventricular dyssynchrony. Interventricular dyssynchrony was associated with the following locations of the AP: anteroseptal (four patients), right free wall (three patients), and right posteroseptal (one patient). Among patients with interventricular dyssychrony, the accessory pathway disappeared spontaneously in two cases at the age of 266 and 3028 days, respectively, and ablation was performed in three patients at the age of 10.3, 11.7, and 12.5 years, respectively.

3.2. Resolution of Ventricular Pre-Excitation

During follow-up, spontaneous resolution of VP was observed in 42 (28%) cases. The left-truncated survival analysis curve of manifest VP is depicted in Figure 1. It estimates that the probability of persistence of anterograde conduction is 53.1% (40.0–70.2) at one year of life, 40.7% (29.4–56.5) at 8 years, and 33.8% (23.7–48.4) at 16 years.

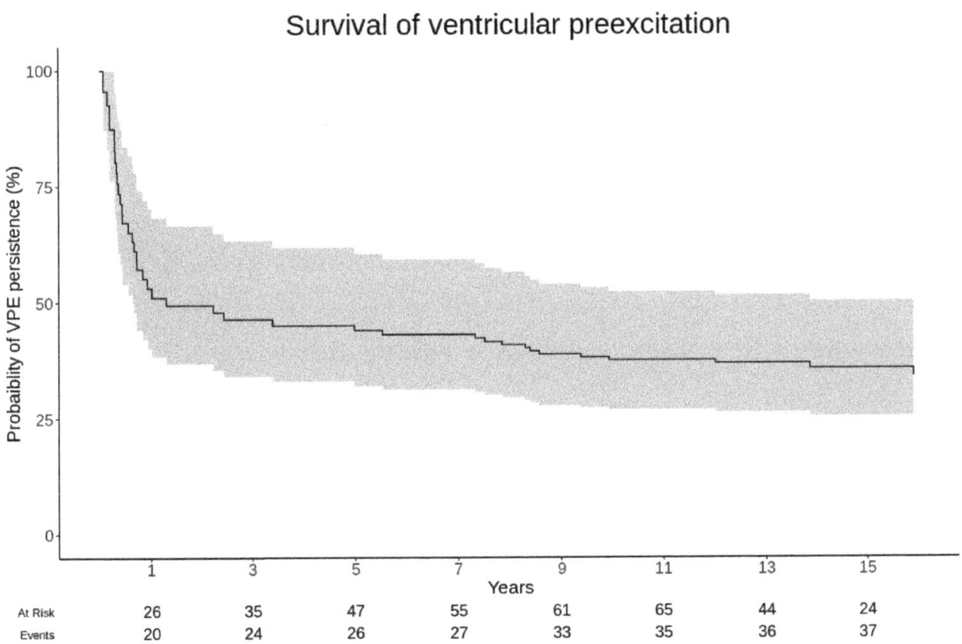

Figure 1. The left-truncated survival analysis curve of manifest pre-excitation.

Sex, AP localization, "low risk" characteristics at non-invasive risk stratification tests, ECG documentation of SVT, and the necessity to start chronic pharmacological therapy were not found to be associated with the primary endpoint in univariate and multivariate analyses and Cox regression analysis. However, the evidence of intermittent VP reached statistical significance during multivariate analysis and was associated with a higher probability of spontaneous loss of VP (HR 3.45, CI 1.32–9.05, *p*-value 0.012) (Figure 2). Furthermore, the presence of symptoms was related to a higher risk of persistence of VP during follow-up during both univariate (HR 0.43, CI 0.20–0.93, *p*-value 0.032) and multivariate analyses (HR 0.15, CI 0.03–0.68, *p*-value 0.014), as described in Table 2 and

Figures S1–S3. Notably, palpitations were reported by 76% of patients with persistent VP and 25% of those with spontaneous loss of VP ($p < 0.001$), regardless of ECG evidence of SVT.

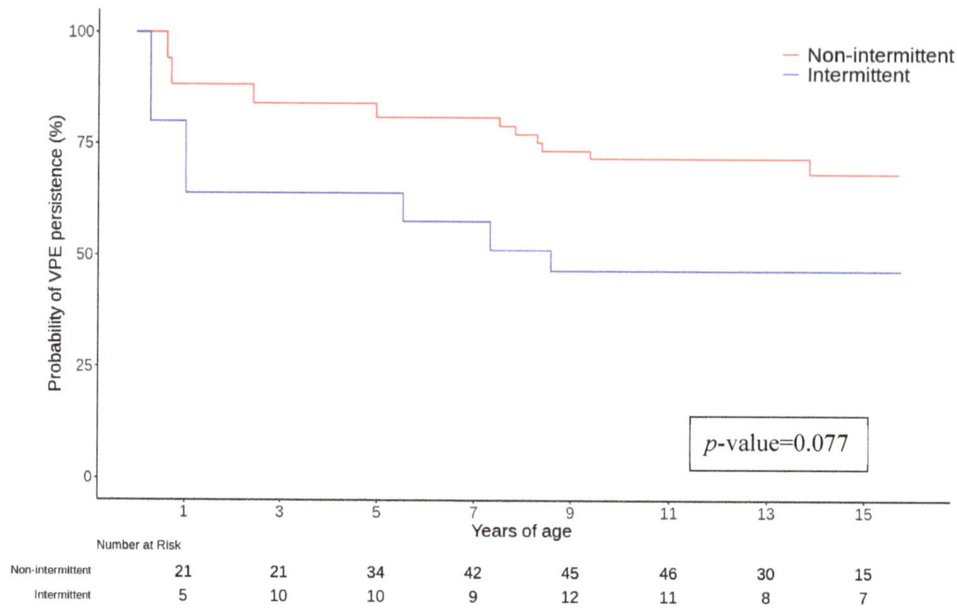

Figure 2. Kaplan–Meier survival curves for VP persistence.

Table 2. Univariate and multivariate analyses.

Variants	Univariable Crude HR (95% CI)	Crude *p*-Value	Multivariable Adjusted HR (95% CI)	Adjusted *p*-Value
Female sex	1.22 (0.66–2–24)	0.522		
Intermittent VP	2.36 (0.91–6.12)	0.077	3.45 (1.32–9.05)	0.012
Non-invasive "low risk" characteristics	2.40 (0.79–7.26)	0.122		
Presence of symptoms	0.43 (0.20–0.93)	0.032	0.15 (0.03–0.68)	0.014
SVT	0.75 (0.35–1.64)	0.473		
Chronic drug therapy	0.82 (0.36–1.84)	0.619		
Left free wall AP	0.96 (0.43–2.15)	0.922		
Left and right free wall AP	0.93 (0.42–2.09)	0.866		
Free walls + epicardial AP	1.05 (0.51–2.17)	0.896		

At the end of the follow-up, none of the children experienced any major arrhythmic event, and all were alive at the end of the study.

3.3. Risk Stratification

Non-invasive risk stratification was performed in 112 (73.2%) patients, and an invasive stratification study was performed in 46 (30%) patients. In total, 67 (43.8%) children presented low-risk characteristics during the non-invasive risk stratification tests. Among them, 1 (1.5%) patient experienced SVT during the follow-up period and 16 (23.9%) patients received treatment. Among patients deemed to be at high risk, five (11.1%) experienced SVT, and four (8.9%) received chronic treatment.

Additionally, 46 patients (30%) underwent an electrophysiological study, with 9 patients undergoing a transesophageal electrophysiological study (EPS) and 42 undergoing an intracardiac EPS. Unfortunately, electrophysiological data were available for only 20 patients, among whom 11 had high-risk characteristics, making this dataset uninformative regarding the overall outcome. The selection between transesophageal and intracavitary EPS was primarily influenced by patient age and cooperation, as transesophageal EPS was preferred for younger or less cooperative children to minimize the invasiveness of the procedure. In contrast, intracavitary EPS was directly performed in patients at high arrhythmic risk to allow for a more comprehensive evaluation of accessory pathway conduction properties and, when indicated, facilitate ablation within the same procedure.

3.4. Chronic Drug Therapy

Twenty-seven symptomatic children required chronic antiarrhythmic therapy. The first therapeutic strategy was adequate in controlling the symptoms in 74% of cases. If the first therapy was ineffective, a second (22.3%) and possibly a third strategy (3.7%) were attempted. Flecainide was the most prescribed drug, alone or in combination (75% of treated patients), at a median age of 6.1 years. Flecainide was the first-line treatment in most cases, while beta-blockers, primarily propranolol, were preferred for younger children. In more complex cases, amiodarone and sotalol were considered as second- or third-line options. In cases where the first treatment failed to achieve adequate symptom control, additional therapeutic combinations were explored, including beta-blockers such as propranolol or atenolol, amiodarone in selected cases with careful monitoring for potential side effects, and sotalol for patients with recurrent, high-risk supraventricular tachycardia (SVT). Overall, approximately 26% of patients required a change in therapy after the initial treatment due to insufficient symptom control. A complete list of the treatments is summarized in Table 3.

Table 3. Other assessments ("d" stands for "days", whereas the rest of the variables are expressed in years).

	Total (n = 153)	VP Persistence (n = 111)	VP Loss (n = 42)	*p*-Value
Non-invasive risk stratification (n, %)	112 (73.2)	93 (83.8)	19 (45.2)	<0.001
ECG Holter monitoring only (n, %)	61 (39.9)	48 (43.2)	13 (30.9)	
Exercise test only (n, %)	2 (1.3)	2 (1.8)	0 (0)	
Holter monitoring and ET (n, %)	49 (32)	43 (38.7)	6 (14.3)	
"Low risk" (n, %)	67 (43.8)	52 (46.8)	15 (35.7)	0.057
VP loss during exercise (n, %)	45 (29.4)	38 (34.2)	7 (16.7)	0.718
Intermittent VP (n, %)	22 (14.4)	14 (12.6)	8 (19)	0.005
AP localization				0.262
Right free wall (n, %)	33 (21.6)	26 (23.4)	7 (16.7)	
Right posteroseptal (n, %)	33 (21.6)	27 (24.3)	6 (14.3)	
Left posteroseptal (n, %)	6 (3.9)	6 (5.4)	0 (0)	
Anteroseptal (n, %)	19 (12.5)	11 (9.9)	8 (19.0)	
Left free wall (n, %)	21 (13.6)	17 (15.4)	4 (9.5)	
Epicardial (n, %)	12 (7.8)	9 (8.1)	3 (7.1)	
Indeterminate (n, %)	29 (18.9)	15 (13.5)	14 (33.4)	
Chronic drug strategy tested	27 (17.7)	20 (18.0)	7 (16.7)	0.845
None (n, %)	126 (82.3)	91 (82)	35 (83.4)	
1 strategy (n, %)	20 (13.1)	15 (13.5)	5 (11.8)	
2 strategies (n, %)	6 (3.9)	4 (3.6)	2 (4.8)	
3 strategies (n, %)	1 (0.7)	1 (0.9)	0 (0)	

Table 3. *Cont.*

	Total (n = 153)	VP Persistence (n = 111)	VP Loss (n = 42)	p-Value
Treatment starting age (years)	6.1 (27 d–11.1)	3.9 (22 d–11.1)	6.1 (1.1–11.1)	0.083
Invasive risk stratification (n, %)	46 (30)	41 (36.9)	5 (11.9)	0.002
Transoesophageal EPS (n, %)	9 (5.9)	9 (8.2)	0 (0)	0.056
Transvenous EPS (n, %)	42 (27.5)	37 (33.3)	5 (11.9)	0.080
Ablation (n, %)	30 (19.6)	30 (27)	0 (0)	
Ablation age (years)	12.7 (11.5–14.5)	12.7 (11.5–14.5)		
Major procedural complications	0 (0)	0 (0)		
Major arrhythmic events	0 (0)	0 (0)	0 (0)	

3.5. Catheter Ablation

Catheter ablation was performed in 30 (19.6%) subjects and effective in 23/30 (76.6%), with the earliest ablation performed at 6.6 years, apart from an urgent procedure attempted in a 2-year-old child with acute heart failure due to drug-refractory SVT. The median time from diagnosis to ablation was 5.1 years (2.7–6.1). The indications were symptoms for 6 patients, high-risk characteristics at invasive stratification in 14, SVT in 6, and the presence of interventricular dyssynchrony in 3.

4. Discussion

The best management strategy for VP in childhood remains unresolved. Therefore, understanding the probability of spontaneous loss of anterograde conduction along the AP is of the utmost importance in decision-making for this cohort of patients. Moreover, little is known about the natural history of VP in this period of life. Our study showed that the probability of spontaneous loss of VP is high in the first year of life (47%). Even though the odds are lower in the subsequent years, they are not null (up to 66% at 16 years of age in the entire population). In addition, the absence of symptoms and an intermittent VP were associated with a higher likelihood of spontaneous loss of VP, even after correction for age.

An important consideration is that not all accessory pathways behave similarly, particularly in their ability to regress over time. It has been hypothesized that APs responsible for SVT possess stronger antegrade conduction properties and shorter refractory periods, making them less likely to regress spontaneously. This may explain why symptomatic patients, irrespective of ECG evidence of SVT, in our study had a lower probability of VP resolution, reinforcing the notion that AP conduction properties influence its natural history. These findings align with prior observations suggesting that APs with higher conduction capacities and lower refractory periods are more resistant to spontaneous resolution.

Our use of the left-truncated Kaplan–Meier method offers a nuanced view that accounts for the time-dependent nature of the condition, enhancing our understanding of the natural resolution rates of VP across different ages. It suggests a more continuous assessment of risk, which is crucial for developing long-term management strategies in pediatric patients diagnosed with WPW syndrome. These results significantly add new insights for the management of children with VP detected in very early childhood. Differing from previous studies, we enrolled consecutive patients with a mean age of 5 years without severe CHD, referred to two tertiary care hospitals in the last 30 years and treated following the most recent evidence. We report the youngest median age ever presented in the literature: Santinelli et al. enrolled patients aged between 5 and 8 years old (median age 10 years) [9]; Cain et al. [20] enrolled around 30% of pts under 1 year of age, but the average age at diagnosis was 7 years. The remaining studies primarily involved an adult population. Another peculiarity is that the intentional exclusion of complex CHD helped to outline the survival profile of VP in the normal heart. These population characteristics, along with the relatively small sample size, may explain the absence of AF, syncope, and SCD. The rarity of SCD and the safety of treatment has already been described in several previous small studies [17].

Our results align closely with subgroup analysis in Cain et al.'s and Benson et al.'s studies, where patients enrolled at an age younger than three months experienced a disappearance of VP in around 35% of patients with a shorter follow-up. In other studies, the percentage of spontaneous resolution was found to be lower as a consequence of enrolment at school age or later and due to a shorter follow-up.

Perry et al. examined the phenomenon of early disappearance and late recurrence of WPW syndrome in children, highlighting that supraventricular tachycardia associated with WPW syndrome that begins in the first year of life may disappear in 93% of cases; however, there is a risk of recurrence later in childhood, typically after 8 years of age. This study involved a significant proportion of patients with CHD (37%), 23% of whom had Ebstein's anomaly, underscoring the varied clinical trajectories in this population. These findings align with our observations and emphasize the necessity of prolonged monitoring and reassessment in managing pediatric patients with VP [21].

Similarly, Benson et al. evaluated the spontaneous resolution of VP using trans-esophageal electrophysiological studies in a small cohort of very young infants, initially assessed at 2 months of age and followed up for an average of 12 months. They observed a rate of spontaneous resolution in the accessory pathways within the first year of life consistent with our data. However, Benson et al. did not evaluate the electrophysiologic properties of accessory pathways beyond early infancy into late childhood or adolescence. This gap highlights the need for further longitudinal studies to explore the persistence or resolution of these pathways over a more extended period [22].

Cain et al. employed a dichotomous statistical analysis to divide their pediatric WPW syndrome population into groups based on age at diagnosis and the presence of associated heart disease. While this method provides valuable insights into differences between these groups, particularly in risk stratification for SCD, it may not fully capture the dynamic nature of VP resolution over time [20]. The use of a statistical analysis that considers the left truncation of the data allowed us to depict for the first time a "real survival" curve of the anterograde conduction of the AP seen at ECG, from birth to 16 years of age. Left truncation correction is a statistical technique used in survival analysis that reduces the selection bias occurring when individuals who experienced the event prior to the beginning of the study (the age of diagnosis in this study) are not included in the study (left truncated data). This can occur when studying a time-dependent condition, such as the persistence of VP. This correction was used since most patients were recruited after the first days of life, which should be the right starting point for observing the persistence of VP, with VP being a congenital condition. Without accounting for left truncation data, the estimated "survival" probabilities would have been greatly overestimated, leading to incorrect conclusions about the persistence of VP over time.

More recently, Yammine et al. [23] retrospectively analyzed a single-center population of 67 patients with an accessory pathway who underwent invasive risk assessment with an electrophysiological study. They showed that 68.7% exhibited high-risk EP parameters. Moreover, there was no significant difference in AVRT inducibility between patients at high risk compared to those at low risk, and patients with significantly shorter AP ERP were more likely to be asymptomatic. On the basis of these data, they concluded that every pediatric patient with AP should be invasively evaluated.

However, some fundamental differences between their population and that of our study must be taken into account. First of all, the average age of our population is extremely low (even if in their population the age at diagnosis is not described), and the highest propensity for spontaneous disappearance of pre-excitation was in fact observed in our population at a much lower age than the average age analyzed by them. Secondly, their population was not analyzed in terms of evolution over time to assess any disappearance of pre-excitation; moreover, in our population, only 30% had undergone invasive assessment, so a direct comparison of the electrophysiological characteristics between the two populations is not feasible.

While catheter ablation can eliminate the risk of SCD, referring every child for an ablation could result in serious and potentially life-threatening complications [13,24]. Moreover, the assessment of AP conduction properties is more challenging and may potentially involve higher procedural risk [5,24]. The latest Consensus Statement on the management of this group of patients dates to 2012 but refers only to asymptomatic patients aged 8–21 years [13]. The most recent 2019 ESC guidelines on supraventricular tachycardia confirm previous 2012 indications [4]. Accordingly, in children over 8 years of age, non-invasive risk stratification with ECG monitoring and exercise testing is suggested and invasive assessment by means of transoesophageal and transvenous electrophysiological study is recommended for those deemed at higher risk. Recent findings further emphasize the limitations of non-invasive tests like the exercise stress test (EST) in accurately stratifying risk, demonstrating low sensitivity and negative predictive value in identifying high-risk accessory pathways, regardless of symptom presence. Their study advocates for the necessary inclusion of electrophysiological studies (EPSs) with the use of isoproterenol to improve diagnostic accuracy, aligning with the call for more definitive assessment techniques in high-risk pediatric cases [14,23,25].

In our population, excluding one patient who underwent ablation for refractory and hemodynamically impairing tachycardias, invasive evaluation or treatment was safely delayed after the age of 6, with an antiarrhythmic drug (mostly flecainide) being started when needed.

Our data significantly reinforce the hypothesis that conservative management should be the preferred choice in this group of patients, especially if diagnosed in the first years of life in asymptomatic and/or in patients with intermittent VP. In symptomatic younger children (below the age of 8 years), a pharmacological approach can be safely performed, postponing an invasive evaluation at an age when procedural risks are significantly reduced.

5. Limitations

The study's limitations mainly lie in its retrospective nature, confounding factors, differential losses to follow-up, and incomplete data that could have altered the analysis results. The majority of VPs were detected following screening ECGs, thus limiting the applicability of our conclusions to children with tachycardia as the initial presentation. Moreover, the study could have been more precise with a higher number of patients recruited before the first year of life. However, the complexities of planning a prospective study are not negligible, as patients should be identified in the neonatal and infant period and followed for a long time frame. APs that lost anterograde conduction may maintain retrograde conduction properties, making them prone to maintaining AV orthodromic re-entry tachycardia. Lastly, it is important to note that it was not possible to exclude that some of our VP mechanisms may involve benign fasciculoventricular fibers that carry no risk of tachycardia or MAEs.

6. Conclusions

The management of VP in childhood remains challenging. Our study offers a unique insight into the natural history of VP from birth to adolescence. The probability of spontaneous resolution of VP during childhood is high, mostly in the first years of life. This suggests that conservative management should be preferred, especially in asymptomatic patients and those with intermittent VP. Our study highlights the rarity of major arrhythmic or life-threatening events in non-invasively treated patients, reinforcing this approach as a safe and viable option. However, the limitations of our retrospective study should be considered, and a larger prospective study would be needed to further validate these findings.

Supplementary Materials: The following supporting information can be downloaded at: https://www.mdpi.com/article/10.3390/jcm14072367/s1, Figure S1. Kaplan-Meier survival curves for VP persistence stratified by the presence of symptoms. Figure S2. Kaplan-Meier survival curves for VP persistence stratified by the presence of baseline risk assessment at non invasive risk stratification. Figure S3. Kaplan-Meier survival curves for VP persistence stratified by gender.

Author Contributions: Conceptualization, A.S. (Antonio Sanzo), A.S. (Alessandro Seganti), A.C.C., B.P., A.B., R.R. and S.M.; methodology, R.S.F., I.R., A.C.C., R.R. and S.M.; validation, A.S. (Antonio Sanzo), A.S. (Alessandro Seganti), A.D., R.S.F. and B.P.; formal analysis, A.S. (Antonio Sanzo); investigation, A.D.; Data curation, A.S. (Antonio Sanzo), A.S. (Alessandro Seganti), I.R. and S.M.; writing—original draft, A.S. (Antonio Sanzo) and R.R.; writing—review & editing, A.S. (Antonio Sanzo), A.S. (Alessandro Seganti), A.D., R.S.F., I.R., A.C.C., B.P., A.B., R.R. and S.M.; project administration, R.R. and S.M. All authors have read and agreed to the published version of the manuscript.

Funding: This research received no external funding.

Institutional Review Board Statement: Ethical review and approval were waived for this study due to as explained in the text (methods section) the review board of both Hospitals approve the publication of anonymized retrospective data of patients using information collected for routine clinical practice and waive the requirement for a specific informed consent or a specific ethical committee approval.

Informed Consent Statement: Patient consent was waived due to the retrospective nature of the study.

Data Availability Statement: Our data can be shared upon reasonable request made to our corresponding author (Dr. Rordorf).

Conflicts of Interest: None of the authors have anything to declare. Dr Rordorf received speaking fees from Abbott and Boston Scientific. The remaining authors have no disclosures to report, as explained in the text (Section 2). The review boards of both hospitals approved the publication of anonymized, retrospective data of patients, using information collected for routine clinical practice, and waived the requirement for specific informed consent or specific ethical committee approval.

Abbreviations

AF	Atrial fibrillation
AP	Accessory pathway
AV	Atrioventricular
CHD	Congenital heart disease
CI	Confidence interval
ECG	Electrocardiogram
EST	Exercise stress test
MAE	Major arrhythmic event
SCD	Sudden cardiac death
SD	Standard deviations
SPERRI	Shortest pre-excited RR interval
SVT	Supraventricular tachycardia
VP	Ventricular pre-excitation
WPW	Wolf–Parkinson–White

References

1. Hiss, R.G.; Lamb, L.E. Electrocardiographic findings in 122,043 individuals. *Circulation* **1962**, *25*, 947–961. [PubMed]
2. Pærregaard, M.M.; Hartmann, J.; Sillesen, A.S.; Pihl, C.; Dannesbo, S.; Kock, T.O.; Pietersen, A.; Raja, A.A.; Iversen, K.K.; Bundgaard, H.; et al. The Wolff-Parkinson-White pattern in neonates: Results from a large population-based cohort study. *Europace* **2023**, *25*, euad165. [PubMed]
3. Klein, G.J.; Bashore, T.M.; Sellers, T.D.; Pritchett, E.L.; Smith, W.M.; Gallagher, J.J. Ventricular fibrillation in the Wolff-Parkinson-White syndrome. *N. Engl. J. Med.* **1979**, *301*, 1080–1085. [CrossRef] [PubMed]
4. Calkins, H. The 2019 ESC Guidelines for the Management of Patients with Supraventricular Tachycardia. *Eur. Heart J.* **2019**, *40*, 3812–3813. [CrossRef]
5. Telishevska, M.; Hebe, J.; Paul, T.; Nürnberg, J.H.; Krause, U.; Gebauer, R.; Gass, M.; Balmer, C.; Berger, F.; Molatta, S.; et al. Catheter ablation in ASymptomatic PEDiatric patients with ventricular preexcitation: Results from the multicenter "CASPED" study. *Clin. Res. Cardiol.* **2019**, *108*, 683–690. [CrossRef]
6. Philip Saul, J.; Kanter, R.J.; Abrams, D.; Asirvatham, S.; Bar-Cohen, Y.; Blaufox, A.D.; Cannon, B.; Clark, J.; Dick, M.; Freter, A.; et al. PACES/HRS expert consensus statement on the use of catheter ablation in children and patients with congenital heart disease: Developed in partnership with the Pediatric and Congenital Electrophysiology Society (PACES) and the Heart Rhythm Society (HRS). Endorsed by the governing bodies of PACES, HRS, the American Academy of Pediatrics (AAP), the American Heart Association (AHA), and the Association for European Pediatric and Congenital Cardiology (AEPC). *Heart Rhythm.* **2016**, *13*, e251–e289. [CrossRef]
7. Munger, T.M.; Packer, D.L.; Hammill, S.C.; Feldman, B.J.; Bailey, K.R.; Ballard, D.J.; Holmes, D.R.; Gersh, B.J. A population study of the natural history of Wolff-Parkinson-White syndrome in Olmsted County, Minnesota, 1953–1989. *Circulation* **1993**, *87*, 866–873. [CrossRef]
8. Deal, B.J.; Keane, J.F.; Gillette, P.C.; Garson, A. Wolff-Parkinson-White syndrome and supraventricular tachycardia during infancy: Management and follow-up. *J. Am. Coll. Cardiol.* **1985**, *5*, 130–135. [CrossRef]
9. Santinelli, V.; Radinovic, A.; Manguso, F.; Vicedomini, G.; Gulletta, S.; Paglino, G.; Mazzone, P.; Ciconte, G.; Sacchi, S.; Sala, S.; et al. The natural history of asymptomatic ventricular pre-excitation a long-term prospective follow-up study of 184 asymptomatic children. *J. Am. Coll. Cardiol.* **2009**, *53*, 275–280. [CrossRef]
10. Inoue, K.; Igarashi, H.; Fukushige, J.; Ohno, T.; Joh, K.; Hara, T. Long-term prospective study on the natural history of Wolff-Parkinson-White syndrome detected during a heart screening program at school. *Acta Paediatr.* **2000**, *89*, 542–545. [CrossRef]
11. Goudevenos, J.A.; Katsouras, C.S.; Graekas, G.; Argiri, O.; Giogiakas, V.; Sideris, D.A. Ventricular pre-excitation in the general population: A study on the mode of presentation and clinical course. *Heart* **2000**, *83*, 29–34. [CrossRef] [PubMed]
12. Arruda, M.S.; McClelland, J.H.; Wang, X.; Beckman, K.J.; Widman, L.E.; Gonzalez, M.D.; Nakagawa, H.; Lazzara, R.; Jackman, W.M. Development and validation of an ECG algorithm for identifying accessory pathway ablation site in Wolff-Parkinson-White syndrome. *J. Cardiovasc. Electrophysiol.* **1998**, *9*, 2–12. [CrossRef] [PubMed]
13. Cohen, M.I.; Triedman, J.K.; Cannon, B.C.; Davis, A.M.; Drago, F.; Janousek, J.; Klein, G.J.; Law, I.H.; Morady, F.J.; Paul, T.; et al. PACES/HRS expert consensus statement on the management of the asymptomatic young patient with a Wolff-Parkinson-White (WPW, ventricular preexcitation) electrocardiographic pattern: Developed in partnership between the Pediatric and Congenital Electrophysiology Society (PACES) and the Heart Rhythm Society (HRS). Endorsed by the governing bodies of PACES, HRS, the American College of Cardiology Foundation (ACCF), the American Heart Association (AHA), the American Academy of Pediatrics (AAP), and the Canadian Heart Rhythm Society (CHRS). *Heart Rhythm.* **2012**, *9*, 1006–1024. [CrossRef] [PubMed]
14. De Ponti, R.; Marazzi, R.; Doni, L.A.; Cremona, V.; Marazzato, J.; Salerno-Uriarte, J.A. Invasive electrophysiological evaluation and ablation in patients with asymptomatic ventricular pre-excitation persistent at exercise stress test. *Europace* **2015**, *17*, 946–952. [CrossRef]
15. Etheridge, S.P.; Escudero, C.A.; Blaufox, A.D.; Law, I.H.; Dechert-Crooks, B.E.; Stephenson, E.A.; Dubin, A.M.; Ceresnak, S.R.; Motonaga, K.S.; Skinner, J.R.; et al. Life-Threatening Event Risk in Children With Wolff-Parkinson-White Syndrome: A Multicenter International Study. *JACC Clin. Electrophysiol.* **2018**, *4*, 433–444. [CrossRef]
16. Escudero, C.A.; Ceresnak, S.R.; Collins, K.K.; Pass, R.H.; Aziz, P.F.; Blaufox, A.D.; Ortega, M.C.; Cannon, B.C.; Cohen, M.I.; Dechert, B.E.; et al. Loss of ventricular preexcitation during noninvasive testing does not exclude high-risk accessory pathways: A multicenter study of WPW in children. *Heart Rhythm.* **2020**, *17*, 1729–1737. [CrossRef]
17. Brugada, J.; Blom, N.; Sarquella-Brugada, G.; Blomstrom-Lundqvist, C.; Deanfield, J.; Janousek, J.; Abrams, D.; Bauersfeld, U.; Brugada, R.; Drago, F.; et al. Pharmacological and non-pharmacological therapy for arrhythmias in the pediatric population: EHRA and AEPC-Arrhythmia Working Group joint consensus statement. *Europace* **2013**, *15*, 1337–1382. [CrossRef]
18. DeBaun, M.R.; Ghafuri, D.L.; Rodeghier, M.; Maitra, P.; Chaturvedi, S.; Kassim, A.; Ataga, K.I. Decreased median survival of adults with sickle cell disease after adjusting for left truncation bias: A pooled analysis. *Blood* **2019**, *133*, 615–617. [CrossRef]
19. Cain, K.C.; Harlow, S.D.; Little, R.J.; Nan, B.; Yosef, M.; Taffe, J.R.; Elliott, M.R. Bias due to left truncation and left censoring in longitudinal studies of developmental and disease processes. *Am. J. Epidemiol.* **2011**, *173*, 1078–1084. [CrossRef]

20. Cain, N.; Irving, C.; Webber, S.; Beerman, L.; Arora, G. Natural history of Wolff-Parkinson-White syndrome diagnosed in childhood. *Am. J. Cardiol.* **2013**, *112*, 961–965. [CrossRef]
21. Perry, J.C.; Garson, A. Supraventricular tachycardia due to Wolff-Parkinson-White syndrome in children: Early disappearance and late recurrence. *J. Am. Coll. Cardiol.* **1990**, *16*, 1215–1220. [CrossRef] [PubMed]
22. Benson, D.W.; Dunnigan, A.; Benditt, D.G. Follow-up evaluation of infant paroxysmal atrial tachycardia: Transesophageal study. *Circulation* **1987**, *75*, 542–549. [CrossRef] [PubMed]
23. Yammine, M.L.; Tamborrino, P.P.; Flore, F.; Di Mambro, C.; Pazzano, V.; Di Marzio, S.; Drago, F. Intermittent ventricular preexcitation in children: Not always a low-risk condition. *Europace* **2024**, *26*, euae250. [PubMed]
24. Van Hare, G.F.; Javitz, H.; Carmelli, D.; Saul, J.P.; Tanel, R.E.; Fischbach, P.S.; Kanter, R.J.; Schaffer, M.; Dunnigan, A.; Colan, S.; et al. Prospective assessment after pediatric cardiac ablation: Demographics, medical profiles, and initial outcomes. *J. Cardiovasc. Electrophysiol.* **2004**, *15*, 759–770. [CrossRef]
25. Jemtrén, A.; Saygi, S.; Åkerström, F.; Asaad, F.; Bourke, T.; Braunschweig, F.; Carnlöf, C.; Drca, N.; Insulander, P.; Kennebäck, G.; et al. Risk assessment in patients with symptomatic and asymptomatic pre-excitation. *Europace* **2024**, *26*, euae036. [CrossRef]

MDPI AG
Grosspeteranlage 5
4052 Basel
Switzerland
Tel.: +41 61 683 77 34

Journal of Clinical Medicine Editorial Office
E-mail: jcm@mdpi.com
www.mdpi.com/journal/jcm

www.ingramcontent.com/pod-product-compliance
Lightning Source LLC
Chambersburg PA
CBHW062042220926
51850CB00010B/2639
9783725863822